S0-BIL-958

GIS in Public Health Practice

Edited by
Ravi Maheswaran
Massimo Craglia

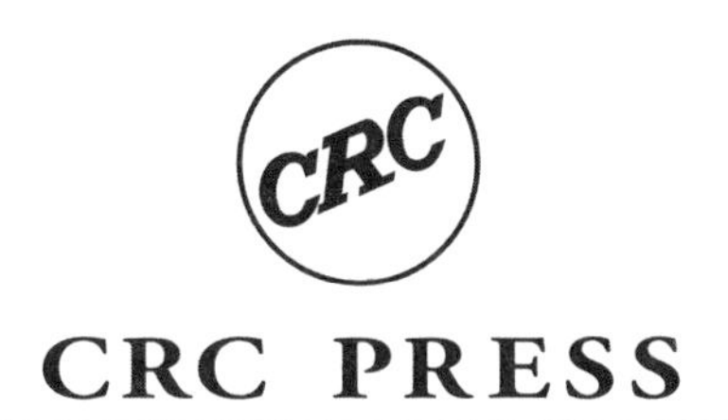

CRC PRESS
Boca Raton London New York Washington, D.C.

Library of Congress Cataloging-in-Publication Data

GIS in public health practice / edited by Ravi Maheswaran, Massimo Craglia.
p. cm.
Includes bibliographical references and index.
ISBN 0-415-30655-8 (alk. paper)
1. Public health--Research--Methodology. 2. Geographic information systems. 3. Public health--Geographic information systems. 4. Public health--Information services. 5. Medical geography--Methodology. I. Maheswaran, Ravi. II. Craglia, Massimo
[DNLM: 1. Topography, Medical--methods. 2. Geographic Information Systems--utilization. 3. Public Health Informatics--methods. WB 700 G531 2004]
RA440.85.G57 2004
614.4--dc22 2003069767

International Standard Book Number 0-415-30655-8
Library of Congress Card Number 2003069767
Printed in the United States of America 2 3 4 5 6 7 8 9 0
Printed on acid-free paper

Preface

Public health has been defined as the "science and art of prolonging life, preventing disease, and promoting health through organized efforts of society." The geographical perspective is a key aspect of public health. Populations and communities are geographically distributed and communities tend to have their own defining characteristics. Factors influencing health are commonly classified under four groups:

1. Inherited conditions
2. Environment, which includes both physical (i.e., air quality, water quality, soil characteristics, radiation) and socioeconomic aspects
3. Lifestyle
4. Healthcare

Each of these factors may have marked geographical variation. The practice of key elements of public health, including communicable disease control, environmental health protection, health needs assessment, planning and policy, surveillance, monitoring and evaluation, and operational public health management, is often explicitly geographical in nature. In addition, resource allocation at the macro and micro levels has a strong geographical component based on demography, health needs, existing provisions, and other factors. GIS, the definition of which has evolved from geographic information systems to geographic information science, involves a scientific problem-solving approach, encompassing the development and application of scientific methods to solve societal problems. It, therefore, has become an integral and essential part of public health research and practice.

Significant advances in scientific approaches to evaluating and using geographic information are taking place. Health information at a fine spatial resolution has become widely available; the same can be said for mapping technology. These developments enable public health practitioners to link and analyze data in new ways at the international, regional, and even street levels. As part of the drive to promote the use of GIS within public health, the European Commission supported the First European Conference on Geographic Information Sciences in Public Health held in Sheffield, United Kingdom, in September 2001. The scientific program drew upon many of the leading public health researchers and practitioners in this area. The breadth of knowledge and expertise at the conference and the clear interest in the field from practitioners from a wide variety of specialisms led us to believe that a book that recognized the breadth of the field would be useful. For this book, specifically selected expanded contributions were invited from participants to illustrate particular areas of application or address issues pertinent to the field. Further chapters were sought from other specialists to cover specific aspects. Many of the chapters have a United Kingdom or European focus, but the principles, issues, and methods discussed should be equally relevant beyond Europe. Although this is not the first book on GIS and public health, we believe it is the first to treat GIS as more than a technology in relation to public health practice. We hope it will be of benefit to practitioners, researchers, and students with an interest in public health.

Dr. Ravi Maheswaran, MD, MRCP, MFPHM
Clinical Senior Lecturer in Public Health Medicine

Dr. Massimo Craglia, PhD, MRTPI
Senior Lecturer in Town and Regional Planning

Acknowledgments

We would like to thank Jane Shields for providing administrative support and preparing the manuscript. We would also like to thank all the contributors for their efforts and support. Acknowledgments of permission to reproduce published material are provided in the corresponding chapters. The Public Health GIS Unit at the University of Sheffield was established with core funding from Trent Regional Health Authority. The unit received a grant from the European Commission's Fifth Framework Programme for promoting collaborative work in the public health GIS field, which included hosting the First European Conference on Geographic Information Sciences in Public Health in 2001.

Contributors

Alessandro Annoni
Institute for Environment and Sustainability
Joint Research Centre of the European Commission
Ispra (VA), Italy

Paul Aylin
Department of Epidemiology and Public Health
Imperial College School of Medicine
London, United Kingdom

Deryck Beyleveld
Department of Law
University of Sheffield
Sheffield, United Kingdom

Alex Bottle
Department of Epidemiology and Public Health
Imperial College School of Medicine
London, United Kingdom

David Briggs
Department of Epidemiology and Public Health
Imperial College School of Medicine
London, United Kingdom

Paul Brindley
Sheffield Centre for Geographic Information and Spatial Analysis
University of Sheffield
Sheffield, United Kingdom

Samantha Cockings
Department of Geography
University of Southampton
Southampton, United Kingdom

Massimo Craglia
Department of Town and Regional Planning
University of Sheffield
Sheffield, United Kingdom

Kees de Hoogh
Department of Epidemiology and Public Health
Imperial College School of Medicine
London, United Kingdom

Gregory A. Elmes
Department of Geology and Geography
West Virginia University
Morgantown, West Virginia

Robert P. Haining
Department of Geography
University of Cambridge
Cambridge, United Kingdom

Robin Haynes
School of Environmental Sciences
University of East Anglia
Norwich, United Kingdom

John Holmes
Public Health South
Dunedin, New Zealand

Edmund Jessop
Department of Public Health
West Surrey Health Authority
Surrey, United Kingdom

Thomas Kistemann
Institute for Hygiene and Public Health
University of Bonn
Bonn, Germany

Andrew B. Lawson
Department of Epidemiology and Biostatistics
School of Public Health
University of South Carolina
Columbia, South Carolina

Andrew Lovett
School of Environmental Sciences
University of East Anglia
Norwich, United Kingdom

Markku Löytönen
Department of Geography
University of Helsinki
Helsinki, Finland

Ravi Maheswaran
Public Health GIS Unit
Section of Public Health
School of Health and Related Research
University of Sheffield
Sheffield, United Kingdom

Tim Pearson
Public Health GIS Unit
Section of Public Health
School of Health and Related Research
University of Sheffield
Sheffield, United Kingdom

Angela Queste
WHO Collaborating Centre for Health Promoting Water Management and Risk Communication
Institute for Hygiene and Public Health
University of Bonn
Bonn, Germany

Clive E. Sabel
Department of Geography
University of Canterbury
Christchurch, New Zealand

Darren Shickle
Section of Public Health
School of Health and Related Research
University of Sheffield
Sheffield, United Kingdom

Ralph Smith
West Midlands Cancer Intelligence Unit
University of Birmingham
Birmingham, United Kingdom

Rupert Suckling
Section of Public Health
School of Health and Related Research
University of Sheffield
Sheffield, United Kingdom

Gilla Sünnenberg
School of Environmental Sciences
University of East Anglia
Norwich, United Kingdom

David Townend
Department of Law
University of Sheffield
Sheffield, United Kingdom

Susan Wallace
Section of Public Health
School of Health and Related Research
University of Sheffield
Sheffield, United Kingdom

Stephen Wise
Sheffield Centre for Geographic Information and Spatial Analysis
University of Sheffield
Sheffield, United Kingdom

Contents

SECTION 4 Data Protection and E-Governance Issues in Public Health

1 Introduction and Overview

Ravi Maheswaran and Massimo Craglia

CONTENTS

1.1 INTRODUCTION

Public health has been defined as "the science and art of preventing disease, prolonging life, and promoting health through the organized efforts of society." This definition was arrived at in the inquiry established to consider the future development of the public health function including the control of communicable disease in England (Acheson, 1988). The inquiry was set up following failures in the system to protect the health of the public from two major outbreaks of communicable disease caused by salmonella and Legionnaires' disease. Since then, a number of health scares have highlighted the need for continuing improvements in public health protection systems. Recent high profile examples include the outbreak of severe acute respiratory syndrome (SARS) and variant Creutzfeldt-Jakob disease, the human form of bovine spongiform encephalopathy commonly known as mad cow disease. The description of disease epidemiology typically has three elements: time, place, and person. Describing the outbreak and spread of a communicable disease therefore explicitly includes a spatial component. Although this has long been recognized (e.g., the investigation of cholera outbreaks in London by John Snow), an important barrier to examining the spatial element of disease outbreaks has been the lack of both digitized spatial data and the computer tools for mapping and spatial analysis.

Environmental health issues have been gaining importance both scientifically and in terms of public concern. These issues range from the global scale — for example, in terms of the health effects of climate change — to the local level where

0-415-30655-8/04/$0.00+$1.50

there may be concern about an increase in cancer around a chemical factory. The interaction between environment and health outcomes is being increasingly recognized at the international level by major organizations including the World Health Organization (WHO) and the European Commission. For example, a recent report for the European Commission estimated that up to 20 percent of ill health might be due to environmental factors, with air pollution being the worst culprit (Commission of the European Communities, 2003). It was estimated that 10 percent of children in Europe have asthma, with a higher incidence in Western Europe than in accession countries, indicating a complex mix of environmental, social, and lifestyle factors. This is not just an environmental and social problem, but also an economic one. In the United Kingdom alone, the total annual cost of asthma is estimated at over EUR 3.9 billion (van Tongelen, 2003).

Understanding the complex relationships between combined exposure over time to a cocktail of chemicals and emissions and health outcomes is becoming a top priority in Europe, requiring integrated research programs with greater availability of shared information and geographically referenced information systems. In addition, there are increased concerns to the public, organizations, and governments of the risks to health posed by the potential of bioterrorism following the events of September 11, 2001. Health protection establishments have been strengthened in numerous countries throughout the world and part of the requirement for active surveillance is the temporal-spatial component for early warning systems.

Although the potential benefits of spatial information and analysis are immediately apparent in the communicable disease and environmental health fields, there are major and not fully recognized benefits to be gained in relation to policy and planning in the health and healthcare fields. The basic elements of work in this branch of public health work include health needs assessment, planning and implementation, and monitoring and evaluation. Related and overlapping aspects include resource allocation, surveillance, and health impact assessment.

There are a number of approaches to health needs assessment (Stevens and Raftery, 1997). Epidemiologically based needs assessment combines epidemiological approaches, including health status assessments, with assessment of the effectiveness and cost effectiveness of interventions. Comparative needs assessment involves comparing levels of service utilization between different populations while corporate needs assessment incorporates obtaining the views of professionals, patients, and other interested and relevant parties. There is a clear spatial element to population-based health needs assessment and the use of Geograhic Information Systems (GIS) in this field will bring many potential benefits. These include resource allocation based on need, and current practice in resource allocation in most countries already includes a geographical element based on regions or smaller areas.

Following a population-based needs assessment, the next step in public healthcare management is to plan and implement strategies and interventions to meet these needs to improve health and well-being. If the health needs assessment has a detailed spatial element, then appropriate geographical targeting of interventions or tailoring interventions to meet varying geographical factors could substantially improve the effectiveness of interventions and efficiency in the use of scarce resources. The interventions may be at the structural level, such as building new healthcare facilities, or at the human resource level, such as increasing the number of specialists per head of population. Interventions to increase geographical access may include the provision of community transport services. Geographical techniques, such as spatial decision support systems, are currently already widely deployed in the commercial and retail sectors. Tailoring interventions may be improved by detailed spatial analysis of existing referral patterns and care pathways, though the latter may pose challenges in the representation of relevant spatial and temporal information within a Geographic Information System (GIS). The need for targeted assessment and policy action is also particularly important given the widely acknowledged relationship between poor health and socioeconomic conditions (see, for example, Acheson, 1998).

The logical step that follows intervention is monitoring and evaluation to ensure that the intervention is achieving the desired goal. Again, the spatial element may dictate that goals should be set at appropriate levels for different geographical areas. Monitoring and evaluation is often underresourced as there is a tendency to move on quickly to a "new" initiative to satisfy political requirements, rather than undertaking careful assessment of the effectiveness of existing policies and interventions. Although cognizant of the political environment in which health policy is couched, we cannot but stress the importance of this part of the policy cycle and the contribution that a spatial perspective brings, particularly when looking at the cumulative effects of cross-sectoral policies.

Health impact assessment has been defined as the estimation of the overall effects of a specified action on the health of a defined population (Scott-Samuel, 1998). These actions may range from something specific such as a new municipal incinerator or landfill site to much larger and complex projects, programs and policies such as housing development projects, urban regeneration programs, and integrated transport policies. GIS has a useful role to play in health impact assessment, both in terms of descriptive and analytical work and in terms of visual presentation of information and evidence to a wider audience to promote public participation. The importance of health impact assessment is being increasingly recognized internationally, including at the European level with the launch by the European Commission of the Integrated Impact Assessment Tool in 2003 (see Chapter 14).

Public need for information is also on the increase and can be supported by the greater availability of information and communication technologies and the Internet in particular. Health-related information has been identified as one of the main application areas for E-government strategies across the world. Although some online services providing general health information (e.g., information on symptoms and potential treatments) are not location specific, there is a wide range of services underpinned by geography, such as the location of the nearest pharmacy, health center or dental practice.

Current policy pressures and requirements indicate that the geographical dimension of public health research and practice is being increasingly recognized. This converges with another set of developments from the technological and geographical information communities. We can distinguish here three main developments. From a technological perspective, there is increasing diffusion of the Internet and related technologies and these have started to become embedded into organizational processes and the daily lives of millions of individuals worldwide. There are therefore increased opportunities for information sharing and dissemination in every field including health. In parallel, we are seeing increased availability of geographically referenced information from public and private sectors, facilitating data acquisition, visualization, and analysis. Again, this is a generic trend supported by policies such as E-government and more generally the development of the Information Society, across Europe, for example (see Chapter 14 for a discussion of this phenomenon). Internet services that deliver maps are enjoying significant increases in popularity across Europe and are set to increase. A report in April 2003 in Italy, for example, highlighted several Web sites with maps that had double-figure increases in the number of hits over a three-month period.[1]

Specific technologies to integrate, analyze, and display geographic information i.e., GIS) have become much more widespread. Systems that until 15 years ago were still very expensive and within the domain of a few experts have now become much cheaper and widely available, spawning an industry estimated to turn over approximately US$1 billion per annum worldwide (www.daratech.com) in software sales alone. Thus, the basic techniques of geographical query and analysis have become available to many and in some instances directly available from basic spreadsheet software packages. This is reflected in the increased use of GIS in public health practice, a response to the requirements and needs identified above.

Against these opportunities, a number of important constraints need to be recognized. First, in spite of the increased technological prowess of current systems, there are still major inequalities in the opportunities to access information (i.e., physical access) and make effective use of it (i.e., social access requiring knowledge and skills). The digital divide is in many instances increasing and cannot be underestimated. Second, although information in general and geographic information in particular is becoming more widely available, it has also been constrained by lack of interoperability (different geographical scales, formats, definitions, and so on). This is particularly acute at the transnational level, with policy frameworks defining conditions of access that are often opaque and unduly restrictive. Furthermore, most organizations in both public and private sectors have yet to come to grips with the full impact of having digital information, as opposed to paper records, and have yet to revise their policies and operations to move into the digital age. For example, most government organizations have yet to define consistent and transparent access and pricing policies and continue to live in a culture of "my" information that undermines information sharing needs. Although this applies to all types of information, geographic and health information pose particular challenges. Geographic information is an expensive commodity to collect and maintain and therefore raises potential conflicts between the pursuit of social objectives, which call for wide dissemination, and economic objectives that call for profit maximization. Health information may be of a very sensitive nature and its use and misuse could lead to substantial problems if appropriate safeguards are not in place to protect confidentiality.

---

[1] Nielsen Netratings, press release for Italy 20/05/2003, http://www.nielsen-netratings.com/pr/pr_030520_italy.pdf.

The wide range of issues highlighted above and the convergence between public health requirements and GIS opportunities are at the origin of this book. It takes a broad view of GIS, not confined to the technology perspective (the S in GIS), but couched in recent views of GIS as a science: a body of knowledge and theory regarding geographic information (Goodchild, 1992; Longley et al., 2001). GIS addresses important issues and questions (e.g., issues of representation, relationships, data models and structures, visualization) in an application-orientated setting and the technology is only part of the approach toward finding solutions to the problems at hand. A wide range of disciplines including epidemiology, statistics, biomedical science, sociology, management science, and health economics underpins public health itself. Other subjects relevant to public health research and practice include ethics, law, and public policy. Hence the intersection between GIS (as a science) and public health requires, in our view, a broad treatment to explore a variety of issues and not be confined to a purely application view of the problem (as seen from a GIS perspective) or a spatial perspective of the subject (as seen from the public health angle). With these considerations in mind, this book is structured into four sections addressing the following sets of issues:

1. Disease mapping and spatial analysis
2. GIS applications in communicable disease control and environmental health protection
3. GIS applications in healthcare planning and policy
4. Data protection and E-governance issues in public health

This book focuses on some of the issues and topics particularly pertinent to current research and practice in the public health GIS field and presents examples that illuminate useful applications in this area of work. It is aimed at practitioners and researchers in the public health field and all sections have strong input from practitioners or academics working in practice. In addition, this book should appeal to a wider audience of people with multidisciplinary interests in health outcomes, policy, and practice. This book will also be relevant to students in masters and doctorate programs in public health and epidemiology. Public health practitioners will be especially interested in the methods used in the different applications, but also in getting a critical appraisal of some of the limitations, including issues of data availability, data protection, and impacts of current policy initiatives to provide an increasing number of services via the Internet.

Throughout this book, the acronym GIS is used interchangeably, referring to geographic information system (or systems) or to geographic information science (or sciences), the latter acknowledging the range of sciences underpinning public health that have a geographical perspective. This book complements others in the GIS and public health field (Cromley and McLafferty, 2002; de Lepper et al., 1995; Melnick, 2002). Existing books focus on technical aspects of GIS, while this book views the subject from a broader perspective as described above. In particular, the sections on disease mapping and spatial analysis and data protection and E-governance issues, described below, cover aspects that a focus on GIS as a technology would traditionally exclude.

1.1.1 Disease Mapping and Spatial Analysis

This first section of this book has a strong methodological flavor and contains three chapters. Chapter 2 by Ravi Maheswaran and Robert P. Haining describes basic elements of geographical analysis, including an introduction to data types and models and issues of data quality. It then provides an overview of cartographic operations relevant to public health and defines the key elements and techniques of exploratory spatial data analysis and ecological studies. The importance of understanding data before using it comes out as a strong message from this chapter.

Chapter 3 by Andrew B. Lawson is a detailed description of disease mapping from a statistical perspective. The chapter moves logically from basic representations of disease distribution to the calculation of rates and standardized rates, interpolation methods and models. The latter section includes a useful discussion of basic likelihood models, random effects, Bayesian models and other more recent developments in disease mapping. An important message from this chapter is the need to be aware of the potential for misrepresentation inherent in some of the most widely available and commonly used "simple" methods of data analysis.

In Chapter 4, Clive E. Sabel and Markku Löytönen focus on disease clusters and methods for detecting clustering, making a useful distinction between the two. This is a good review of the strengths and weaknesses of alternative methods, some of which are illustrated with examples from Finland. The challenges identified by the authors include the need to integrate space and time into public health GIS research and to find appropriate ways to integrate comprehensive individual-level data, such as that available in some of the Nordic countries, into spatial analytical frameworks.

1.1.2 GIS Applications in Communicable Disease Control and Environmental Health Protection

This second section introduces an important application area with contributions from both researchers and practitioners. Chapter 5 by Thomas Kistemann and Angela Queste is an overview of GIS applications in communicable disease control, made all the more topical since the SARS outbreak in early 2003. It traces the historical routes to the spatial analysis of communicable disease and describes the opportunities for using GIS for the prevention, surveillance, and control of communicable diseases. Some of the pitfalls highlighted included the lack of robust statistical methods embedded within widely available standard GIS software and the lack of trained staff.

Chapter 6 by John Holmes provides a good example of the added value of a spatial perspective in outbreak investigation. It describes the analysis of recurrent outbreaks of *Salmonella* Brandenburg in sheep and humans over a five-year period in New Zealand. In this practical application, we see the opportunity afforded by GIS not only in terms of spatial analysis and visualization but also as a platform to enable the integration of data from different sources. As a result of the analysis, educational and other preventative measures have been put in place that have reduced considerably the extent and effects of such outbreaks, demonstrating the value of this type of analysis in a practical situation.

Chapter 7 is contributed by Kees de Hoogh, David Briggs, Samantha Cockings, and Alex Bottle of the Small Area Statistics Unit at Imperial College, London. The chapter draws on the experiences of this unit to illustrate a range of methods, packed with examples, to assess environmental exposure. The benefits of GIS are clear from these examples, as well as new challenges lying ahead with respect to the need to model individuals rather than areas and to develop dynamic rather than static models.

Chapter 8 by Paul Brindley, Ravi Maheswaran, Tim Pearson, Stephen Wise, and Robert P. Haining provides a good example of using modeled outdoor air pollution data for health surveillance based on a project they undertook in Sheffield. The chapter contains a detailed discussion of data interpolation methods for linking modeled air pollution estimates to areas and their populations to enable the assessment of the health impact of air pollution. It also addresses the issue of data quality of the modeled pollution estimates.

Chapter 9 by Paul Aylin and Samantha Cockings describes the value of establishing a rapid inquiry facility for the rapid initial assessment of apparent disease clusters and of the health impacts of point sources of environmental pollution in the United Kingdom. The chapter then presents preliminary experiences from the European Health and Environment Information System project, which involves setting up similar facilities in other European countries.

1.1.3 GIS Applications in Healthcare Planning and Policy

The focus on practical applications continues in this section with four chapters on healthcare planning and policy. Ralph Smith in Chapter 10 provides a valuable practitioner's perspective of the importance of regional structures for supporting GIS-based analysis for the National Health Service in the United Kingdom. The regional dimension is important with respect to the stability of institutions, availability of critical skills, data integration, and data analysis across counties and districts. This dimension is well recognized across Europe where regions play a very important role. This chapter adds weight to current debates in the United Kingdom and elsewhere on devolution and regional structures of governance.

Chapter 11 by Edmund Jessop continues the theme but from a smaller territorial entity: the district. The use of GIS in practice at this level is described well. What is important here is not technical sophistication of the methods deployed but the real issues that need addressing, from boundary maps and changes to travel time zones, as well as the practical use of some of the techniques described earlier in the book. Practitioners at the local level will find this chapter valuable for describing what GIS could do to their work.

Andrew Lovett, Gilla Sünnenberg, and Robin Haynes in Chapter 12 focus on one of the key aspects of public health research and practice: access to services. Using work undertaken by the authors in East Anglia, they present a clear view of the potential of GIS to evaluate accessibility to services using both public and private transport. The chapter discusses data issues and devotes most of its contents to the discussion of methods for data analysis. The value of calculating accessibility across the network rather than in straight lines is confirmed. The chapter discusses challenges in evaluating the complex mix of options and modes of travel currently available at different times of the day and days of the week.

Although the chapters thus far in this section have provided a United Kingdom perspective, Chapter 13 by Gregory A. Elmes gives an incisive overview of recent trends and developments in the use of GIS for public health practice in the United States. The chapter describes some of the broad characteristics of the U.S. health system and its use of GIS in public health planning with several examples of programs and initiatives at federal and state levels. The many opportunities for wider use of GIS in public health in the United States are reviewed and in many ways are similar to the situation in Europe. Against these opportunities, Gregory Elmes does well to warn the reader about the highly politicized nature of the healthcare system that may well inhibit the smooth integration of GIS into day-to-day practice.

1.1.4 Data Protection and E-Governance Issues in Public Health

Although the first three sections of the book have addressed broad methodological issues and applications, the four chapters in this section provide four complementary perspectives on policy, the legal framework, trust, and technology, respectively.

Chapter 14 by Massimo Craglia and Alessandro Annoni sets GIS and public health within the wider perspective of the development of the Information Society and E-government and the increasing focus on the complex relationships between environment and health across Europe. With particular regard to the initiatives launched by the European Commission, the chapter reviews current environmental and health policy requirements and the development of an infrastructure for spatial information in Europe. The conclusion to this chapter draws attention to the legal frameworks necessary to ensure data sharing and flows as well as confidentiality of the individual. It also emphasizes the importance of maintaining the trust of citizens and patients in their relationships with the healthcare system and more generally with the system of government.

The 1995 European Data Protection Directive provides a key aspect of the legal framework within which all GIS and health practitioners in the European Union have to operate. Deryck Beyleveld and David Townend discuss this directive in detail in Chapter 15. The authors introduce the directive and its objectives, requirements and exemptions, with a particular focus on informed consent. The important issue of anonymous data is discussed together with differences between the European Directive and its transposition into U.K. law.

Obtaining informed consent is crucial not only to respect the law but also to develop and maintain the relationship of trust with the data subjects, such as patients. The risks are otherwise incalculable for both researchers and the citizens themselves. Rupert Suckling, Darren Shickle, and Susan Wallace address this important issue in Chapter 16. Reviewing existing international literature, the authors analyze several aspects of public attitudes to the use of health information. Knowledge of existing rights is explored together with the extent to which health professionals are perceived as requiring access to sensitive information. The findings of this review are potentially constrained by the U.S. bias of available literature but provide a benchmark against which more recent studies (e.g., Spadaro, 2003) can be assessed.

Chapter 17 by Markku Löytönen and Clive E. Sabel reflects on the opportunities and limitations of recent technological advances in a range of fields including mobile telephony, remote sensing, and positioning systems. Their combination into a new generation of technologies and services is explored through speculative scenarios that ought to add to the debate about the boundaries between what is technologically possible and what is socially desirable.

Chapter 18 by the editors draws together the many threads of the four sections through an analysis of the strengths, weaknesses, opportunities, and threats facing GIS in public health.

References

Acheson, D. (chair of committee), 1988, Public health in England: The report of the Committee of Inquiry into the future development of the public health function, Cmnd 289, London: HMSO.

Acheson, D., 1998, *Independent Inquiry into Inequalities in Health,* London: HMSO.

Commission of the European Communities, 2003, A European environment and health strategy, COM(2003) 338, Brussels: European Commission.

Cromley, E.K. and McLafferty, S.L., 2002, *GIS and Public Health,* New York: Guilford Press.

de Lepper, M.J.C., Scholten, H.J., and Stern, R.M., Eds., 1995, *The Added Value of Geographical Information Systems in Public and Environmental Health*, Dordrecht, Netherlands: Kluwer Academic Publishers.

Goodchild, M.F., 1992, Geographical information science, *International Journal of Geographical Information Systems,* 6, 1, 31–45.

Longley, P. et al., 2001, *Geographic Information Systems and Science*, Chichester, U.K.: Wiley.

Melnick, A.L., 2002, *Introduction to Geographic Information Systems in Public Health,* Gaithersburg, MD: Aspen Publishers.

Scott-Samuel, A., 1998, Health impact assessment: Theory into practice, *Journal of Epidemiology and Community Health,* 52, 74–75.

Spadaro, R., 2003, European Union citizens and sources of information about health, Eurobarometer 58, March 2003. Survey of the European Opinion Research Group for DG SANCO, Brussels: EORG.

Stevens, A. and Raftery, J., 1997, *Health Care Needs Assessment,* 2nd series, Oxford: Radcliffe Medical Press.

van Tongelen, B., 2003, Personal communication from European Commission's DG Environment, 13 June 2003.

Section 1

Disease Mapping and Spatial Analysis

2 Basic Issues in Geographical Analysis

Ravi Maheswaran and Robert P. Haining

CONTENTS

2.1 INTRODUCTION

The purpose of this chapter is to consider basic issues in relation to the geographical analysis of public health data. The chapter is divided into two parts. The first part examines basic aspects of geographical data. It addresses spatially referenced data issues, including classification of data and assessment of data quality. The second part of the chapter is more technical in content. It describes the approaches to geographical analysis and focuses on cartographic operations, exploratory spatial data analysis, and ecological studies.

Cartographic operations are described briefly followed by a more detailed description of exploratory spatial data analysis. The section on ecological studies focuses on epidemiological and conceptual issues. Several of the later chapters in this book illustrate and expand on the data issues and some of the methods described in this chapter.

2.2 DATA ISSUES

The term data in the geographical context refers to both the attribute (e.g., a health outcome or a socioeconomic attribute) and the location identifier for the attribute (e.g., an address, a postcode or a census enumeration district). Since every

0-415-30655-8/04/$0.00+$1.50

measurement occurs at some point or during an interval of time, then any item of spatial data consists of the triple attributes: value (what), location (where) and time (when). The distribution of an attribute in geographical space is conceptualized as either a continuous surface or field or as a collection of discrete point, line and area objects in the study area. Air pollution across a region would be conceptualized as a field, the set of houses, roads or urban places as objects. An attribute like population is an exception to the suggestion of a unique conceptualization because it can be treated either as a field (e.g., a population density map) or as a collection of objects (e.g., a dot map of addresses).

For the practical purpose of storing either type of spatial data in a (finite) data matrix, which is a prerequisite for many areas of spatial data analysis, the analyst must choose a particular finite, discrete representation for the data. Spatial data are represented as points, lines, or areas. Points can be used to represent a field variable (e.g., a sample of points from the field) or point objects (e.g., an incinerator chimney). Lines can be used to represent boundaries on a surface (e.g., contours) or linear objects. Areas can be used to represent aggregations of a field variable, aggregations of point objects (e.g., census tracts) or areal objects. Often areas are artificial constructions that are unrelated to the underlying spatial variability in the attribute that is recorded (e.g., a ward). Areas can be in the form of a regular grid or in the form of irregular areas, such as enumeration districts or wards. In GIS, the terms raster and vector are used to distinguish these different forms of area representation.

Raster data are essentially gridded data (equivalent to a bitmap) with an attribute value attached to each cell of the grid. This may be the average level of pollution in an area. A polygrid is a similar concept where a range of attribute values is attached to each cell. Vector data are essentially data related to coordinates. These may be coordinates (x and y coordinates) of a point location or the longitude and latitude of that location. The point location may be that of a house or the postcode centroid. Vector data also commonly represent lines, where each line is represented by a series of point coordinates. Coordinates for the ends of the line can represent a straight line, while a curved line is approximated by a number of short straight segments and represented by a series of point locations. The vector database can also hold information on relationships (e.g., the left and right of a line). A series of lines joined together in a closed loop will form a polygon (e.g., the boundary of an electoral ward). These aspects of spatial data are described in detail elsewhere (Longley et al., 2001; Wise, 2002).

The term attribute data is sometimes used to refer to attribute information that may be attached to a spatial location or object. For example, at a point location such as a postcode centroid, we may have information on the number of households, people, age distribution, and other factors associated with that postcode. Similarly, there will be information on linear structures such as roads (e.g., type of road, traffic flow along the road) and polygons (e.g., census-based characteristics of an electoral ward).

A limited range of locational spatial data is often sufficient for routine public health work. The common ones are point locations (e.g., addresses, postcode centroids) and polygons (e.g., health authority boundaries, census ward boundaries).

Linear spatial information is often related to potential sources of exposure (e.g., roads, overhead power lines) or used to calculate road travel distances and times. Once georeferenced, the major interest for public health purposes relates to the attribute data. The classification of attribute data can be done in a number of ways. A formal way is to classify attribute data in terms of the level of measurement (nominal, ordinal, interval, or ratio), which is important since it specifies what mathematical operations are permissible on the data and hence what types of statistical tests can be performed. A substantive approach that is important with respect to public health applications is to classify it as data related to compositional attributes such as age and sex, exposures or risk factors, socioeconomic attributes (including confounders such as deprivation in a dose–response model) and data related to health outcomes. The exposure data may be classified conceptually as point, line, or area exposures. Examples of point and line sources of exposure include incinerators (points) and power lines (lines). Although area implies a continuous exposure, this may in practice be represented by a raster dataset with pollution values for each cell or as a vector dataset with polygons (e.g., water quality indicators for water supply zones). A range of census variables is commonly used to measure compositional and confounder attributes (e.g., percentage of owner-occupied houses, unemployment rate).

Health outcome data may be obtained from routine data sources or from specifically collected datasets. Routine data tends to refer to data routinely collected for mainly administrative and management purposes, but which may be used for public health analysis. The main examples are mortality data, hospital admission data, cancer registration data, and congenital malformation data.

Often, analysis in public health is based on areas rather than point locations because data confidentiality means point location (individual level) analysis is not possible. Analysis may be based on geographical units of varying sizes. A key requirement for this type of analysis is an appropriate denominator population for the calculation of rates. This commonly comes from census-derived information. Censuses are carried out periodically, not infrequently at ten-year intervals; they provide detailed information at the small-area level regarding the age-sex composition of the resident population. However, the denominator becomes progressively less reliable the further it is from the last census. Often, midyear estimates take into account births, deaths, and migration. These estimates are produced for larger administrative areas, such as local government or health authority areas. National or government bodies may carry out such estimates but in some areas, local authorities also produce their own estimates using additional local information (e.g., the development of new housing estates).

In the United Kingdom, an alternative source of denominator population information increasingly used is patient registration data from general practices. This information may be aggregated to the postcode level and subsequently to higher levels of aggregation. This information potentially provides an up-to-date denominator database for calculation of rates. In some other countries, administrative records are maintained at very detailed levels such as by household, so the denominator can be aggregated and used for calculation in very flexible ways (e.g., street-level rates).

Factors that influence health may be classified in a number of ways. A simple and useful classification uses four headings: genetic and inherited, environment, lifestyle and healthcare. The environment may be further classified into physical (air, soil, water, and radiation), socioeconomic and psychosocial, with the built environment as an additional category incorporating characteristics such as type of housing and degree of open space. The ways in which these factors are used in public health analyses are varied. There may be a simple spatial description of the distribution of these factors. On the other hand, the association between these factors and health outcomes may be examined. In some cases, one of these factors may be the main exposure of interest (e.g., effect of air quality on respiratory disease) and other factors (e.g., smoking) may be treated as confounders or covariables in the analysis. Another approach would be to see if the effect of the main factor of interest on the outcome varies with the level of another factor (e.g., socioeconomic deprivation). In this latter analysis, the technical term is effect modification or interaction. There are a number of issues related to both the conceptual and statistical aspects of interaction and these are addressed in detail elsewhere (Rothman and Greenland, 1998).

A common problem regarding factors that influence health is the availability of data for geographical analysis. Data on the physical environment are becoming increasingly available often through remote sensing technology, although there are still considerable barriers to obtaining exposure data at a fine spatial resolution. Socioeconomic data may be available from censuses and other sources (e.g., claims for unemployment benefit, free school meals). Often the data may be available in some parts of the system (e.g., within social services departments) but there are strong barriers to data sharing due to real or perceived confidentiality and data protection issues. Another issue is the level at which these data are georeferenced and the accuracy of this georeferencing. Data on the psychosocial environment are not normally available through any routine sources and are usually obtained through special surveys. Similarly, data on lifestyle factors (e.g., smoking, alcohol consumption, physical exercise) are usually obtained through surveys. Such surveys are normally conducted for other purposes but could be used for geographical analysis providing there is appropriate spatial stratification. An important limitation often is the sparsity of data at a small area level. An alternative approach to analysis would be to examine these data at the individual level using cohort or case-control methodologies rather than ecological analysis.

Data on healthcare factors may be available through routine health information systems that collect data for administrative purposes. Such data may include numbers of beds available, numbers of consultants and other specialist staff, bed occupancy rates or provision of specialist services, for example. Information that is more detailed will usually require additional efforts to gather such as policies for treatment and referral or care pathways. These data will then usually need to be converted to rates (e.g., specialists per 1000 population) for comparison across areas and for use in ecological analyses. To do this, the population being served by the staff or facilities will need to be determined. If service provision areas have been clearly agreed upon, then calculation of rates is straightforward, based on the resident population in these areas. Otherwise, catchment populations will need to be estimated and this is not always easy. In some cases, the local geography will mean that virtually all the local population will attend the main hospital for a town. However, in larger urban conurbations, with a number of provider hospitals, determining the catchment population could be more difficult. A common approach is to allocate a geographical unit to the healthcare facility that the majority of referrals or admissions from that area attend.

Spatial data quality may be considered in terms of accuracy, resolution, completeness, and consistency. These four dimensions can be related to the three components of a single item of spatial data: attribute, location, and time (Haining, 2003; Veregin and Hargitai, 1995). For example, if a study is being carried out to examine the association between overhead power lines and cancer, high levels of spatial resolution of locations is needed as the electromagnetic fields decrease very rapidly with increasing distance from power lines. This high level of resolution is important for both the point location of cases and controls (or the denominator population) and for the power lines. If, however, postcode centroids are used to link cases and controls to exposure to different levels of drinking water constituents and the latter data are for water supply zones with several thousand people per zone, then lower levels of location resolution for postcode centroid georeferencing will be acceptable.

The quality of health data has received much attention in epidemiological and public health circles. With regard to routinely collected health data, such as mortality and hospital admission data, coding of cause of death or admission may or may not be accurate. Mortality coding may become progressively less specific with increasing age. A further issue is the contribution of multiple pathologies to the cause of death in very elderly people. There are agreed systems of coding such as the International Classification of Disease but there may still be variations in interpretation of the guidelines for coding and classification.

Several factors may affect the interpretation of hospital admissions statistics (Anderson, 1978). The etiology of the disease determines the underlying levels of morbidity; however, underlying morbidity is not all observed or known about. This will depend on a range of factors including medical practice, illness behavior and the organization of medical care. These factors also influence admission to hospital and admission criteria. Diagnostic coding and even fashion influence the recording of hospital statistics. A further issue is identifying readmissions, which require a unique patient identifier. Errors and biases at several stages in the process generating hospital admissions data would lead to variations in data quality that need to be taken into account when interpreting the data.

Although death registration is mandatory and recording of hospital admissions is firmly governed by administrative systems, cancer registration often relies on a voluntary system. Thus, in addition to the issues related to diagnosis and coding, there may be major discrepancies in completeness of data capture across geographical areas. It should also be noted that even when recording is mandatory there might still be significant underreporting and a good example is in relation to notifiable diseases.

The quality of denominator data also needs careful consideration. Censuses may not reliably enumerate the entire population for various reasons, including misconceptions about the use of census data, concerns about privacy and negative publicity.

In the U.K. 1991 census, there was substantial underenumeration partly related to the perception that census data would not be confidential and could be used for surveillance, including identifying individuals for taxation purposes. Some sections of the population might be more likely to be underenumerated, such as young men, refugees, and ethnic minority groups. Alternative sources for the denominator population, such as general practice registered populations, are also potentially problematic. List inflation is a recognized problem, especially in areas where there is a highly mobile population and people who have left the area may not be removed from general practice lists. Underregistration may also be a problem, especially of young adults, refugees, and homeless people. The place of registration of students is also potentially problematic as they can be registered either with their general practice near their home address or with student medical services at their higher education institution. This is also a problem with censuses and needs careful consideration in geographical studies with regard to the denominator population at risk (e.g., geographical studies of the incidence of sexually transmitted disease, leukemias, and lymphomas).

2.3 GEOGRAPHICAL ANALYSIS

There are a number of ways of classifying geographical analysis. One approach is to distinguish between cartographic operations, spatial data analysis, and mathematical modeling. Cartographic operations include buffering, overlay, geometric (as opposed to statistical) forms of spatial interpolation and regionalization. These are described in the following section on cartographic operations.

Spatial data analysis is usually divided into two sections: exploratory spatial data analysis and confirmatory spatial data analysis. Exploratory spatial data analysis may be purely descriptive or may involve an element of hypothesis testing where no model is proposed for the alternative hypothesis, such as testing for significant clusters of cases of a disease (as described in Chapter 4). Exploratory spatial data analysis has numerical and visualization aspects. It is described in detail in the section on exploratory spatial data analysis.

Confirmatory spatial data analysis is concerned with inference and hypothesis testing. A model is proposed to represent variation in the data, which is then used for the purposes of hypothesis testing. A typical example would be the investigation of an association between an exposure and a health outcome, with the term exposure being used in a broad sense to include any factor that may affect a health outcome. The term health outcome may also be viewed more generally and could be substituted with proxies for health outcomes or intermediate process measures. The main type of epidemiological study used to test hypotheses in a geographical setting is the ecological study. It is described in detail in the section on ecological studies.

Mathematical modeling includes optimization and models for describing the spread of communicable disease. Optimization involves the process of obtaining the best solution to a problem. One use is identifying locations that are most suitable based on defined criteria. Examples include siting of primary care facilities to maximize geographical access and population coverage and identifying the shortest or quickest routes for travel for emergency ambulances or patient transport vehicles from a variety of locations to healthcare facilities. This chapter does not cover mathematical modeling of spatial data in detail.

2.3.1 Cartographic Operations

Longley et al. (2001) provide a clear and detailed description of cartographic operations and argue that these operations are in many ways the crux of GIS. Cartographic operations often involve map-based or spatial querying of a database to identify properties. They are an important component of what it means to add value to geographic data and we summarize the key features in this section.

One group of cartographic operations has to do with measurement and there are four elements:

1. Distance and length
2. Area
3. Shape
4. Slope and aspect

Measuring distance relies on a metric or rule for determining distance. The simplest and easiest to implement is calculating straight-line distance. When calculating greater distances, the earth's curvature needs to be taken into account. More complicated distance measurements include distance along a road network, often referred to as a stick network because segments of roads are represented as straight lines.

The area of a polygon is measured using the trapezium rule implemented within a GIS. The area measurement in public health applications is often used as part of a calculation, for example, as a denominator for calculating population density. Sometimes it is used to describe the geographical size of a patch served by a healthcare unit such as a psychiatric community outreach team.

The shape of an area is often measured in relation to the compactness of the geographical area. The measurement of shape may be used when creating geographical areas for administrative purposes or for targeting interventions and may be part of the optimization process in constructing regions.

Slope and aspect have clear applications in relation to digital elevation (terrain) models. In the public health field, these measures may be useful in modeling the ecology and climate in relation to communicable disease, such as climate change and changes in the local environment that may enhance the spread of vectors for disease.

Transformations are arguably the key element within a GIS for public health use. Longley et al. (2001) classify transformations under five headings:

1. Buffering
2. Point-in-polygon
3. Polygon overlay
4. Spatial interpolation
5. Density estimation

Buffering is the process by which an area is created around an object such as a 200-meter circle around a point source of pollution. Buffers may be created around line and area sources of pollution. Other examples of use include defining potential catchment areas around healthcare centers.

Point-in-polygon methods are essentially a means of linking points to areas. For instance, all postcodes falling within a geographically defined urban regeneration area will be linked to that area using this GIS process.

Polygon overlay is a method of linking information from two or more sources with boundaries that do not correspond. Reassigning values from one dataset to another may then be carried out (e.g., using an allocation based on proportional area).

Cartographically based methods of spatial interpolation include cell declustering, triangulation, and inverse distance weighting, which are described in detail elsewhere (Isaaks and Srivastava, 1989).

The fifth heading under transformations is density estimation, e.g., estimating population density. There is an important distinction between the last two categories: density estimation creates a field from discrete objects, while for spatial interpolation a field already exists (e.g., outdoor air pollution levels) but we only have samples from this field to work with.

Other elements sometimes included within the list of cartographic operations include the identification of centers and measures of dispersion, spatial dependence and fragmentation and fractional dimension.

Measures of centers include centroids and the point of minimum aggregate travel, both of which are described in detail by Longley et al. (2001). The centroid is the weighted average of x and y coordinates of points (e.g., individuals' addresses) within a given area and is thus a measure of the center of the distribution of these points. It is the point that minimizes the sum of squared distances. Centroids are frequently used in public health GIS work. There are two types: geometric centroids and population weighted centroids. The latter tends to be used more as it reflects the location of the bulk of the population within a geographical area. Population weighted centroids are typically used to attribute an exposure to a population in small geographical areas (e.g., census enumeration districts) or to calculate distances to healthcare locations. Population weighted centroids tend to be used because point locations (of addresses or postcode centroids) are not available for cases and the population at risk within small areas.

Measures of dispersion, spatial dependence, and fragmentation and fractional dimension are described in more detail elsewhere (Longley et al., 2001). They tend not to be used largely within public health GIS analysis although spatial dependence measures, for example, are potentially of use in exploring questions about the infectiousness of some diseases. These are as-yet-unexplored areas of GIS capability in relation to public health questions. They may also overlap with other categories of geographical analysis.

Region building, or zone designing, is the process of partitioning an area into (quasi) homogenous subareas or regions using small areal units as the basic building blocks (e.g., deprivation regions using enumeration districts as the building blocks). One of the purposes of region building is obtaining spatial units in which calculated rates of disease, for example, are of equivalent statistical precision. These regions can subsequently be used in exploratory spatial data analysis to examine patterns because imposing a coarser regional framework is similar to passing a filter across a map thereby smoothing and, providing the filter is not too large, helping to reveal patterns. These regions can also be used in confirmatory spatial data analysis (e.g., to model relationships between health outcomes and socioeconomic deprivation), and in the planning process to inform the targeting of public health interventions.

2.3.2 Exploratory Spatial Data Analysis

2.3.2.1 Purpose and Conduct

The aim of exploratory data analysis (EDA) is to identify data properties for the purposes of detecting patterns within the data, formulating hypotheses from the data and examining some aspects of model assessment (e.g., goodness of fit, identifying data effects on model fit). EDA is based on the use of graphical and visual methods and the use of numerical techniques that are statistically robust (i.e., not much affected by extreme or atypical data values). Hence, the median rather than the mean is used to measure the center of a distribution of values. The emphasis in EDA is on descriptive methods rather than formal hypothesis testing or model building. The approach emphasizes the importance of "staying close to the original data" in the sense of using simple, intuitive methods.

What is exploratory spatial data analysis (ESDA)? It is an extension of EDA to detect spatial properties of data. Additional techniques to those found in EDA are needed for detecting spatial patterns in data, formulating hypotheses based on the geography of the data, and assessing spatial models. It is important to be able to link numerical and graphical procedures with the map and the analyst needs to be able to answer the question: where are those cases on the map? With modern graphical interfaces, this is often done by brushing: cases are identified by brushing the relevant part of a box plot and the related regions are identified on the map.

The link between ESDA and GIS is interesting. Most GIS software has not been developed with ESDA in mind, but rather to support data management (e.g., by utilities that keep track of networks or the location of key sites), cartographic modeling (e.g., whole map operations such as sieve analysis to locate areas) and some selected forms of spatial analysis (e.g., network analysis). Nevertheless, particular GIS products do contain some ESDA-type facilities (for example, see Geostatistical Analyst in ArcGIS® Desktop, Version 8.1). Some have argued that the large datasets now becoming available in GIS require new tools to be developed which can detect patterns and anomalies automatically and that traditional ESDA methods are not appropriate in a GIS context (e.g., Openshaw in Fotheringham and Rogerson, 1994). Others, however, feel there is a role for current statistical methods and that these can be given new power and made more useful and widely available by linking to particular GIS software (Haining, 1996). This is the view taken here and is illustrated by the SAGE software developed by Haining et al. (1996, 1998).

When carrying out a program of ESDA, the analyst may find it useful to have a conceptual data model in mind. There have been a number of suggestions for appropriate conceptual models (see, for example, Haining, 2003). Tukey (1977) suggested for EDA that data be considered as decomposable into rough and smooth elements thus:

DATA = ROUGH + SMOOTH

In the case of bivariate relationships, the best-fit line defines the smooth and the scatter about the best-fit line defines the rough. These elements are specified for each data value. Such a conceptual model can be adapted to the case of spatial data where a spatial trend (e.g., from north to south) represents the smooth and variation around the trend represents the rough.

In ESDA, data properties for a single variable may be classified under nonspatial properties and spatial properties. The nonspatial properties for a single variable may be further subclassified under smooth and rough properties. The smooth nonspatial properties include the center of the distribution (measured by the median), the spread of the distribution (measured by the interquartile range) and the shape of the distribution (depicted by box plots, histograms and smoothed curves if the data takes the form of a sequence of values). The rough nonspatial properties include outliers that are values more than a certain distance above the upper or below the lower quartiles of the distribution (Haining, 1993, 2003).

Spatial properties for a single variable may also be subclassified under smooth and rough properties. The smooth spatial properties include spatial trends or gradients and spatial autocorrelation. The rough spatial properties include spatial outliers that are individual attribute values different in magnitude from their neighboring values.

When carrying out ESDA to examine data properties and relationships between variables, the scatterplot is one of the basic tools used. The scatterplot is used to visualize the relationship between two variables. The best-fit line through the scatterplot identifies the smooth element of the relationship. The residuals from the best-fit line identify the rough element. An outlier is typically defined as a data value more than a certain vertical distance from the best-fit line.

In the classification of ESDA methods, it is useful to distinguish between two classes of ESDA statistics: global and focused. Global or whole map statistics process all the cases for one or more attributes, while focused or local statistics process subsets (windows) of the data one at time and usually involve a sweep through the data looking for evidence of smooth and rough elements of the mapped data. They generate local summaries (means, medians) that may then allow the analyst to fit a locally smoothed surface. This chapter only considers global statistics. The application of ESDA might involve working with windowed subsets of the map (analyst-defined boxes, circles, or polygons). Processing might involve applying global or focused statistics only to cases in the window and executing a spatial query such as "identify all the areas within the window possessing attribute property x."

2.3.2.2 Techniques

The median, quartiles, interquartile spread, and box plots are some of the ESDA techniques for identifying nonspatial properties of a single attribute. All are standard EDA techniques. The link to the map, however, makes them part of ESDA. The median is a measure of the location (or center) of the distribution of attribute values. A typical ESDA query might be "which are the areas with attribute values above (or below) the median?" Quartiles and the interquartile spread are a measure of the spread of values about the median. The corresponding ESDA query might be "which are the areas that lie in the upper (or lower) quartile?" Box plots provide a graphical summary of the distribution of attribute values. ESDA queries might include "where do cases that lie in specific parts of the box plot occur on the map? Are outlier cases located on the map?"

There are several ESDA techniques for describing the spatial properties of an attribute. The techniques described below are in some cases the spatial equivalents of methods developed for nonspatial data (e.g., time series data). As with the techniques above for nonspatial properties, they only apply to a single attribute at a time.

Smoothing is a useful ESDA tool. Where a map consists of many small areas or point samples from a surface it is often helpful to apply simple smoothing methods that, depending on the scale of the smoother, may help to reveal the presence of general patterns that are unclear from the mosaic or sample of values. Local spatial averaging is an example of this technique. This process is carried out by simply taking the attribute value of an area and its neighbors, averaging them and then allocating the average (mean) value to that central area. The process is then repeated for each area using its corresponding neighbors. The median could also be used in this way: instead of calculating the mean of values, the median is calculated. This simple smoothing technique can be applied to standardized mortality (or morbidity) ratios where the sum of observed counts is divided by the sum of expected counts. It can also be applied to rates, for example, to obtain smoothed age-specific rates by dividing the sum of cases by the sum of the denominator population. The smoothed age-specific rates can be applied to a standard population (e.g., the European Standard Population) to produce a map of smoothed directly standardized rates.

A typical question in ESDA is "are there any general trends or gradients in the map distribution of values?" There are a number of ESDA techniques for identifying trends and gradients on the map (e.g., the existence of a general increase in heart disease incidence from southern to northern England):

- Kernel estimation
- Taking transects through the data and plotting with the attribute value on the vertical axis and spatial location on the horizontal axis
- Producing spatially lagged box plots with lag order specified with respect to a particular area or zone
- Applying two-way median polish adapted to nonregular lattice data as suggested by Cressie (1991) and described in Haining (1993)

Spatial autocorrelation is the propensity for attribute values in neighboring areas to be similar. The ESDA technique is to use a scatterplot with the area attribute value on the vertical axis plotted against the average of the attribute values in the adjacent areas on the horizontal axis (Haining, 1993). A scatterplot where there is an upward sloping scatter to the right is indicative of positive spatial autocorrelation (adjacent values tend to be similar). Where the scatter slopes upward to the left, this is indicative of negative spatial autocorrelation (adjacent values tend to be dissimilar).

A spatial outlier is an individual attribute value that is not necessarily extreme in the distributional sense, but is extreme in terms of the attribute values in adjacent areas. The ESDA technique for detecting spatial outliers is to use the scatterplot technique as for spatial autocorrelation and then run a regression line through the plot. Cases with standardized residuals greater than 3.0 or less than –3.0 might be flagged as possible outliers although, for reasons beyond the level of this chapter, the use of least squares estimation for the line will tend to overstate the number of outliers (Haining, 1993).

In addition to describing the spatial and nonspatial properties of attributes, ESDA techniques can be used for model assessment. ESDA is not used for model confirmation in the sense of hypothesis testing. However, ESDA techniques can be used to test model assumptions, as in the case of regression. Regression assumes that model errors are independent. The presence of residual spatial autocorrelation is grounds for believing that this assumption is not met. The ESDA technique is to map the residuals and look for evidence of positive residuals clustering together. The scatterplot method for spatial autocorrelation described above can be applied to the regression residuals. A strong gradient in the scatterplot is indicative of a failure to meet the assumption of independence.

The lack of spatial analytical capability within standard GIS software has been a cause for concern, although several specialist statistical packages are available for advanced spatial analysis (e.g., S-Plus® software with the S+SpatialStats™ add-on, SPLANCS, GeoBUGS). However, the situation is changing. ESRI's ArcGIS incorporates statistical capability with Geostatistical Analyst, which includes tools for exploratory spatial data analysis.

For a more detailed discussion of ESDA, refer to Haining (2003).

2.3.3 Ecological Studies

In this section, we describe some of the basic features of ecological studies, closely following the approach taken by Morgenstern (1995). An ecological study may be defined as a study in which the focus is on the comparison of groups rather than individuals. Usually, the main reason for this focus is that individual level data are missing for the joint distribution of at least two, and perhaps all, variables within each group. Ecological studies may examine associations in terms of place, time or place and time.

There are a number of types of ecological study. Common examples are descriptive studies on the variation in health between populations. These studies include geographical correlation studies (e.g., studies examining the association between socioeconomic deprivation and mortality and studies of the occurrence of disease in relation to spatially defined exposures (e.g., point sources such as nuclear installations, line sources such as high voltage power lines and exposure surfaces such as air pollution). Other examples are studies of disease clusters without an identified exposure and studies more generally of disease clustering. Ecological studies may be used for health surveillance or for examining the effects of health interventions at a community level. Migrant studies at the area level, studies of time trends, time series analyses, and studies of space–time interactions are other examples of different types of ecological studies. Morgenstern (1995) has suggested that ecological studies may be thought of as exploratory when no exposure has been measured or analytical when an exposure or a proxy for exposure has been measured. However, in practice studies are often mixed.

Morgenstern (1995) has proposed a classification for variables in ecological studies: environmental, aggregate, and global. Environmental measures refer to physical characteristics of an area for which there is an equivalent measure at the individual level (e.g., drinking water magnesium level), even though this may not have been measured at the individual level. Aggregate measures are summary measures of variables derived at the individual level and grouped to the area level (e.g., percentage of smokers). A global measure refers to an attribute of the place, which is a contextual attribute, which has no corresponding equivalent at the individual level. Examples are motorcycle helmet laws and social capital. It is important to recognize that all three classes of variables are ecological variables and are therefore properties of areas (or the groups of people living in those areas), whereas individual-level variables are properties of individuals. We mentioned previously that one classification for factors influencing health has four categories: inherited, environmental, lifestyle, and healthcare. Furthermore, in environmental epidemiology, a commonly used classification comprises compositional (e.g., age), environmental (e.g., air quality) and socioeconomic factors (e.g., social class). How do these classifications fit in with that proposed by Morgenstern? Inherited, compositional, lifestyle and some socioeconomic and healthcare factors are individual-level measures that may be aggregated to the area level, while other socioeconomic factors (e.g., social capital) and healthcare factors (e.g., bed occupancy rates) are contextual or global measures.

An important issue in ecological studies is the level of analysis in relation to the level of inference. The level of analysis may be at the individual level or at the ecological (or group) level. For an analysis at the individual level, ecological-level variable values are allocated to all individuals within an area. For an analysis at the ecological level, all individual-level variables are grouped to a common ecological or area level. The unit of analysis is therefore the level to which all variables have been assigned and this may be at the individual or at the area level. Sophisticated approaches are available that take into account information at the individual and area levels (including multiple area levels such as family, neighborhood, and county). The main approaches are multilevel modeling and Bayesian hierarchical modeling.

With respect to interpretation, the underlying objective may be to make inferences about biobehavioral, ecological, and contextual effects on health.

Biological or behavioral effects refer to effects on risks at the individual level; for example, the biological effect of wearing a seat belt on the risk of road-traffic-related injury and death among drivers and passengers.

Ecological effects refer to effects on group rates. For example, the ecological effect of seat belt laws on accident mortality rates in different countries depends not only on the protective effect of the seat belt but also on the degree of compliance with the law in each country. An additional factor may be risk compensation, that is, the tendency to drive faster because drivers feel safer when wearing seat belts.

Contextual effects refer to the effects of an ecological exposure on individual risk, for example, the contextual effect of living in a socioeconomically deprived area on the risk of ill health over and above the effects of deprivation at the individual level. With regard to the seat belt example, the contextual effect might be family or peer pressure to conform to the law.

Another example of the contextual effect comes from communicable disease epidemiology. The risk of contracting a disease is typically dependent on the host, the agent, and the environment. One of the environmental factors is the prevalence of disease in close contacts or the community in which the individual resides. The risk to the individual will increase if the prevalence of disease in close contacts increases. Conversely, if herd immunity is high due to high levels of vaccination coverage, then the risk to individuals within the community, even those unvaccinated, may be low.

As ecological studies are often carried out to draw inferences, it is important to see if the level of inference matches the level of analysis. Not infrequently, analyses are carried out at the ecological level because information on exposures of interest is not available at the individual level or would be too expensive or impractical to collect. The real interest and therefore inference may be at the individual level regarding biological effects, such as the effect of radon exposure on lung cancer. Such cross-level inferences are particularly susceptible to ecological bias.

Ecological studies have a number of advantages. They tend to be inexpensive and are quick to carry out. Routine statistics are frequently available by area and over time. Exposure information is often only or most readily available at the area level (e.g., air pollution measurements from monitoring stations). Random errors are often smaller for populations than for individuals. Differences in exposure between areas may be larger than differences between individuals in the same area. Mapping and spatial analysis of epidemiological data may reveal important features and generate hypotheses to be tested at the individual level. Ecological studies may be entirely appropriate if the interest is in ecological level effects, such as the effectiveness of population interventions or legislation.

Ecological studies, however, have numerous potential disadvantages. Measures of exposure are only surrogates based on the average exposure for a population. The association seen between exposure and outcome at the group level may not be reliably extrapolated to that at the individual level (see ecological bias, discussed later). There may be systematic differences between areas and over time in recording disease frequency, regarding quality of diagnosis, disease classification, completeness of reporting, differential survival and population under- or overenumeration.

There may be systematic differences in the measurement of exposures. Data are often not available for confounding factors and controlling for them may be difficult. Spatial boundaries sometimes artificially divide populations in ways that may obscure the true distribution of exposure and disease risk. There may be significant statistical problems posed by spatial and temporal autocorrelation. There may be unstable estimates of risk in small area studies due to small numbers. Selective migration across groups in small area studies would tend to obscure or exaggerate associations. Routine data are usually collected for mortality statistics rather than for estimation of incidence. There may also be the issue of temporal ambiguity unlike cohort studies where we can usually be confident that disease did not precede exposure. A number of covariates, particularly demographic, socioeconomic, and environmental factors, tend to be more highly correlated with each other than they are at the individual level. This problem with colinearity tends to make it very difficult to separate their effects statistically.

A major limitation of ecological analysis for making causal inferences is ecological bias: the failure of ecological effect estimates to reflect the biological effect at the individual level. Ecological bias occurs when the measure of association found at the group level is a distortion of the association that exists at the individual level. To assume that grouped results apply to individuals could result in the ecological fallacy. A famous example is the correlation between suicide rates and religion in regions in Prussia. The relative risk of suicide among Protestants was estimated to be 7.6 at the ecological level, but only 2 at the individual level (Morgenstern, 1995). Ecological bias can arise from several sources. Confounding, bias or misclassification may alter the association between an exposure and a health outcome within areas. If there were a bias in the same direction in most areas, the ecological estimate of the association would also be biased. Nonlinear relationships at the individual level will affect the ecological estimate of the association. Important sources of ecological bias are those that result from the phenomena referred to as confounding by group and effect modification by group. Confounding by group occurs when the background rate of disease in the population varies across areas. For example, heart disease mortality rates may be higher in regions with higher levels of air pollution. However, the higher rates in the populations within these regions may be due to other factors such as genetically determined risk levels. Confounding by group occurs in this situation even when there is no association between exposure to air pollution and genetically determined risk at the individual level within areas. Effect modification by group occurs if the effect of exposure on risk at the individual level varies across areas. For example, the effect of exposure to high levels of grass pollen on asthma might be more marked within a region where the individuals are more susceptible to the adverse effects of pollen, perhaps due to genetic or dietary factors, than in a region where they are not. The ecological estimate of the effects of pollen on asthma across these regions would not reflect the biological effect at the individual level.

For an in-depth discussion of epidemiological and statistical issues in ecological studies, refer to other sources (Elliott et al., 2000; Lawson et al., 1999).

2.4 CONCLUSIONS

In this chapter, we have examined a number of the issues regarding data used for geographical analysis. It is clear that there are many facets to both the location and attribute aspects of spatial data. An important message is that data quality should be explicitly considered as any analysis and interpretation will depend on the quality of data used. Uncritical use of spatial data should be avoided, as there are numerous potential pitfalls.

The chapter has also described cartographic operations, which are a special feature of GIS. A substantial amount of public health information has an intrinsic spatial component, which is often not realized. The use of GIS and cartographic operations is strongly recommended to bring an added dimension to public health intelligence.

ESDA and ESDA techniques have been described. Some forms of ESDA can be implemented in standard GIS software and can be implemented using database and spreadsheet software in conjunction with GIS. We recommend that public health analysts, particularly those involved in public health observatory and surveillance-type work, become familiar with and utilize at least the basic methods available. Ecological studies are more the domain of the public health researcher and, aside from the limitations, can be useful tools for public health research.

References

Anderson, H.R., 1978, The epidemiological value of hospital diagnostic data, in Bennett, A.E., Ed., *Recent Advances in Community Medicine*, Edinburgh: Churchill Livingstone.

Cressie, N., 1991, *Statistics for Spatial Data,* New York: Wiley.

Elliott, P. et al., Eds., 2000, *Spatial Epidemiology: Methods and Applications,* Oxford: Oxford University Press.

Fotheringham, A.S. and Rogerson, P., 1994, Eds., *Spatial Analysis and GIS,* London: Taylor and Francis.

Haining, R.P., 1993, *Spatial Data Analysis in the Social and Environmental Sciences*, Cambridge: Cambridge University Press.

Haining, R.P., 1996, Designing a health needs GIS with spatial analysis capability, in Fischer, M., Scholten, H., and Unwin, D., Eds., *Spatial Analytical Perspectives on GIS,* London: Taylor and Francis.

Haining, R.P., 2003, *Spatial Data Analysis: Theory and Practice,* Cambridge: Cambridge University Press.

Haining, R.P., Wise, S.M., and Ma, J., 1996, The design of a software system for interactive spatial statistical analysis linked to a GIS, *Computational Statistics,* 11, 449–466.

Haining, R.P., Wise, S.M., and Ma, J., 1998, Exploratory spatial data analysis in a GIS environment, *The Statistician*, 47, 457–469.

Isaaks, E.H. and Srivastava, R.M., 1989, *An Introduction to Applied Geostatistics*, Oxford: Oxford University Press.

Lawson, A. et al., Eds., 1999, *Disease Mapping and Risk Assessment for Public Health,* Chichester, U.K.: Wiley.

Longley, P.A. et al., 2001, *Geographic Information Systems and Science,* Chichester, U.K.: Wiley.

Morgenstern, H., 1995, Ecologic studies in epidemiology: Concepts, principles, and methods, *Annual Review of Public Health,* 16, 61–81.

Rothman, K.J. and Greenland, S., 1998, *Modern Epidemiology,* Philadelphia: Lippincott-Raven.

Tukey, J.W., 1977, *Exploratory Data Analysis,* Reading, MA: Addison-Wesley.

Veregin, H. and Hargitai, P., 1995, An evaluation matrix for geographical data quality, in Guptill, S.C. and Morrison, J.L., Eds., *Elements of Spatial Data Quality,* Oxford: Elsevier Science.

Wise, S., 2002, *GIS Basics*, London: Taylor and Francis.

3 Disease Mapping: Basic Approaches and New Developments

Andrew B. Lawson

CONTENTS

3.1 INTRODUCTION

The representation and analysis of maps of disease-incidence data is a basic tool in the analysis of regional variation in public health. The development of methods for mapping disease incidence has progressed considerably in recent years. One of the earliest examples of disease mapping is the map of the addresses of cholera victims related to the locations of water supplies by John Snow in 1854. In that case, the street addresses of victims were recorded and their proximity to putative pollution sources (water supply pumps) was assessed (Snow, 1854).

The subject area of disease mapping has developed considerably in recent years. This growth in interest has led to a greater use of geographical or spatial statistical

0-415-30655-8/04/$0.00+$1.50

tools in the analysis of data both routinely collected for public health purposes and in the analysis of data found within ecological studies of disease relating to explanatory variables. The study of the geographical distribution of disease can have a variety of uses. The main areas of application can be conveniently broken down into the following classes:

- Disease mapping
- Disease clustering
- Ecological analysis

In the first class — disease mapping — usually the object of the analysis is to provide (estimate) the true relative risk of a disease of interest across a geographical study area (map), a focus similar to the processing of pixel images to remove noise. Applications for such methods lie in health services resource allocation and in disease atlas construction; e.g., see Pickle et al. (1999).

The second class — disease clustering — has particular importance in public health surveillance, where it may be important to be able to assess whether a disease map is clustered and where the clusters are located. This may lead to examination of potential environmental hazards. A particular special case arises when a known location is thought to be a potential pollution hazard. The analysis of disease incidence around a putative source of hazard is a special case of cluster detection.

The third class — ecological analysis — is of great relevance within epidemiological research, as its focus is the analysis of the geographical distribution of disease in relation to explanatory covariates, usually at an aggregated spatial level. Many issues relating to disease mapping are also found in this area, in addition to issues relating specifically to the incorporation of covariates.

In this chapter, the issues surrounding the first class of problems, namely disease mapping, are the focus of attention. While the focus here is on statistical methods and issues in disease mapping, it should be noted that the results of such statistical procedures are often represented visually in mapped form. Hence, some consideration must be given to the purely cartographic issues that affect the representation of geographical information. The method chosen to represent disease intensity on the map, be it color scheme or symbolic representation, can dramatically affect the resulting interpretation of disease distribution. It is not the purpose of this review to detail such cognitive aspects of disease mapping, but the reader is directed to some recent discussions of these issues (Pickle and Hermann, 1995; Walter, 1993).

3.2 DISEASE MAPPING AND MAP RECONSTRUCTION

To begin, we consider two different mapping situations that clearly demarcate approaches to this area. The form of the mapped data that arises in such studies defines these situations. First, the lowest level of aggregation of data observable in disease incidence studies is the case itself. Its geographical reference (georeference), usually the residential address of the case, is the basic mapping unit. This type of data is often referred to as case event data. We usually define a fixed study area within which case events occur. The second type of data commonly found in such studies is a count of disease cases within arbitrarily defined administrative regions (tracts), such as census tracts, electoral districts, or health authority areas. Essentially the count is an aggregation of all the cases within the tract. Therefore, the georeference of the count is related to the tract location, where the individual case spatial references (locations) are lost. Often this latter form of data is more commonly available from routine data sources such as government agencies than the first form. Confidentiality can limit access to the case event realization. Figure 3.1 and Figure 3.2 display examples of such data formats.

The first example is the address locations of cancer of the larynx cases in southern Lancashire, England, for the period of 1974 to 1983. The second example is of 26 enumeration districts (census tracts) in central Falkirk, Scotland, in which were collected the respiratory cancer disease counts for the period of 1978 to 1983. Figure 3.3 highlights the correspondence between case event and count data.

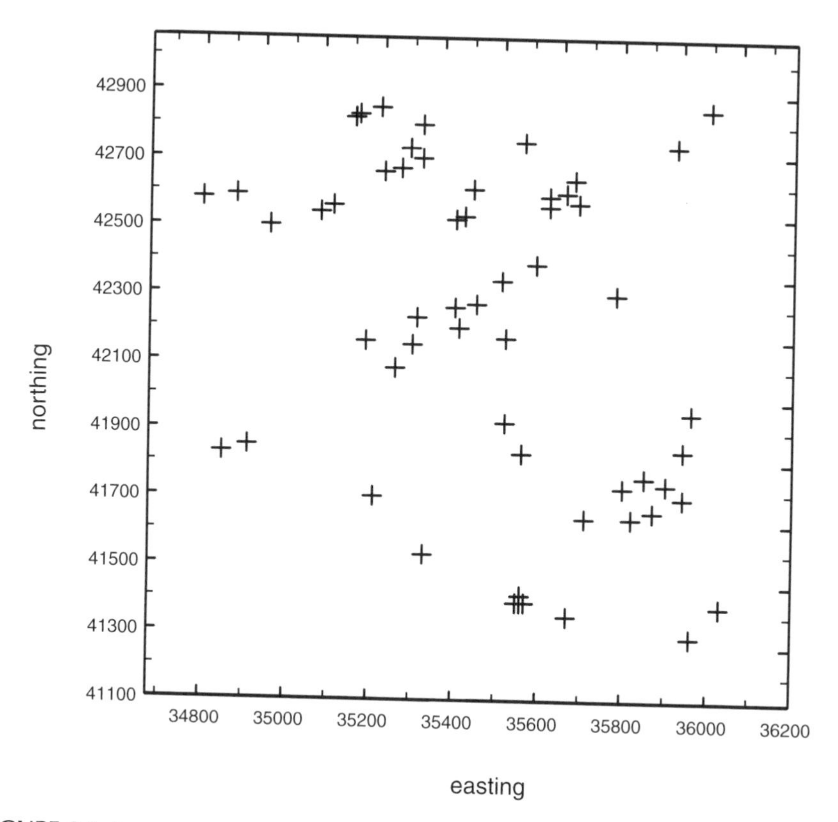

FIGURE 3.1 Larynx cancer case event map, Lancashire, England, 1974 to 1983. *Source*: Lawson, A.B., 2001, *Statistical Methods in Spatial Epidemiology*, New York: Wiley. With permission.

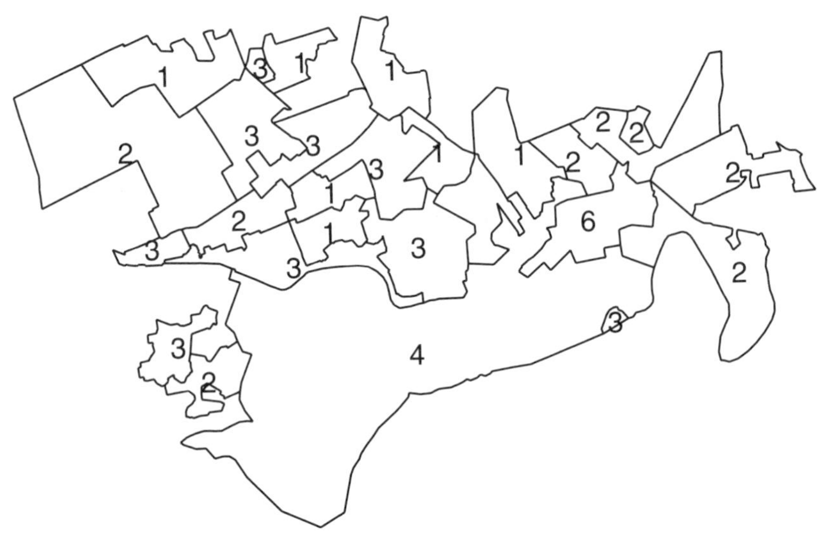

FIGURE 3.2 Respiratory cancer counts in 26 census tracts in Falkirk Central, Scotland, 1978 to 1983. *Source*: Lawson, A.B., 2001, *Statistical Methods in Spatial Epidemiology,* New York: Wiley. With permission.

3.3 DISEASE MAP RESTORATION

3.3.1 Simple Statistical Representations

The representation of disease-incidence data can vary from simple point object maps for cases and pictorial representation of counts within tracts, to the mapping of estimates from complex models purporting to describe the structure of the disease events. This section and Section 3.3.2 describe the range of mapping methods from simple representations to model-based forms. The geographical incidence of disease has as its fundamental unit of observation, the address location of cases of disease. The residential address (or possibly the employment address) of cases of disease contains important information relating to the type of exposure to environmental risks. Often, however, the exact address locations of cases are not directly available and instead one must use counts of disease in arbitrary administrative regions, such as census tracts or postal districts. This lack of precise spatial information may be due to confidentiality constraints relating to the identification of case addresses or may be due to the scale of information gathering.

3.3.1.1 Crude Representation of Disease Distribution

The simplest possible mapping form is the depiction of disease rates at specific sets of locations. For case events, this is a map of case event locations. For counts within tracts, this is a pictorial representation of the number of events in the tracts plotted at

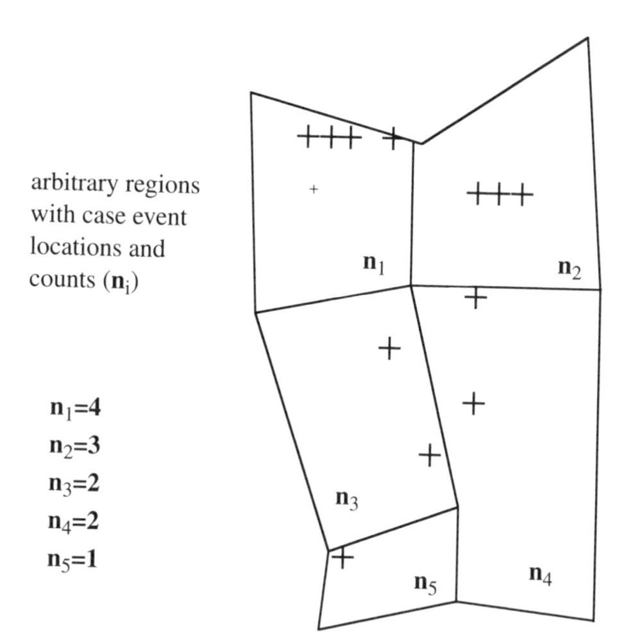

FIGURE 3.3 Case event map with arbitrary regions superimposed. *Source*: Lawson, A.B. and Cressie, N., 2000, Spatial statistical methods for environmental epidemiology, in Rao, C.R. and Sen, P.K., Eds., *Handbook of Statistics: Bio-Environmental and Public Health Statistics*, Vol. 18, New York: Elsevier.

a suitable set of locations (e.g., tract centroids). The locations of case events within a spatially heterogeneous population can display a small amount of information concerning the overall pattern of disease events within a window. Ross and Davis (1990) provide an example of such an analysis of leukemia cluster data. However, any interpretation of the structure of these events is severely limited by the lack of information concerning the spatial distribution of the background population that might be at risk from the disease of concern. This population also has a spatial distribution and failure to take account of this spatial variation severely limits the ability to interpret the resulting case event map. In essence, areas of high density of at-risk populations would tend to yield a high incidence of case events and so, without taking account of this distribution, areas of high disease intensity could be spuriously attributed to excess disease risk. Figure 3.4 displays an example of a case address map for Humberside, U.K., for cases of childhood leukemia and lymphoma in a fixed period.

For counts of cases of disease within tracts, similar considerations apply when crude count maps are constructed. Here, variation in population density also affects the spatial incidence of disease. It is also important to consider how a count of cases could be depicted in a mapped representation. Counts within tracts are totals of events from the whole tract region. If tracts are irregular, then a decision must be made to either locate the count at some tract location (e.g., tract centroid, however defined) with suitable symbolization or to represent the count as a fill color or shade over the whole tract (choropleth thematic map). In the former case, the choice of

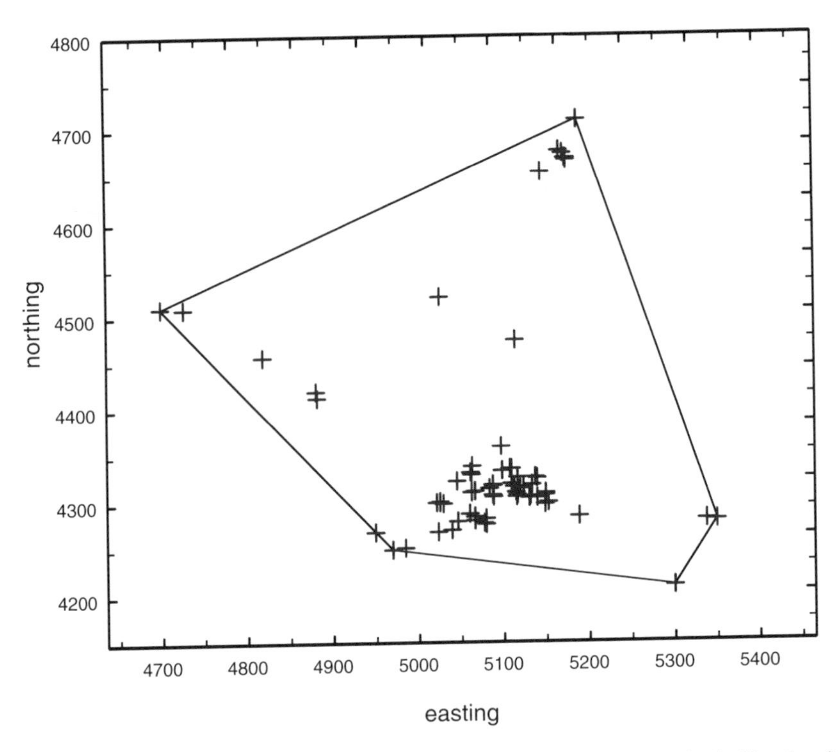

FIGURE 3.4 Case address locations of childhood leukemia and lymphoma in the Humberside region of the United Kingdom, within a fixed time period. *Source*: Lawson, A.B., 2001, *Statistical Methods in Spatial Epidemiology*, New York: Wiley. With permission.

location will affect interpretation. In the latter case, symbolization choice (shade or color) could also distort interpretation although an attempt to represent the whole tract may be attractive.

In general, methods that attempt to incorporate the effect of the background at-risk population are to be preferred. These are discussed in the next section.

3.3.1.2 Standardized Mortality/Morbidity Ratios and Standardization

To assess the status of an area with respect to disease incidence, it is convenient to attempt to first assess what disease incidence should be locally expected in the tract area and then to compare the observed incidence with the expected incidence. This approach has been traditionally used for the analysis of counts within tracts and can be applied to case event maps.

3.3.1.2.1 Case Events

Case events can be mapped as point-event locations. For the purposes of assessment of differences in local disease risk, it is appropriate to convert these locations into a continuous surface describing the spatial variation in intensity of the cases. Once this surface is computed, then a measure of local variation is available at any spatial location within the observation window: the intensity surface (IS). This surface can be formally defined as the first-order intensity of a point process (e.g., see Lawson and Waller, 1996) and can be estimated by a variety of methods including density estimation (Härdle, 1991). To provide an estimate of the at-risk population (ARP) at spatial locations, it is necessary first to choose a measure that will represent the intensity of cases expected at such locations. Two possibilities can be explored. First, it is possible to obtain rates for the case disease from either the whole study window or a larger enclosing region. Often, these rates are available only at an aggregated level (e.g., census tracts). The rates are obtained for a range of subpopulation categories that are thought to affect the case disease incidence. For example, the age and sex structure of the population or the deprivation status of the area (e.g., see Carstairs, 1981) could affect the amount of population at risk from the case disease. The use of such external rates is often called external standardization (Inskip et al., 1983). It should be noted that rates computed from aggregated data would be less variable than would rates based on density estimation of case events. An alternative method of assessing the at-risk population structure is to use a case event map of another disease, which represents the background population but is not affected by the etiological processes of interest in the case disease. For example, the spatial distribution of coronary heart disease (CHD: ICD 9 code, List A 410–414) could provide a control representation for respiratory cancer (ICD 9 code, List A 162) when the latter is the case disease in a study of air pollution effects, as CHD is less closely related to air pollution insult. Other examples of the cited use of a control disease are:

- Larynx cancer (case) and lung cancer (control) (Diggle, 1990) (however, this control is complicated by the fact that lung cancer is also related to air pollution risk)
- Lower body cancers (control) and gastric cancer (case) where lower body organs may only be affected by specific pollutants (e.g., nickel) (Lawson and Williams, 2000)
- Birth defects (case) and live births (control)

While exact matching of diseases in this way will always be difficult, there is an advantage in the use of control diseases in case event examples. If a realization of the control disease is available in the form of a point-event map, then it is possible to compute an estimate of the first-order intensity of the control disease. This estimate can be used directly to compare case intensity with background intensity. Note that the ARP can be estimated, equally, from census-tract standardized rates (e.g., see Lawson and Williams, 1994).

The comparison of estimates of the intensity surface (IS) and ARP can be made in a variety of ways. First, it is possible to map the ratio of IS/ARP over the whole area. Bithell (1990) first suggested this. Modifications to this procedure have been proposed by Lawson and Williams (1993) and Kelsall and Diggle (1995). Care must be taken to consider the effects of study/observation window edges on the interpretation of the ratio. Some edge-effect compensation should be considered when there is a considerable influence of window edges in the final interpretation of the map. A detailed discussion of edge effects can be found elsewhere (Lawson et al., 1999).

Apart from ratio forms, it is also possible to map transformations of ratios (e.g., log transforms) or to map differences. The choice of ratio or difference will depend on the underlying model assumed for the excess risk. This is discussed in Section 3.3.2.

In all the approaches above to the mapping of case event data, some smoothing or interpolation of the event or control data has to be made. The statistical properties of this operation depend on the method used for estimation of each component of the map. Optimal choices of the smoothing constant (i.e., bandwidth) are known for density estimation and kernel smoothing (e.g., see Härdle, 1991).

3.3.1.2.2 Tract Counts

As in the analysis of case events, it is usual to assess maps of count data by comparison of the observed counts to those counts expected to arise given the at-risk population structure of the tract. Traditionally, the ratio of observed to expected counts within tracts is called a Standardized Mortality/Morbidity Ratio (SMR) and this ratio is an estimate of relative risk within each tract (i.e., the ratio describes the odds of being in the disease group rather than the background group). The justification for the use of SMRs can be supported by the analysis of likelihood models with multiplicative expected risk (e.g., see Breslow and Day, 1987). Figure 3.5 displays the SMR thematic map for the Falkirk example, based on expected rates calculated from the local male and female population counts and the Scottish respiratory cancer rate for the period.

Then the SMR is defined as the ratio of observed count (O) to expected count (E): O/E in each region.

The alternative measure of relation between observed and expected counts, which is related to an additive risk model, is the difference: O–E.

In both cases, the comments made in Section 3.1 and Section 3.2 about mapping counts within tracts apply. In this case, it must be decided whether to express the ratio or difference as fill patterns in each region or to locate the result at some specified tract location, such as the centroid. If it is decided that these measures should be regarded as continuous across regions then some further interpolation of the ratio or difference must be made (e.g., see Breslow and Day, 1987). This is discussed briefly in the next section.

SMRs are commonly used in disease map presentation, but have many drawbacks. First, they are based on ratio estimators; hence, they yield large changes in estimate with relatively small changes in expected value. In the extreme, when a (close to) zero expectation is found, the SMR will be very large for any positive count; in addition, the zero SMRs do not distinguish variation in expected counts and the SMR variance is proportional to 1/E in each region. The SMR is essentially a saturated estimate of relative risk and hence is not parsimonious.

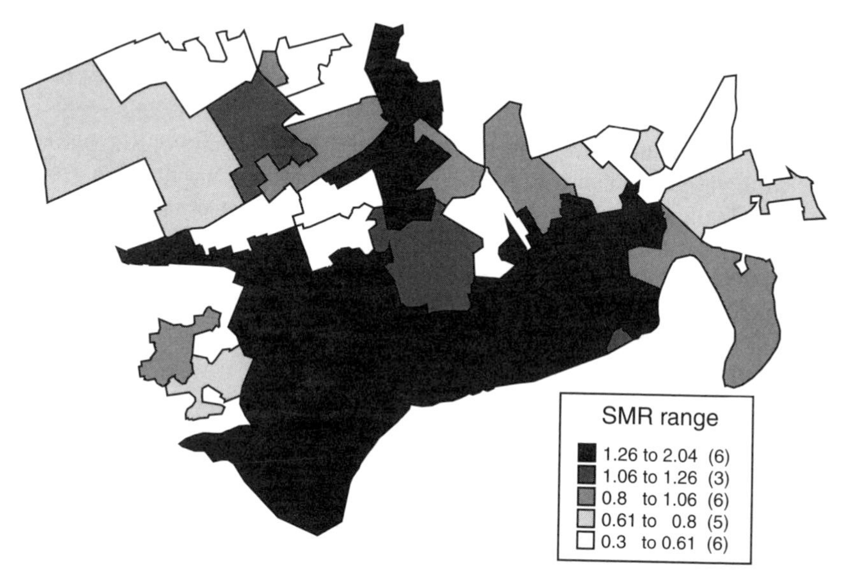

FIGURE 3.5 Falkirk respiratory cancer SMR map.

3.3.1.3 Interpolation

In many of the mapping approaches mentioned above, interpolation methods must be used to provide estimates of a surface measure at locations where there are no observations. For example, we may wish to map contours of a set of tract counts if we believe the counts to represent a continuously varying risk surface. For the purposes of contouring, a grid of surface interpolant values must be provided. Smoothing of SMRs has been advocated by Breslow and Day (1987). Those authors employ kernel smoothing to interpolate the surface (in a temporal application). The advantage of such smoothing is that the method preserves the positivity condition of SMRs, that is, the method does not produce negative interpolants (which are invalid), unlike kriging methods (e.g., see Lawson and Cressie, 2000, for discussion of this issue). Other interpolation methods also suffer from this problem. Many mapping packages utilize interpolation methods to provide gridded data for further contour and perspective view plotting (e.g., SAS™, S-Plus® software). However, often the methods used are not clearly defined or they are based on mathematical rather than statistical interpolants (e.g., the Akima or Delauney interpolators). ArcGIS® with Geostatistical Analyst provides a range of kriging methodologies that could be applied within the small area health context if suitable transformations are employed.

Note that the comments above also apply directly to case-event density estimation. The use of kernel density estimation is recommended, with edge correction as appropriate. For ratio estimation, Kelsall and Diggle (1995) recommend the joint estimation of a common smoothing parameter for numerator and denominator when a control-disease realization is available.

3.3.1.4 Exploratory Methods

The discussion above, concerning the construction of disease maps, could be considered as exploratory analysis of spatial disease patterns. For example, the construction and mapping of ratios or differences of case and background measures is useful for highlighting areas of incidence requiring further consideration. Contour plots or surface views of such mapped data can be derived. Comments concerning the psychological interpretation of mapped patterns also apply here; e.g., see Ripley (1981) and Walter (1993). However, inspection of maps of simple ratios or differences cannot provide accurate assessment of the statistical significance of, for example, areas of elevated disease risk. Proper inference requires statistical models and that is the subject of the next section.

3.3.2 Basic Models

In the previous section, the use of primarily descriptive methods in the construction of disease maps was discussed. These methods do not introduce any particular model structure or constraint into the mapping process. This can be advantageous at an early or exploratory stage in the analysis of disease data but, when more substantive hypotheses or greater amounts of prior information are available concerning the problem, it may be advantageous to consider a model-based approach to disease map construction. Model-based approaches can also be used in an exploratory setting and if sufficiently general models are employed then this can lead to better focusing of subsequent hypothesis generation. Likelihood models for case event data are considered below, followed by a discussion regarding the inclusion of extra information in the form of random effects.

3.3.2.1 Basic Likelihood Models

3.3.2.1.1 Case Event Data

Usually the basic model for case event data is derived from the following three assumptions:

1. Individuals within the study population behave independently with respect to disease propensity, after allowance is made for observed or unobserved confounding variables.
2. The underlying at risk population intensity has a continuous spatial distribution, within specified boundary vertices.
3. The case events are unique, in that they occur as single spatially separate events.

Assumption 1 allows the events to be modeled via a likelihood approach, which is valid conditional on the outcomes of confounder variables. Further, Assumption 2, if valid, allows the likelihood to be constructed with a background continuous modulating intensity function (the ARP) representing the at-risk population. The uniqueness of case event locations is a requirement of point process theory (the property called orderliness; e.g., see Daley and Vere-Jones, 1988), which allows the application of Poisson-process models in this analysis. Assumption 1 is generally valid for noninfectious diseases. It may also be valid for infectious diseases if complete information about current infectives were known at given time points. Assumption 2 will be valid at appropriate scales of analysis. It may not hold when large areas of a study window include zones of zero population (e.g., harbors/industrial zones). Often models can be restricted to exclude these areas however. Assumption 3 usually holds for relatively rare diseases, but it may be violated when households have multiple cases that occur at coincident locations. This may not be important at more aggregate scales, but could be important at a fine spatial scale. Remedies for such nonorderliness are the use of declustering algorithms (which perturb the locations by small amounts) or analysis at a higher aggregation level. Note that it is also possible to use a conventional case-control approach to this problem (Diggle et al., 2000).

Given the assumptions above, it is possible to specify that the case events arise as a realization of a Poisson point process, with first-order multiplicative intensity so that two components combine multiplicatively to give the local disease risk. The IS and ARP estimates are used to represent these two components.

In this definition, the IS can include a function of confounder variables as well as location, a parameter (vector) and the overall constant rate of the process. The confounder variables can be widely defined however. For example, a number of random effects could be included to represent unobserved effects, as well as observed covariates, as could functions of other locations. The inclusion of random effects could be chosen if it is felt that unobserved heterogeneity is present in the disease process. This could represent the effect of known or unknown covariates that are unobserved.

For suitably specified IS, a variety of models can be derived. In the case of disease mapping, where only the background intensity is to be accounted for, a reasonable approach to intensity parameterization is IS/ARP over the whole study window. The preceding definition can be used as an informal justification for the use of intensity ratios in the mapping of case event data; such ratios represent the local extraction of at risk background, under a multiplicative hazard model. On the other hand, under a pure additive model, differencing the two estimated rates would be supported.

3.3.2.1.2 Tract Count Data

In the case of observed counts of disease within tracts, the Poisson-process assumptions given above imply that the counts are Poisson distributed with, for each tract, a different expectation based on the integral of the overall model intensity over the small area.

Often a parameterization is assumed where, as in the case event example, the intensity is defined as a simple multiplicative function of the background ARP. An assumption is often made at this point that the expectation can be regarded as a parameter within a model hierarchy. This assumption leads to considerable simplifications, but at a cost. The effect of such an approximation should be considered in any application example, but is seldom considered in the existing literature; Marshall (1991) and Lawson et al. (1999) provide reviews.

The mapping of extracted intensities for case events or modified SMRs for tract counts is based on the view that once the at-risk background is extracted from the observed data, the resulting distribution of risk represents a clean map of the ground truth. Of course, as the background function, ARP must usually be estimated, and some variability in the resulting map will occur by inclusion of different estimators. For tract count data, the use of external standardization alone to estimate the expected counts within tracts may provide a different map from that provided by a combination of external standardization and measures of tract-specific deprivation, e.g., deprivation indices (Carstairs, 1981). If any confounding variables are available and can be included within the estimate of the at-risk background, then these should be considered for inclusion. Examples of confounding variables could be found from national census data, particularly relating to socioeconomic measures. These measures are often defined as deprivation indicators or related to lifestyle choices. For example, the local rate of car ownership or percentage unemployed within a census tract or other small area could provide a surrogate measure for increased risk, due to correlations between these variables and poor housing, smoking lifestyles, and ill health. Hence, if it is possible to include such variables in the estimation of ARP, then any resulting map will display a close representation of the true underlying risk surface.

When it is not possible to include such variables within ARP it is sometimes possible to adapt a mapping method to include covariables of this type by inclusion within the IS itself.

3.3.2.2 Random Effects and Bayesian Models

3.3.2.2.1 Random Effects

In the previous sections, some simple approaches to mapping intensities and counts within tracts have been described. These methods assume that once all known and observable confounding variables are included within the ARP estimation then the resulting map will be clean of all artifacts and hence depicts the true excess risk surface. However, it is often true that unobserved effects are thought to exist within the observed data. These effects should be included within the analysis. These effects are often termed random effects and their analysis has provided much literature both in statistical methodology and in epidemiological applications; e.g., see Manton et al. (1981), Tsutakawa (1988), Marshall (1991), Devine and Louis (1994), and reviews given in Lawson (2001) and Elliott et al. (2000). Within the literature on disease mapping, there has been a considerable growth in recent years in modeling random effects of various kinds. In the mapping context, a random effect could take a variety of forms. In its simplest form, a random effect is an extra quantity of variation (or variance component) that is estimable within the map and which can be ascribed a defined probabilistic structure. This component can affect individuals or can be associated with tracts or covariables. For example, individuals vary in susceptibility to disease and hence individuals who become cases could have a random component relating to different susceptibility. This is sometimes known as frailty. Another example is the interpolation of a spatial covariable to the locations of case events or tract centroids. In that case, some error will be included in the interpolation process and could be included within the resulting analysis of case or count events; in addition, the locations of case events might not be precisely known or subject to some random shift, which may be related to uncertain residential exposure. (However, this type of uncertainty may be better modeled by a more complex integrated intensity model, which no longer provides an independent observation model.) Finally, within any predefined spatial unit, such as tracts or regions, it may be expected that there could be components of variation attributable to these different spatial units. These components could have different forms depending on the degree of prior knowledge concerning the nature of this extra variation. For example, when observed counts, thought to be governed by a Poisson distribution, display greater variation than expected (i.e., variance greater than the mean), it is sometimes described as overdispersion. This overdispersion can occur for various reasons. Often it arises when clustering occurs in the counts at a particular scale. It can also occur when considerable numbers of cells have zero counts (sparseness), which can arise when rare diseases are mapped. In spatial applications, it is important furthermore to distinguish two basic forms of extra variation. First, as in the aspatial case, a form of independent and spatially uncorrelated extra variation can be assumed. This is often called uncorrelated heterogeneity (e.g., see Besag et al., 1991). Another form of random effect is that which arises from a model where it is thought that the spatial unit (such as case events, tracts, or regions) is correlated with neighboring spatial units. This is often termed correlated heterogeneity. Essentially, this form of extra variation implies that there exists spatial autocorrelation between spatial units; e.g., see Cliff and Ord (1981) for an accessible introduction to spatial autocorrelation. This autocorrelation could arise for a variety of reasons. First, the disease of concern could be naturally clustered in its spatial distribution at the scale of observation. Many infectious diseases display such spatial clustering and a number of apparently noninfectious diseases also cluster; e.g., see Cuzick and Hills (1991) and Glick (1979). Second, autocorrelation can be induced in spatial disease patterns by the existence of unobserved environmental or frailty effects. Hence, the extra variation observed in any application could arise from confounding variables that have not been included in the analysis. In disease mapping examples, this could easily arise when simple mapping methods are used on SMRs with just basic age–sex standardization.

In the discussion on heterogeneity, it is assumed that a global measure of heterogeneity applies to a mapped pattern. That is, including a general heterogeneity term in the mapping model can capture any extra variation in the pattern. However, often spatially specific heterogeneity may arise where it is important to consider local effects as well as, or instead of, general heterogeneity. To differentiate these two approaches, we use the terms specific and nonspecific heterogeneity. Specific heterogeneity implies that spatial locations are to be modeled locally; for example, clusters of disease are to be detected on the map. In contrast, nonspecific describes a global approach to such modeling, which does not address the question of the location of effects. In this definition, it is tacitly assumed that the locations of clusters of disease can be regarded as random effects themselves. Hence, there are strong parallels between image processing tasks and the tasks of disease mapping.

Random effects can take a variety of forms and suitable methods must be employed to provide correctly estimated maps under models including these effects. In this section, we discuss simple approaches to this problem from a Bayesian viewpoint.

3.3.2.2.2 Bayesian Approach

There is a variety of approaches to random effects modeling. Some are nonparametric or approximate. Multilevel modeling makes some simplifying assumptions that lead to approximate inference (see Leyland and Goldstein, 2001). However, it is natural to consider modeling random effects within a Bayesian framework. Primarily, random effects naturally have prior distributions and the joint distribution of the data and the prior distributions of the parameters are examined together for estimation. The product of the data likelihood and the prior distributions is called the posterior distribution. Hence, the development of full Bayes and empirical Bayes (posterior approximation) methods has developed naturally in the field of disease mapping. The prior distribution(s) for the parameters in the intensity specification have parameters themselves called hyperparameters (in a Poisson-gamma example, these would be the scale and shape parameters of the gamma: a, b, etc.). These hyperparameters can also have distributions, which are known as hyperprior distributions. The distributions chosen for these parameters depend on the application. In the full Bayesian approach, inference is based on the posterior distribution of the parameters given the data. However, it is possible to adopt an intermediate approach where the posterior distribution is approximated in some way and subsequent inference may be made via estimation of parameters or by computing the approximated posterior distribution. In the tract count example, approximation via intermediate prior parameter estimation would involve the estimation of a and b (in the gamma example), followed by inference on the estimated posterior distribution; e.g., see Carlin and Louis (2000).

Few examples exist of simple Bayesian approaches to the analysis of case event data in the disease mapping context. One approach, described by Lawson et al. (1996), can be used with simple prior distributions for parameters and the authors provide approximate empirical Bayes estimators based on tile area integral approximations. For count data, a number of examples exist where independent Poisson distributed counts (with constant within tract rate) are associated with prior distributions with varying complexity. The earliest examples of such a Bayesian mapping approach can be found in Manton et al. (1981) and Tsutakawa (1988). In addition, Clayton and Kaldor (1987) developed a Bayesian analysis of a Poisson likelihood model where the tract count has an expectation that is a product of the relative risk and ARP. They found that the relative risk prior distribution given by gamma (a, b) led to the posterior expectation where the numerator of the SMR is augmented by a and the denominator by b. Hence, one could map directly these Bayes estimates.

3.3.3 Advanced Bayesian Models

Many of the models discussed above can be extended to include the specification of prior distributions for parameters and hence can be examined via Bayesian methods. In general, one can distinguish between empirical Bayes methods and full Bayes methods on the basis that any method that seeks to approximate the posterior distribution is regarded as empirical Bayes. All other methods are regarded as full Bayes.

The most important of these full Bayes methods was that of Besag et al. (1991) — BYM — that allows the inclusion of both trend effect and uncorrelated and correlated heterogeneity within the relative risk model. This model requires special posterior sampling methods (Gibbs sampling) for its implementation. The model can be fitted on the package WinBUGS, as can simpler relative risk models. Figure 3.6 displays the BYM posterior expected relative risks for the Falkirk map. Note that the resulting estimates are smoother than the SMR map.

3.4 NEW DEVELOPMENTS

In recent years there have been a number of notable new approaches to disease mapping. One of the most notable developments has been the use of mixture models and partition models; e.g., see Denison and Holmes (2001), Knorr-Held and Rasser (2000), and reviews in Lawson and Denison (2002). The idea behind mixture models is that the observed data arises from more than one distribution. For example, it might be assumed there is a small set of components from which the true risk is derived and the observed data is a random variation around these components. Hence, what is observed is an overlaying of these components. These models can be useful in providing a map of partitioned components of risk (which are discrete) or could provide a type of nonparametric smoothing of the risk map. They can also be used to allow discontinuities in the relative risk surface not admitted by the Besag et al. approach. Lawson and Clark (2002) proposed a different mixture approach for discontinuities, which is programmable in WinBUGS.

Only little attention has been paid to the analysis of multiple maps of disease. Knorr-Held and Best (2001) proposed an analysis based on a linkage parameter, while a competing risk approach was adopted by Lawson and Williams (2000). Spatiotemporal mapping has received greater attention and is likely to receive much more due to the needs of health surveillance. Most models in this area have focused on simple types of space–time interaction, although Knorr-Held (2000) examined a greater range of interaction effects. A recent review of these models appears in Lawson (2001).

The real-time or near real-time analysis of mapped data is little developed and is likely to be of great import following the events of September 11, 2001. Real-time analysis has received little attention so far. In addition, the important issues, such as early detection of outbreaks (syndromic surveillance) and the tools best suited to the earliest detection of outbreaks must be addressed. Some recent approaches to this appear in Brookmeyer and Stroup (2003).

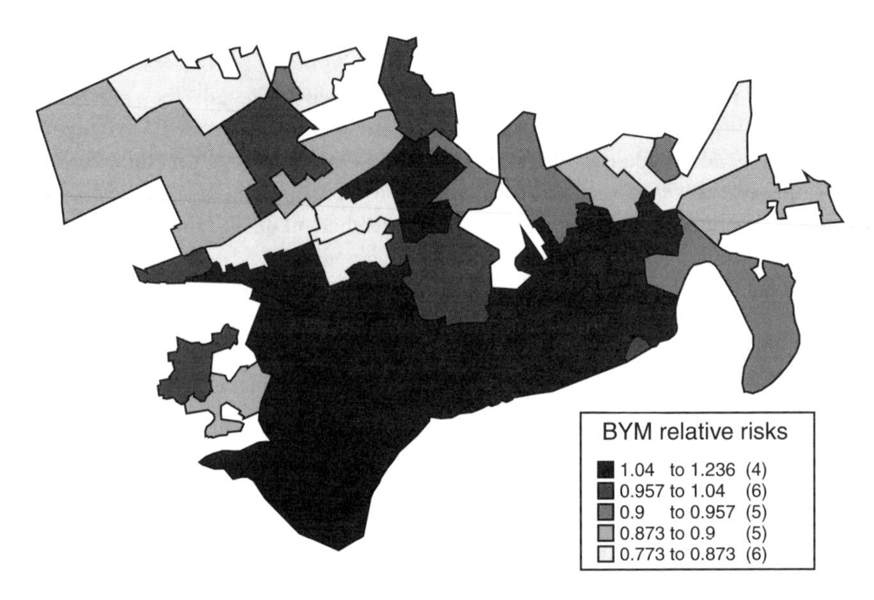

FIGURE 3.6 Falkirk BYM full Bayes relative risk estimates.

3.5 DISCUSSIONS AND CONCLUSIONS

This chapter has focused on the issue of disease mapping, i.e., the production of clean maps of the geographical distribution of disease (incidence or prevalence). An example of the application of a variety of methods, ranging from likelihood to full Bayes methods has been examined with a simple data set (Figure 3.5 and Figure 3.6). The results of this application tend to highlight a variety of issues, which commonly arise in such applications. First, crude SMR relative risk estimates often contain artifacts that relate to the method of estimation as well as unobserved heterogeneity in the data. These artifacts can be partially removed by the inclusion of random effects. Under Bayesian models, these random effects can be posterior-sampled and the associated relative risk estimates can be averaged to produce a posterior-average relative risk. Approximate methods that seek to directly estimate the prior distribution parameters in these setups lead to empirical Bayes methods. Finally, the incorporation of both uncorrelated and correlated heterogeneity can be modeled within the full Bayesian posterior sampling framework.

It is clear that, while empirical Bayes methods lead to relatively simple estimators of relative risk, other methods provide greater flexibility in the choice of model and hence possibilities for analysis. While empirical Bayes methods can be implemented more easily, the use of full Bayesian methods has many advantages, not least of which is the ability to specify a variety of components and prior distributions in the model setup. Sampling of posterior distributions is now easily achieved with software such as WinBUGS that provides Gibbs sampling for a variety of hierarchical Bayesian models.

In public health applications, it may be important to provide some guidance as to the use of such methods and to recommend relatively simple methods to be used by practitioners in such areas. From a variety of studies, it would appear that the simplest approach to the problem lies in the use of empirical Bayes estimators (e.g., gamma-Poisson model) as these can be computed relatively easily and appear to be reasonably robust. However, a full Bayesian approach has many benefits, although it may not be easily implemented by nonstatisticians. The use of crude SMR maps cannot be recommended and if employed, as is commonly the case in practice, should be accompanied by maps of variability. Indeed, it is to be recommended that all relative risk mapping exercises should include small area variability estimates as standard output. Of course, even when good methods of estimation are adopted, there remains the issue of visual interpretation of mapped results that adds a further stage of processing to the spatial information.

References

Besag, J., York, J., and Mollie, A., 1991, Bayesian image restoration with two applications in spatial statistics, *Annals of the Institute of Statistical Mathematics,* 43, 1–59.

Bithell, J., 1990, An application of density estimation to geographical epidemiology, *Statistics in Medicine,* 9, 691–701.

Breslow, N. and Clayton, D., 1993, Approximate inference in generalised linear mixed models, *Journal of the American Statistical Association*, 88, 9–25.

Breslow, N. and Day, N., 1987, The design and analysis of cohort studies, in *Statistical Methods in Cancer Research,* Vol. 2, Lyon, France: International Agency for Research in Cancer.

Brookmeyer, R. and Stroup, D., Eds., 2003, *Statistical Principles and Methods in Public Health Surveillance*, London: Oxford University Press.

Carlin, B. and Louis, T., 2000, *Bayes and Empirical Bayes Methods for Data Analysis,* 2nd ed., London: CRC/Chapman & Hall.

Carstairs, V., 1981, Small area analysis and health service research, *Community Medicine,* 3, 131–139.

Clayton, D. and Kaldor, J., 1987, Empirical Bayes estimates of age-standardised relative risks for use in disease mapping, *Biometrics,* 43, 671–691.

Cliff, A. and Ord, K., 1981, *Spatial Processes: Models and Application,* London: Pion.

Cuzick, J. and Hills, M., 1991, Clustering and clusters: Summary, in Draper, G., Ed., *Geographical Epidemiology of Childhood Leukemia and Non-Hodgkin's Lymphomas in Great Britain 1966–1983,* London: HMSO.

Daley, D. and Vere-Jones, D., 1988, *An Introduction to the Theory of Point Processes,* New York: Springer Verlag.

Denison, D.G.T. and Holmes, C.C., 2001, Bayesian partitioning for estimating disease risk. *Biometrics*, 57(1): 143–149.

Devine, O. and Louis, T., 1994, A constrained empirical Bayes estimator for incidence rates in areas with small populations, *Statistics in Medicine,* 13, 1119–1133.

Diggle, P., 1990, A point process modeling approach to raised incidence of a rare phenomenon in the vicinity of a prespecified point, *Journal of the Royal Statistical Society A,* 153, 349–362.

Diggle, P., Morris, S., and Wakefield, J., 2000, Point-source modelling using matched case-control data, *Biostatistics,* 1, 1–17.

Elliott, P. et al., 2000, *Spatial Epidemiology: Methods and Applications*, Oxford: Oxford University Press.

Ferriera, J., Denison, D., and Holmes, C., 2002, Partition modelling, in Lawson, A. and Denison, D., Eds., *Spatial Cluster Modelling,* London: CRC/Chapman & Hall.

Glick, B. J., 1979, The spatial autocorrelation of cancer mortality, *Social Science Medicine,* 13D, 123–130.

Härdle, W., 1991, *Smoothing Techniques: With Implementation in S,* New York: Springer Verlag.

Inskip, H. et al., 1983, Methods for age-adjustment of rates, *Statistics in Medicine,* 2, 483–493.

Kelsall, J. and Diggle, P., 1995, Non-parametric estimation of spatial variation in relative risk, *Statistics in Medicine*, 14, 2335–2342.

Knorr-Held, L., 2000, Bayesian modelling of inseparable space-time variation in disease risk, *Statistics in Medicine*, 19, 2555–2567.

Knorr-Held, L. and Best, N., 2001, A shared component model for detecting joint and selective clustering of two diseases, *Journal of the Royal Statistical Society A,* 164, 73–85.

Knorr-Held, L. and Rasser, G., 2000, Bayesian detection of clusters and discontinuities in disease maps, *Biometrics*, 56, 13–21.

Lawson, A.B., 2001, *Statistical Methods in Spatial Epidemiology,* New York: Wiley.

Lawson, A.B. and Clark, A.B., 2002, Spatial relative risk mixture models in disease mapping, *Statistics in Medicine,* 21, 359–370.

Lawson, A.B. and Cressie, N., 2000, Spatial statistical methods for environmental epidemiology, in Rao, C.R. and Sen, P.K., Eds., *Handbook of Statistics: Bio-Environmental and Public Health Statistics*, Vol. 18, New York: Elsevier.

Lawson, A.B. and Denison, D., Eds., 2002, *Spatial Cluster Modelling,* London: CRC/Chapman & Hall.

Lawson, A.B. and Waller, L., 1996, A review of point pattern methods for spatial modeling of events around sources of pollution, *Environmetrics,* 7, 471–488.

Lawson, A.B. and Williams, F., 1993, Applications of extraction mapping in environmental epidemiology, *Statistics in Medicine*, 12, 1249–1258.

Lawson, A.B. and Williams, F., 1994, Armadale: A case study in environmental epidemiology, *Journal of the Royal Statistical Society A,* 157, 285–298.

Lawson, A.B. and Williams, F., 2000, Spatial competing risk models in disease mapping, *Statistics in Medicine,* 19, 2451–2468.

Lawson, A.B., Biggeri, A., and Lagazio, C., 1996, Modelling heterogeneity in discrete spatial data models via MAP and MCMC methods, in Forcina, A., Marchetti, G., Hatzinger, R., and Galmacci, G., Eds., *Proceedings of the 11th International Workshop on Statistical Modelling,* Graphos: Citta di Castello.

Lawson, A.B. et al., 1999, *Disease Mapping and Risk Assessment for Public Health,* New York: Wiley/WHO.

Leyland, A. and Goldstein, H., 2001, *Multilevel Modelling of Health Statistics,* New York: Wiley.

Manton, K., Woodbury, M., and Stallard, E., 1981, A variance components approach to categorical data models with heterogeneous mortality rates in North Carolina counties, *Biometrics,* 37, 259–269.

Marshall, R., 1991, A review of methods for the statistical analysis of spatial patterns of disease, *Journal of the Royal Statistical Society A,* 154, 421–441.

Pickle, L. and Hermann, D., 1995, Cognitive Aspects of Statistical Mapping, Technical Report 18, Washington, DC: NCHS Office of Research and Methodology.

Pickle, L. et al., 1999, Exploring spatial patterns of mortality: The new atlas of United States mortality, *Statistics in Medicine*, 18, 3211–3220.

Ripley, B., 1981, *Spatial Statistics,* New York: Wiley.

Ross, A. and Davis, S., 1990, Point pattern analysis of the spatial proximity of residences prior to diagnosis of persons with Hodgkin's disease, *American Journal of Epidemiology,* 132, Suppl., 53–62.

Snow, J., 1854, *On the Mode of Communication of Cholera,* 2nd ed., London: Churchill Livingstone.

Tsutakawa, R., 1988, A mixed model for analyzing geographic variability in mortality rates, *Journal of the American Statistical Association,* 83, 37–42.

Walter, S.D., 1993, Visual and statistical assessment of spatial clustering in mapped data, *Statistics in Medicine*, 12, 1275–1291.

4 Clustering of Disease

Clive E. Sabel and Markku Löytönen

CONTENTS

4.1 DISEASE CLUSTERS AND CLUSTERING

In these times of increased public awareness of and concern toward sources of environmental pollution and their potential links to disease, reports of a cluster or hot spot of disease in a particular area are commonplace. These concerns have no doubt been heightened, in the United Kingdom at least, by public health issues such as the so-called childhood leukemia cluster around the Sellafield nuclear reprocessing plant in northwest England (Gardner, 1993), over bovine spongiform encephalopathy (popularly known as mad cow disease), and more recently, the foot and mouth disease outbreak in 2001. Much of the controversy surrounding clustering lies in the difficulty in providing an adequate definition. To remove any potential for confusion, we draw the reader's attention to the distinction between the identification of disease clusters, the topic of this chapter, and the entirely separate statistical technique of cluster analysis, which aims to aggregate variables with similar characteristics in a dataset together to simplify subsequent analysis.

0-415-30655-8/04/$0.00+$1.50

Cluster detection methods can be classified into either global or local tests. Global tests detect the presence or absence of clustering over the whole study region without specifying spatial location. Local tests additionally specify the location and, if extended to consider temporal patterns, can specify spatiotemporal clusters. A special case of local tests is the focused test, which is used to detect raised incidence of disease around some prespecified source, such as an incinerator. In this chapter, we concentrate on local tests because we are concerned with locating disease clustering spatially and temporally.

In general lay conversation, the terms cluster and clustering are used interchangeably, usually applied loosely to mean any unusual collection of events. The Centers for Disease Control (CDC) discuss "any unusual aggregation of health events, real or perceived." Diggle, however, suggests that there are three distinct and separate problems in spatial epidemiology, namely cluster detection, clustering, and spatial variation in risk, but acknowledges that the distinctions between them are often blurred (Diggle, 2000). Cluster detection, according to Diggle, might be better named anomaly detection or surveillance, whereas clustering is a departure from complete spatial randomness (i.e., the hypothesis that cases occur independently of each other), which, he suggests, invites an interpretation in terms of genetic susceptibility or infectious transmission. Here it is useful to acknowledge that aggregation can occur by random processes, but cluster investigations seek to identify excess aggregation. For a lucid, diagrammatic presentation of the statistical model of complete spatial randomness, the reader may wish to consult Waller (2000). Spatial variation in risk is a departure from the hypothesis that all members of the population are at equal risk, which Diggle (2000) suggests invites an environmental interpretation. Wakefield et al. (2000) also discuss the underlying risk surface and suggest a wider definition with a cluster corresponding to an area and time period in which the (residual) risk surface is elevated (after adjusting for known risk factors), i.e., excess disease risk. Risk surfaces have the additional advantage of potentially highlighting areas of apparent low risk, which may be of value etiologically.

Clustering, however, according to Alexander and Cuzick (1992), might be defined as "a more heterogeneous and clumped distribution of disease cases than would be expected from the variations in the population density and chance fluctuations." It is thus important to recognize the distinction between the notion of an individual cluster and the concept of a general tendency for clustering.

Knox (1989) suggests three alternative definitions, with a cluster being a geographically or temporally bounded group of occurrences:

1. Of a disease already known to occur characteristically in clusters
2. Of sufficient size and concentration to be unlikely to have occurred by chance
3. Related to each other through some social or biological mechanism, or having a common relationship with some other event or circumstance

The second of Knox's definitions introduces the important concept of significance testing and begs the question of possible etiology; whereas the third definition relies on some notion of causation. The utility of cluster studies might thus be summarized as the identification, statistical confirmation or rejection, and the suggestion of potential clues as to etiology.

4.2 WHY INVESTIGATE DISEASE CLUSTERING?

The detection and investigation of disease clusters has a long and controversial history in the field of spatial epidemiology. The basic interest in analyzing disease patterns is in determining whether the observed events exhibit any systematic pattern as opposed to being distributed at random over the study region. Wartenberg and Greenberg (1993) consider cluster studies to be a form of preepidemiology, placing them in an investigative niche prior to confirmatory epidemiological studies. Questions that one might wish to pose include:

- Is the observed clustering due mainly to natural background variation in the at-risk population from which events arise?
- Over what scale does any clustering occur?
- Are clusters merely a result of some obvious *a priori* heterogeneity in the study region?
- Are clusters associated with proximity to other features of interest, such as transport arteries or possible point sources of pollution?
- Are events that aggregate in space also clustered in time?

Disease clustering investigations might be used to generate ideas and hypotheses regarding disease etiology, but perhaps also to calm public fears of a local excess. Wartenberg (2001) suggests that public concern (often based on personal tragedy, perhaps with a specific point-source environmental contaminant in mind, but involving perhaps only a few cases), cannot and should not simply be dismissed as "lying within acceptable statistical limits" or explained away with demographic, statistical, or sampling error fluctuations. Reassurance is often required, which can be established via a carefully designed investigation.

Rothman (1990) has suggested that the payoff from clustering research comes from specific hypotheses that emerge to explain the observed pattern of excess occurrence. Whether infectious agents, genetic susceptibilities, or environmental pollutants, determining mechanisms is the goal, but only rarely have etiological insights resulted from cluster investigations.

Disease clustering investigations may prove most useful, however, in actively identifying outbreaks, particularly for infectious diseases. There have been attempts to establish national active-cluster surveillance programs, which might regularly scan register-based data for evidence of elevated risk. However, investigating incidence data over a relatively large population systematically is costly and so most investigations are more passive and are often the result of an initial request from a member of the public. For example, in the United Kingdom, the Rapid Inquiry Facility developed by the Small Area Health Statistics Unit (SAHSU) (Aylin et al., 1999) aims to produce a report within three days of a request by routinely collecting morbidity, mortality, and population data at a small spatial scale in anticipation of requests for an investigation.

4.3 CHOOSING BETWEEN METHODS

What is an appropriate public health and scientific response to a report of a suspected disease cluster? Great care needs to be taken in the presentation and interpretation of results to avoid unwarranted alarm among local residents, while not diminishing the importance of a real and observed public health concern. Obviously, the response varies depending on whether we are concerned with infectious diseases, typically operating over relatively short time scales, or noninfectious diseases with processes operating, say, over many decades. Naturally, disease can cluster spatially, temporally, or spatiotemporally. Particularly with infectious diseases, it is important to adopt methods that simultaneously test spatial and temporal clustering.

As with all research, one should establish what the research question is prior to considering what approach to take, what limitations the data impose, and whether there are other external factors to be taken into consideration. Then specific methods for the analysis can be selected.

There are two critical aspects — statistical power and confounding — to consider when selecting an appropriate method for the task at hand (Wartenberg and Greenberg, 1993). Statistical power is the ability to detect a real effect. The reader will become acquainted in the literature with the ability of methods to identify true clusters (true positives), but also the frequency with which the methods report clusters falsely (false positives). Comparative evaluations of statistical power, often by running competing cluster methods against a set of simulated data with known properties, can provide guidance in the choice and application of particular methods. Confounding is the distortion of the apparent effect of an exposure on risk brought about by the association of the exposure with other factors that can influence the outcome. In this situation, confounding may be the erroneous attribution of a disease cluster to the exposure under study, but the cluster has in fact been caused by a confounding factor associated with the exposure and independently influences disease outcome. It might be as simple as a change in background population density or involve known demographic factors such as age, gender, or ethnicity. Methods that can control for known confounding effects should be used in the first instance.

Wartenberg and Greenberg (1993) suggest that the scattered scientific literature on the evaluation of cluster methodology shows little consistency and thus has limited utility for the public health researcher seeking to distinguish between methods. Dozens of methods exist in the literature for the detection of spatial clustering over and above that due to the natural distribution of the population. Only a subset is regularly used, often due to the complexity of the methods and perhaps a lack of direction about the relative benefits of each and when it is appropriate to apply which method, because different methods suit different scenarios. Wartenberg and Greenberg suggest that users, when confronted with the multitude and complexity of methods available, often select methods arbitrarily basing choices on software availability or ease of implementation. Consideration of the statistical power and ability to adjust for potential confounding effects in differing tests are overlooked.

Wakefield et al. (2000) have devised a useful classification of methods, separated into four groups which we shall mention briefly:

1. Traditional methods
2. Distance/adjacency methods
3. Moving windows methods
4. Risk surface estimation methods

The first group — traditional methods — primarily detects overdispersion in areally aggregated data. They are global tests and hence do not provide an indication of location, but detect the presence or absence of clustering over the whole study region. Examples of such tests are Pearson's chi-squared statistic and the Potthoff and Whittinghill's method.

The second group — distance/adjacency methods — consists of global tests that assess the spatial dependence in a set of data. Here one considers such techniques as autocorrelation statistics (among the most common of which are Moran's I and Geary's c), Whittemore's method, Tango's method, and K-functions.

The third group — moving windows — has been developed since the mid-1980s and has been designed to assess whether the number of cases within a window exceeds that expected by chance. A window can be defined in a number of ways, such as a circle of a particular radius or a 3-×-3 grid in which observations are assessed. The window moves systematically throughout the study region. These are local tests with the ability to detect spatial locations of excess. Here Wakefield et al. consider Openshaw's method, Besag and Newell's method, scan statistics, and Cuzick and Edwards's method. Scan methods are particularly recommended where there are sparse data (Wartenberg and Greenberg, 1993).

The fourth group concerns risk surface estimation. Here such methods include kernel estimation, generalized additive models, and geostatistical methods. In these relatively recently developed techniques, the emphasis is less on hypothesis testing and more on estimation of the underlying residual risk surface. These methods can potentially offer more insight into the nature of the clusters since they produce continuous surfaces of risk across the whole study region and not just the statistically identified clusters. The downside of risk surfaces is a less well-developed statistical understanding and often the necessity for the use of specialized software. They do also tend to be computationally expensive and more difficult to implement.

For further details on the methods discussed in these four groups, we refer the reader to Bailey and Gatrell (1995) and Fotheringham et al. (2000). For further discussion of the relative merits of the alternative clustering methods, see Alexander and Boyle (1996), Alexander and Cuzick (1992), Elliott et al. (2000), Kulldorff (1998), Lawson and Kulldorff (1999), and Wakefield and Elliott (1999).

Spatial statisticians often perform analyses within specialist statistical software such as S-Plus or using homegrown code, rather than within GIS. This undoubtedly is because proprietary GIS lacks real statistical modeling sophistication, despite some advances recently such as the ArcGIS® Geostatistical Analyst. Other products such as CDC's Epi Info™ 2002 (including its allied mapping product, Epi Map) have little to no cluster detection functionality.

4.4 SOME ACCESSIBLE METHODS

A daunting number of methods exist from which investigators need to select a method suitable for their specific circumstances. In this section, we concentrate on three of the most common local cluster methods accessible to GIS users, because intuitively we feel pinpointing the location of clusters is of greater utility in this context than global tests that merely detect the presence or absence of clustering in the study region. We also look for methods that are methodologically sound and can control for covariates.

4.4.1 Openshaw's Method

Within the GIS community, probably the best known is Openshaw's Geographical Analysis Machine (GAM) (Openshaw et al., 1987). GAM is freely available on the Internet together with a comprehensive user guide. GAM is an exploratory cluster detection approach, which works by examining a large number of overlapping circles at a variety of scales and assesses the statistical probability of the number of events occurring by chance. Where the number of observations is statistically significant, a circle is plotted, which results in a visual impression of where clusters might occur. A more recent generation — GAM/K — makes use of kernel estimation to display the results of the iterative process. Openshaw et al. (1999) compared the performance of several exploratory geographical methods to identify patterns spatially and temporally. The aforementioned GAM/K worked well with spatially distributed data and the GAM/K-T (GAM/K plus time) method correctly identified temporal clustering. However, Openshaw's method has been heavily criticized in the literature, largely due not only to the multiple testing problems where there were a large number of tests, but also due to the dependency of the test. The original version was also heavily computer intensive.

4.4.2 Kulldorff's Spatial Scan Statistic

A method gaining increasing attention is Kulldorff's Spatial Scan Statistic (SaTScan) (Kulldorff, 2002). SaTScan™ software is freely available over the Internet, but is installed locally on a user's PC. The spatial scan statistic has been used to test for disease clustering in a number of recent studies, including:

- A focused test investigating potential clusters of soft-tissue sarcoma and non-Hodgkin's lymphoma around a solid waste incinerator in France (Viel et al., 2000)
- Childhood leukemia in Sweden (Hjalmars et al., 1996)
- Breast cancer in the United States (Kulldorff et al., 1997)
- Amyotrophic lateral sclerosis (ALS) birthplace clustering in Finland (Sabel et al., 2003)

The scan statistic is a spatial, temporal, or spatiotemporal, local cluster detection method for aggregated data. It can be applied to both focused and nonfocused investigations and, importantly, adjusted for confounders, including adjusting for a heterogeneous background population density. The method imposes a circular scanning window on the map and lets the center of the circle move over the study area so that at each position the window includes different sets of neighboring administrative areas. For each circle centroid, the radius varies continuously from zero to a user-defined maximum. Although the choice of maximum cluster circle size is somewhat arbitrary, and there are no clear guidelines for its choice, it is important to make the choice of maximum cluster size *a priori* to avoid the problems of multiple hypothesis testing. The test statistic adopted is the likelihood ratio, which is maximized over all the windows to identify the most likely disease clusters. A criticism of the test is that it has good power to report clusters in approximate circular forms, but poor power to detect linear clusters that perhaps follow rivers or overhead power lines. If one does not know, *a priori,* what shape a cluster might form, the test will impose a circular one regardless. Kulldorff argues, however, that it is not the exact borders of the cluster that one is most interested in, but rather the general area and centroid. Unlike some other techniques such as Openshaw's GAM, the test statistic does take into account the problem of multiple hypothesis testing and reports the significance of each reported cluster.

Sabel et al. (2003) used the scan statistic to analyze the impact of residential migration between places of birth and death for the rare neurological disease ALS in Finland for deaths between 1985 and 1995. In Figure 4.1, we present an adapted figure from this paper using a maximum cluster size of 20 percent of the total population. Background population-at-risk data was taken from the population census in 1990 for each municipality. Both significant and nonsignificant clusters are highlighted, reflecting the full output from SaTScan. The figure shows significant and widespread clustering at time of death in two areas of the south and southeast of the country, indicating areas to investigate further.

From Table 4.1, where all nine clusters are detailed, one can see that the first two clusters have a p value of less than 0.05, which might be interpreted as being significant. Cluster 1 and Cluster 2 each comprise more than 100 cases and have relative risk (RR) estimates of 1.79 and 1.32, respectively. Cluster 3 through Cluster 9 all have higher RRs, but note the small numbers of cases involved; hence, the lack of significance of these areas.

4.4.3 Kernel Estimates

A solution of how to estimate spatial variation in relative risk was first proposed in an epidemiological setting by Bithell (1990). He proposed adopting probability density estimation techniques of which kernel estimation is the most commonly used and most well understood statistically. Bithell's ideas have been developed by Kelsall and Diggle (1995) and Sabel (1999). Sabel et al. (2000) extended them to deal with the temporal component on the third dimension by weighting each location by a value representing the length of residence at that location. Sabel et al. (2000) also investigated space–time interaction by creating separate density estimates of temporal slices of the data, which were then sequenced together in an animation or movie, to enable the authors to obtain a greater understanding of the time lag of the etiology of the disease.

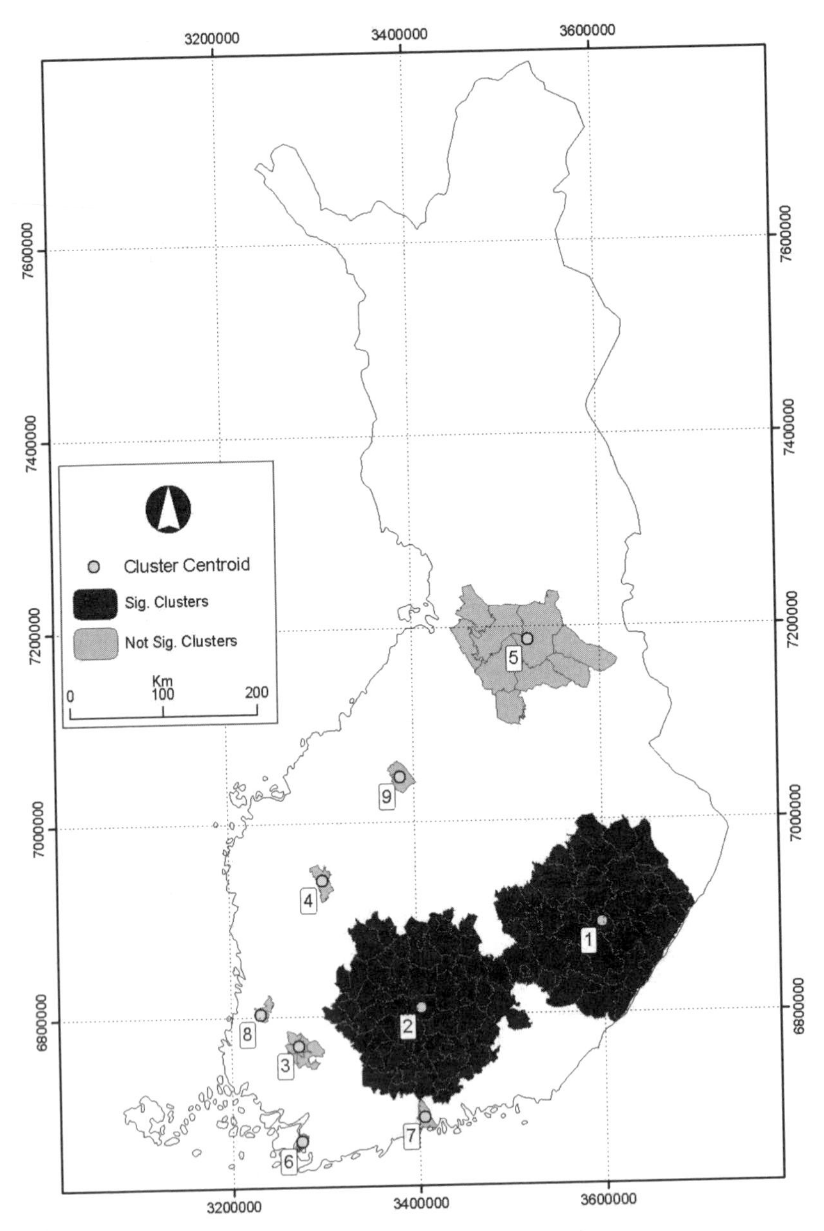

FIGURE 4.1 SaTScan identified clusters. ALS death place clusters in Finland, 1985 to 1990. (Axes labels are in meters.)

Kernel estimation is a statistical technique whereby, in epidemiological applications, a distribution of discrete points or events representing incidence of disease is transformed into a continuous surface of disease risk. Essentially, a moving three-dimensional function (the kernel) of a given radius or bandwidth visits each of the

TABLE 4.1
ALS Death Place Clusters in Finland (1985 to 1995) Using the Spatial Scan Statistic

Cluster	Approximate Location		Cases	Exp	Relative Risk Estimate (RR)	Log Likelihood Ratio (LLR)	*p* value
1	3598250	6893290	120	66.99	1.791	18.49	0.00001
2	3403860	6807980	229	174.13	1.315	9.73	0.013
3	3273130	6769600	10	2.63	3.797	6.00	0.368
4	3301020	6940090	5	0.82	6.105	4.87	0.716
5	3523310	7186900	16	7.59	2.109	3.56	0.983
6	3275130	6670440	2	0.17	11.716	3.09	0.998
7	3405190	6694410	8	2.93	2.731	2.98	0.999
8	3232900	6802670	7	2.51	2.794	2.71	1.000
9	3385530	7046240	2	0.22	8.992	2.62	1.000

points or events in turn and weights the area surrounding the point proportionately to its distance to the event. The sum of these individual kernels is then calculated for the study region and a smoothed surface is produced. Varying the bandwidth determines the degree of smoothing achieved. By taking a ratio of the kernel estimates of case intensity and underlying population, one can produce a map of relative risk, which can be tested statistically using Monte Carlo simulation techniques. Both of ESRI's ArcGIS and ArcView® GIS products include the functionality to calculate kernel estimates.

In Figure 4.2, we demonstrate output from a kernel estimate, using similar data to that shown in Figure 4.1. Here we have adapted output from Sabel et al. (2000) to again show ALS data from Finland. In this analysis, the authors took the place of residence in 1985 of ALS cases to create a relative risk estimate using kernel estimation. Population at risk was estimated by adopting a case control methodology, which has the added advantage of enabling controlling for age, gender and other covariates. A large 60-kilometer bandwidth was chosen to reveal broad trends. Significance of the surface was obtained by running Monte Carlo simulations to produce the 95 percent confidence intervals shown in the figure. Concentrating on the significant highs, a cluster in southeast Finland again manifests itself together with some other smaller areas in low-density locations. Note instances of the small number problem occurring in the north of Finland, where the applied techniques break down when spurious significant lows are shown.

Figure 4.1 and Figure 4.2 are not directly comparable. Apart from different cluster methods adopted, one uses aggregated-level data, while the other uses individual level data. Population at risk is also estimated differently between the two figures. These observations notwithstanding, the presence of the southeast cluster in both analyses suggests areas worthy of follow-up for this disease with unknown etiology.

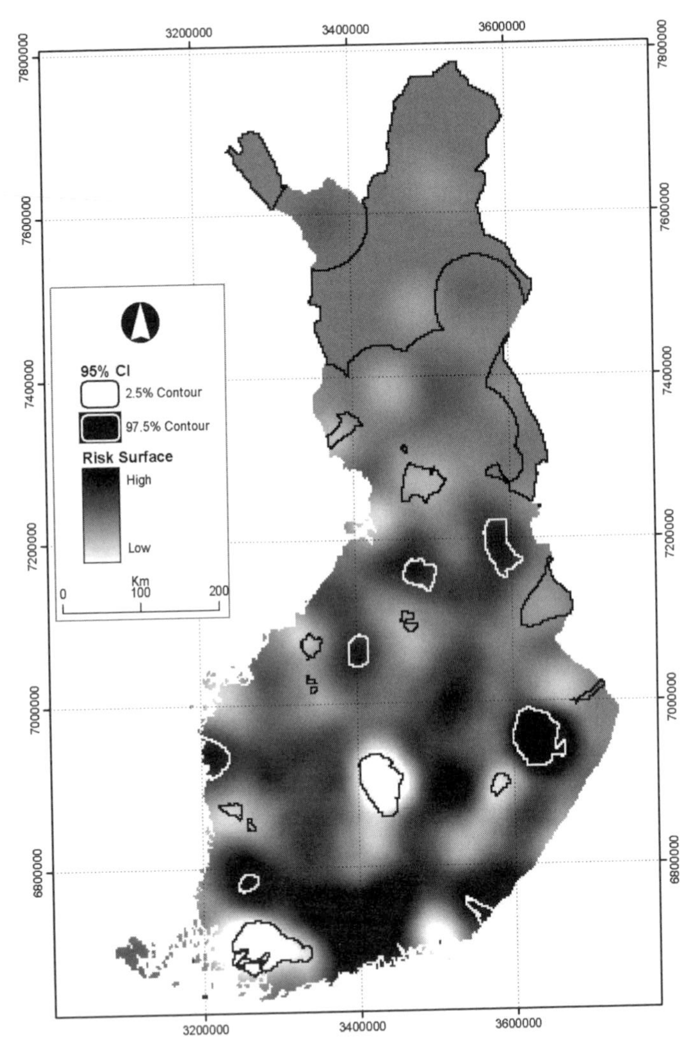

FIGURE 4.2 Relative risk surfaces derived using kernel estimation: ALS case residences, Finland, 1985. (Axes labels are in meters.)

4.5 CONSIDERATIONS AND LIMITATIONS

As important as the choice of the cluster detection test in any analysis are issues concerning data, the scale of analysis, correction for confounders and the underlying background population. It is tempting to conclude that the study of disease clustering involves so many assumptions and caveats that such studies should perhaps be avoided. Indeed, Rothman (1990) has even gone as far as to suggest that searching for individual clusters or indeed overall clustering is of little scientific value due to the (in)accuracy of the methods and the (poor) quality of data.

4.5.1 Mapping and GIS

Recall that the themes running throughout this volume are the possibilities and limitations of the use of GIS in public health. GIS has developed; it is no longer driven from the command line. Instead, it uses Microsoft® Windows®-based user interfaces, which are more intuitive. Although making the discipline less daunting for newcomers, this development risks uncritical and uninformed use of techniques that are now no more than a few clicks away. Here we might be concerned with, and warn against, the problems of naïve disease mapping, such as ignoring basic cartographic principles or, in the case of cluster investigations, adopting methods not suitable for the data being examined.

GIS is very good at exploratory visualization, but confirmatory (analytical) modeling has not developed as fast, which is often why specialized statistical packages are brought in. Ideally, data might be visualized in GIS prior to analysis within specialist cluster-detection software or routines. GIS analysis needs to develop well beyond throwing a few concentric circles or buffers around a site under investigation (Gatrell, 1999), but, dangerously for the newcomer, these are the most accessible tools available.

4.5.2 Data Quality

In studies investigating disease clustering, the quality of incidence data is paramount. Often data collection anomalies, on closer inspection, have been the cause of many clusters. Data might be inaccurate geographically or temporally, biased or missing. In instances where just one or two more cases can alter the result of the statistical test, it goes without saying that capturing all cases is highly desirable, if not a prerequisite. The use of accurate registers of disease or national death certificate registers can greatly help, but again, the quality of registers does differ. In small isolated studies, often triggered by concerns by the public, it is particularly vital to ensure that complete case ascertainment has been achieved.

Although a concern is minimizing false negatives, minimizing false positives through diagnostic inaccuracies is also an issue. This differential diagnosis is not easily handled without closely inspecting the data and perhaps even returning to the case notes of the patients. When studies involve thousands of cases, perhaps diagnosed by hundreds of doctors, this is naturally not practical and it should be noted that for some diseases, diagnosis is not clear-cut. As important as case ascertainment is accurate estimation of the underlying population at risk against which cases are compared. This is a nontrivial problem and is considered in greater depth later in this section.

Once cases have been identified, geocoding or address matching becomes an issue. Here an attempt is made to match as accurately as possible the given address to geographical space, whether latitude and longitude, census areas, or postal or zip codes. Inevitably, errors can be introduced at this stage and some cases will remain unmatched and therefore lost to the analysis.

Balancing the desire to improve healthcare through historical analysis of health events with the individual's right to privacy poses a severe limitation on the types of spatial analysis one can achieve. This fear of violating medical confidentiality often results in individual level data not being released to researchers. In this case, out of necessity, aggregated methods must be used.

4.5.3 Geography

Studies of disease clustering are often criticized due to the way in which boundaries of space and time have been chosen. Methodologies should be adopted that are "as released as possible from preclusions in the shape of artificial spatial and temporal units and population aggregates" (Schærström, 1996). To avoid the problems of "boundary shrinkage" (Openshaw, 1984), geographic scope should be defined at the outset. Otherwise, there is the temptation to fit the study region to the desired result because the tighter the boundaries chosen around the cluster, the higher the risk will be relative to the population at risk.

When considering count or aggregated data, investigators should be aware of the Modifiable Areal Unit Problem (MAUP) (Openshaw, 1984). One component of MAUP is where a possibly false interpretation is made from analyses purely because of arbitrary aggregations of the data. This arises because data is often collected and aggregated for convenience by local administrative, postcodes or zip codes, or health areas, borders that diseases are reluctant to respect. A second issue concerns the scale of aggregation. At one level of aggregation (e.g., postcode sectors of 1000 population), no significant result may be observed, whereas if the data were reaggregated (e.g., to postcode districts of 5000 people), an effect may be observed. The data remains the same, all that changes is the scale of analysis.

Analyzing data at the individual level using point data with no spatial aggregation has obvious advantages in attempting to overcome some of these traditional concerns of MAUP. However, there remain scale issues, such as the degree of smoothing to adopt in point methods such as kernel estimation.

4.5.4 Residential Migration

Many studies examining associations between geographical patterns of disease and causal factors assume that current residence in an area can be equated with exposure to conditions that currently (and historically) pertain there (Bentham, 1998). This is important, since epidemiologists and geographers often adopt the place of residence at the time of diagnosis or death as the location for further analysis of the disease in question. Yet, people move and hence previous exposure to causative agents will not be included in the study. The problems will be greater for diseases such as many cancers that have a long lag or latency period, which allows plenty of time for mobility of the population. By adopting only the current residential address, not only will an individual's migration history be neglected, but also the daily activity spaces of the patient will be ignored, where perhaps occupational exposure might be crucial.

4.5.5 Statistical Issues

In addition to method-specific statistical issues, there remain some generic statistical considerations relevant to all geographical investigations.

A common issue arising in cluster detection is the problem of multiple hypothesis testing. Here, if any chosen method repeatedly tests multiple hypotheses with the same data in the same geographical area, there is a high probability that at least some of the tests will be spuriously significant. For example, if one performed 1000 tests, while adopting a significance level of 0.01, then a false-positive result might be expected to occur ten times. Clearly, this raises the possibility of accepting a falsely positive cluster.

In studies of rare diseases in sparsely populated areas or simply where there are few cases, the small number problem may arise (Kennedy, 1989). This is where a difference of perhaps just one or two cases can make a huge difference to rates. In these cases, cluster methods rarely have enough data with which to generate sufficient power to test specific hypotheses, although some, such as the scanning window type, are better at dealing with sparse data.

Within the medical profession, there is a heavy reliance on formal significance testing. We would like to challenge the statistical fallacy whereby a lack of formal significance is equated with a lack of effect. Ritual testing of hypotheses is often performed without adequate consideration over whether or not this is appropriate (Nester, 1996), which has led to a preoccupation with or blindness toward *p*-values. Scientific method or the biomedical tradition appears to dictate that hypothesis testing is integral to good science; however, is the positivist model of significance testing valid in all disease clustering investigations? In studies with large sample sizes, statistical significance is relatively easy to attain due to its dependence on sample size, making the acceptance of the hypothesis relatively meaningless. Whereas when we have small number problems, say, with three isolated cases of a rare disease in a rural area, significance might well be impossible to achieve. To the concerned local resident, does the "significant" cluster appear any more important than an "insignificant" one that happens to occur in the workplace? It is suggested that estimation of relative risk to examine the strength of the relationship might be a way to proceed.

It is also well worth repeating the mantra that statistically significant findings do not equate with the establishment of causal relationships in cluster detection studies. Most clustering work is essentially exploratory spatial data analysis, where specific causal hypotheses are not even tested. Causal mechanisms can only be established with follow-up studies, perhaps triggered by the initial cluster investigation.

4.5.6 Confounding

Confounding is the single most important problem affecting cluster studies (Wartenberg and Greenberg, 1993). Any spatial or temporal variation of confounders (also known as covariates), such as demographics (e.g., gender, age, ethnicity), lifestyle characteristics (e.g., diet, smoking behavior or physical activity), or simply population density (considered separately later), can mask or exacerbate real disease patterns. To illustrate this concept, consider the idea that people of similar ethnic origin have traditionally tended to live close together, although this is less the case now with increased population migration. Because we know that some diseases are inherited, one would expect to observe spatial clusters of genetic diseases. Thus, studies investigating excess clusters in these diseases would have to examine evidence for clustering over and above that exhibited in the background (ethnically skewed) population, after adjusting for the genetic confounding effect.

Ideally, methods such as Kulldorff's SaTScan should be adopted to adjust for confounding. If a case control-study design is adopted, however, known and unknown confounders could potentially be accounted for at the risk of adjusting for a real-but-unknown etiological effect.

4.5.7 Correcting for Population Density

A special case of confounding concerns the underlying or background population at risk. Correcting for spatial variations in the population at risk is an integral part of spatial epidemiological research, simply because any observed patterning of health events needs to be tempered by the underlying population distribution due to the heterogeneously distributed pattern of population settlement where most individuals congregate together in cities.

The suitable selection of an appropriate correction method is a nontrivial research problem. One often applied method in point-pattern analysis is to define a suitable set of controls from the at-risk population. By comparing the spatial arrangement of the observed cases with that of the controls, a relative risk estimate can be produced that has adjusted for the underlying inhomogeneity. Defining the control set as an accurate sample or representation of the whole underlying population distribution then becomes an issue, because inaccuracies introduced here might reveal false results in the analysis.

A fundamentally different method makes use of cartograms (or density equalized map projections) (Koch and Denike, 2001; Schulman et al., 1988) to correct for the heterogeneity in the background population data. Here, if one were to transform the disease data by the geography of the underlying population density or some measure of the population at risk, one would produce a distorted space map with the disease events still in their relative positions.

With aggregated count data, adjustment for variations in the underlying population density is normally achieved using figures obtained from a population census. In the United Kingdom and United States, the census occurs every ten years and thus may not reflect population changes and migrations between censuses. Censuses are subject to underenumeration, which, if left uncorrected, result in elevated disease risk estimates, particularly among those most difficult to enumerate and most susceptible to disease: the homeless, the most deprived, the young, and the elderly.

4.6 CHALLENGES

This review aimed to highlight major issues regarding cluster detection. It has demonstrated that the discipline remains of great importance in public health studies, with both active surveillance and *post hoc* confirmatory modeling being useful modes of investigation. However, there remain some significant outstanding methodological and technical challenges if the fields of cluster detection and GIS are to develop their relationship beyond anything other than a loose coupling. Here we present our wish list, extending Gatrell (1999) while concentrating on cluster detection.

One key advantage GIS has over bespoke cluster detection software is its ability to integrate complex (environmental) datasets with health data. Where GIS falls down currently is in its ability to assimilate cutting-edge cluster detection models within its framework. Is there merit in attempting to integrate these cluster models within the accepted GIS user interfaces to bring sound methodology to a wider audience?

We have already discussed the validity of the current residential address as an adequate geographical marker for disease exposure. Many, perhaps most, of us spend much time at work or at school and may be as exposed to potential environmental contamination there as at home. The occupational setting may be at least as important as the residential. Historical exposures may be more relevant in diseases with long latency periods. We also need to conduct research that looks at the practicality and the relative merits of collecting and using data on space–time activity on a daily scale. Related to this, we must do much more research that builds knowledge of migration paths into our analyses. We remain convinced that GIS has a role to play here, a view that is endorsed conceptually by Löytönen (1998) and Schærström (1996) and demonstrated technically and empirically by Sabel et al. (2000).

Further work is also needed on the coupling of physical models to GIS, whether concerned with air or water contamination. The key to successful environmental epidemiology is access to good data on the exposure of interest. Too often, such environmental information is only available at a crude geographical scale, which leads to some rather optimistic attempts to link exposure to health outcomes. Remember that disease incidence or exposures may not follow a simple circular pattern (as assumed by many cluster detection methods), but rather may follow air dispersion plumes, drainage basins, or ethnic population boundaries. At the very least, we need as far as possible to collect data on potential confounders; much of this essential information is missing from routine, geocoded databases and is only available via large-scale surveys. It is, however, essential if we are to exploit GIS in an epidemiological context.

We need to be much more sensitive to issues of error and scale and resolution problems. This also ties in with questions of exposure assessment. What error bars are attached to our locational and attribute data, whether the data are environmental or social? At what scale should we conduct our investigations? Are our data available at a suitably fine level of resolution? For example, if we are attempting to investigate the link between radon and lung cancer or electromagnetic fields and childhood leukemia, surely we can only make real progress if data are collected for individuals and properties that have locational coordinates at a resolution of less than ten meters.

Finally, we need to challenge the implicit assumption of cluster studies that single exposures lead to single outcomes. Should we not, as Wartenberg and Greenberg (1993) suggest, consider more realistic situations where single exposures can result in multiple outcomes and in which diseases are considered multifactorial, and thereby adapt our models and conceptual thinking accordingly?

References

Alexander, F.E. and Boyle, P., 1996, *Methods for Investigating Localised Clustering of Disease,* Lyon, France: IARC Scientific Publications.

Alexander, F.E. and Cuzick, J., 1992, Geographical and environmental epidemiology: Methods for small-area studies, in Elliott, P. et al., Eds., *Methods for the Assessment of Disease Clusters*, Oxford: Oxford University Press.

Aylin, P. et al., 1999, A national facility for small area disease mapping and rapid initial assessment of apparent disease clusters around a point source: The U.K. Small Area Health Statistics Unit, *Journal of Public Health Medicine*, 21, 289–298.

Bailey, T.C. and Gatrell, A.C., 1995, *Interactive Spatial Data Analysis,* Harlow, U.K.: Longman.

Bentham, G., 1998, Migration and morbidity: Implications for geographical studies of disease, *Social Science & Medicine*, 26, 49–54.

Bithell, J.F., 1990, An application of density estimation to geographical epidemiology, *Statistics in Medicine*, 9, 691–701.

Diggle, P.J., 2000, Overview of statistical methods for disease mapping and its relationship to cluster detection, in Elliott, P. et al., Eds., *Spatial Epidemiology: Methods and Applications*, Oxford: Oxford University Press.

Elliott, P. et al., Eds., 2000, *Spatial Epidemiology: Methods and Applications,* Oxford: Oxford University Press.

Fotheringham, A.S., Brunsdon, C., and Charlton, M., 2000, *Quantitative Geography: Perspectives on Spatial Data Analysis*, London: Sage Publications.

Gardner, M.J., 1993, Investigating childhood leukaemia rates around the Sellafield nuclear plant, *International Statistical Review*, 61, 231–244.

Gatrell, A.C., 1999, GIS in public and environmental health: Visualisation, exploration and modelling, available at http://geog.queensu.ca/h_and_e/healthandenvir/gatrell.html

Hjalmars, U. et al., 1996, Childhood leukaemia in Sweden: Using GIS and a spatial scan-statistic for cluster detection, *Statistics in Medicine*, 15, 707–715.

Kelsall, J.E. and Diggle, P.J., 1995, Non-parametric estimation of spatial variation in relative risk, *Statistics in Medicine*, 14, 2335–2342.

Kennedy, S., 1989, The small number problem and the accuracy of spatial databases, in Goodchild, M. and Gopal, S., Eds., *Accuracy of Spatial Databases*, London: Taylor and Francis.

Knox, G., 1989, Detection of clusters, in Elliott, P., Ed., *Methodology of Enquiries into Disease Clustering*, London: Small Area Health Statistics Unit.

Koch, T. and Denike, K., 2001, GIS approaches to the problem of disease clusters: A brief commentary, *Social Science & Medicine*, 52, 1751–1754.

Kulldorff, M., 1998, Statistical methods for spatial epidemiology: Tests for randomness, in Gatrell, A.C. and Löytönen, M., Eds., *GIS and Health: GISDATA 6*, London: Taylor and Francis.

Kulldorff, M., 2002, SaTScan v. 3.0: Software for the Spatial and Space-Time Scan Statistics, Information Management Services Inc., Bethesda, MD: National Cancer Institute.

Kulldorff, M. et al., 1997, Breast cancer in northeastern United States: A geographical analysis, *American Journal of Epidemiology*, 146, 161–170.

Lawson, A.B. and Kulldorff, M., 1999, A review of cluster detection methods, in Lawson, A.B. et al., Eds., *Disease Mapping and Risk Assessment for Public Health*, New York: Wiley.

Löytönen, M., 1998, GIS, time, geography and health, in Gatrell, A.C. and Löytönen, M., Eds., *GIS and Health: GISDATA 6*, London: Taylor and Francis.

Nester, M.R., 1996, An applied statistician's creed, *Applied Statistics*, 45, 401–410.
Openshaw, S., 1984, *The Modifiable Areal Unit Problem: CATMOG 38*, Norwich, U.K.: Geo Books.
Openshaw, S. et al., 1987, A Mark 1 geographical analysis machine for the automated analysis of point data sets, *International Journal of Geographical Information Systems*, 1, 335–358.
Openshaw, S. et al., 1999, Testing space-time and more complex hyperspace geographical analysis tools, in *GISRU.K. '99*, Southampton, U.K.: University of Southampton.
Rothman, K.J., 1990, Keynote presentation: A sobering start for the cluster buster's conference, *American Journal of Epidemiology*, 132, S6–13.
Sabel, C.E., 1999, GIS, environmental exposure and health: An exploratory spatial data analysis of motor neurone disease, Ph.D. thesis, Lancaster, U.K.: University of Lancaster.
Sabel, C.E. et al., 2000, Modelling exposure opportunities: Estimating relative risk for motor neurone disease in Finland, *Social Science & Medicine*, 50, 1121–1137.
Sabel, C.E. et al., 2003, The spatial clustering of amyotrophic lateral sclerosis in Finland at place of birth and place of death, *American Journal of Epidemiology*, 157, 10, 898–905.
Schærström, A., 1996, Pathogenic paths? A time geographical approach in medical geography, Ph.D. thesis, Lund, Sweden: Lund University Press.
Schulman, J., Selvin, S., and Merrill, D.W., 1988, Density equalized map projections: A method for analyzing clustering around a fixed point, *Statistics in Medicine*, 7, 491–505.
Viel, J-F., 2000, Soft-tissue sarcoma and non-Hodgkin's lymphoma clusters around a municipal solid waste incinerator with high dioxin emission levels, *American Journal of Epidemiology*, 152, 13–19.
Wakefield, J. and Elliott, P., 1999, Issues in the statistical analysis of small area health data, *Statistics in Medicine*, 18, 2377–2399.
Wakefield, J.C., Kelsall, J.E., and Morris, S.E., 2000, Clustering cluster detection and spatial variation in risk, in Elliott P. et al., Eds., *Spatial Epidemiology: Methods and Applications*, Oxford: Oxford University Press.
Waller, L.A., 2000, A civil action and statistical assessments of the spatial pattern of disease: Do we have a cluster? *Regulatory Toxicology and Pharmacology*, 32, 174–183.
Wartenberg, D., 2001, Investigating disease clusters: Why, when, and how? *Journal of the Royal Statistical Society Series A, Statistics in Society*, 164, 13–22.
Wartenberg, D. and Greenberg, M., 1993, Solving the cluster puzzle: Clues to follow and pitfalls to avoid, *Statistics in Medicine*, 12, 1763–1770.

Section 2

GIS Applications in Communicable Disease Control and Environmental Health Protection

5 GIS and Communicable Disease Control

Thomas Kistemann and Angela Queste

CONTENTS

5.1 INTRODUCTION

This chapter examines how GIS may be used to help in some spatial-dimension aspects of current communicable disease-control problems. Hardware, software, data, and statistical problems are not addressed in detail.

The question might arise, whether it is appropriate to discuss the use of GIS for communicable disease control separately. There are, however, some features unique to communicable diseases (Figure 5.1) (Giesecke, 2001). One of the major objectives of this chapter is to demonstrate that these aspects provide good reasons for the application of GIS in the control of communicable diseases.

0-415-30655-8/04/$0.00+$1.50

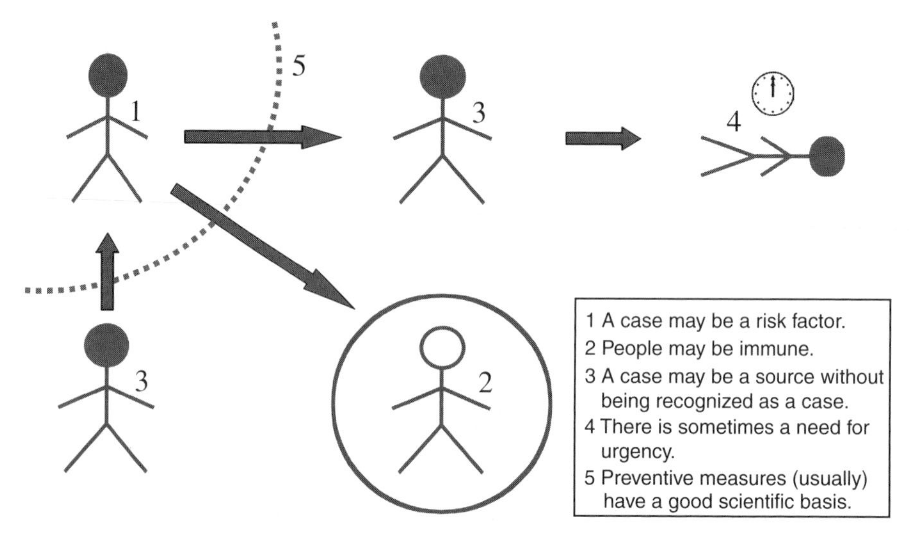

FIGURE 5.1 Some special features of communicable diseases (after Giesecke, J., 2001, *Modern Infectious Disease Epidemiology*, London: Arnold).

5.2 THE STARTING PART: COMMUNICABLE DISEASE MAPPING

Disease mapping has most probably begun with the mapping of communicable diseases, reflecting the importance of this group of diseases in ancient times. The oldest examples known are a world map of diseases drawn up by Finke in 1792 (Barrett, 2000) and a mapping of yellow fever occurrences in the harbor of New York drawn up in 1798 (Stevenson, 1965). In connection with the mapping of the London cholera outbreak in 1854 (Snow, 1855), John Snow has been accredited with the introduction of the map-supported spatiotemporal analysis into inductive infectious disease cause research.

The number of communicable disease maps rapidly increased in the course of the nineteenth century, but they were an incidental supplement rather than an essential part of epidemiological reports. This also applies to the medical topographies, a health description of the population, which started to appear after Johann Peter Frank (1779) had pointed out their importance. The first geographer who devoted his attention to communicable disease mapping was August Petermann (Diesfeld, 1995). When he recorded the cholera epidemics in the British Isles for the years between 1831 and 1833 (Petermann, 1852), the map was his fundamental tool and was of remarkable quality. In the twentieth century, numerous comprehensive communicable disease atlases were published, including the *World Atlas of Infectious Diseases* (Rodenwaldt and Jusatz, 1952–1961) and the *London International Atlas of AIDS* (Smallman-Raynor et al., 1992).

In the past two decades, communicable disease mapping was part of a cartographic revolution that was only possible due to the development of computer cartography. The new cartography is digital, dynamic, and networked, and it can be realized by users themselves (Schweikart, 1999). The automated generation of maps resulting from technical advancements by no means makes use of the full range of possibilities offered by GIS (O'Dwyer, 1998), but today it is the most widespread GIS application in the healthcare research sector (Scholten and de Lepper, 1991). GIS is most frequently used to display and investigate disease distributions by different mapping techniques: dot maps, diagram maps, choropleth maps, probability maps and flow maps. Advanced mapping applications allow for near-to-real-time imaging of epidemic waves and may support public health management during outbreaks and emergencies.

5.3 THE SPATIAL DIMENSION OF THE OCCURRENCE OF COMMUNICABLE DISEASE

Space is, in addition to person and time, the third important factor in the field of communicable disease epidemiology and control. For Robert Koch, mapping the water supply and sewage situation was an important and natural instrument in order to uncover the causes of the huge typhoid fever pandemic in the Ruhr area in 1901 (Figure 5.2).

Every link of an infection chain, from the occurrence of the microbial agent via existence and extension of reservoirs and sources, if need be the occurrence of vectors and hosts, to human cases within populations with specific conditions of

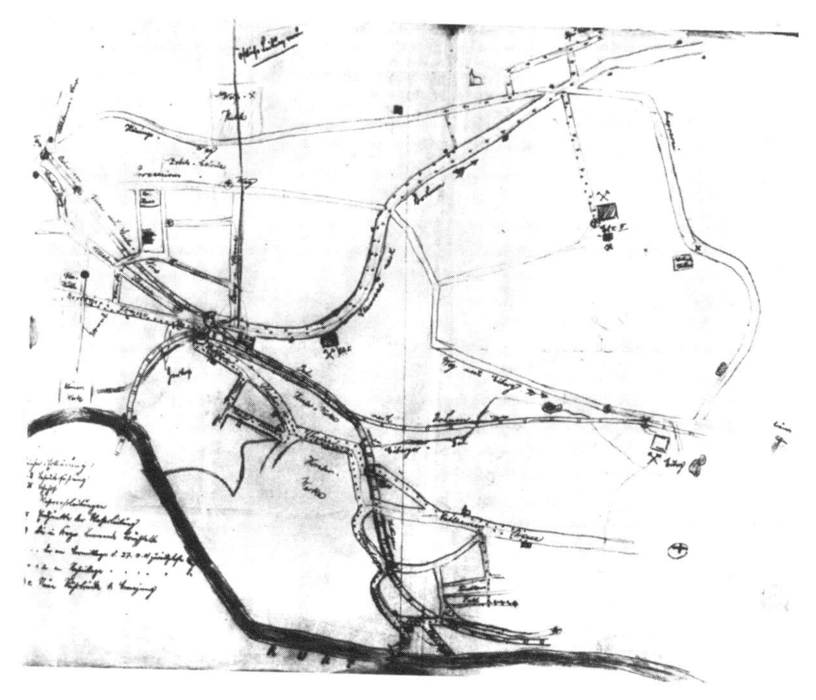

FIGURE 5.2 Robert Koch's hand-drawn map displaying sanitary conditions in relation to a huge outbreak of typhoid fever in the German Ruhrgebiet, 1901.

social interaction (contact patterns), susceptibility or immunity, has its own spatial dimension. It is necessary to compile all these different spatial dimensions to understand fully the occurrence, emergence, and disappearance of communicable diseases.

In the twentieth century, a number of factors have contributed to the fact that the spatial dimension of communicable disease received decreasing attention. The decreased importance of infectious diseases for overall mortality as a consequence of improvements in hygiene and new therapeutic options (antibiotics), a focus on the microbiological-etiologic concept of communicable diseases, and emphasis on the individual-oriented medical approach have in particular encouraged this perspective. However, the widespread idea that communicable diseases in principle could be overcome has had to be revised in the last few years; in addition, in the future infectious diseases will keep their high epidemiological importance worldwide, as demonstrated by the severe acute respiratory syndrome (SARS) outbreak in 2003. Only a few can be eradicated and most can only be kept under control if the most favorable conditions for disease control exist. According to the World Health Organization (WHO), approximately one third of all deaths registered worldwide were due to communicable diseases in 1997. In developed countries, communicable diseases have not lost their epidemiological status as regards morbidity and they constitute a considerable economic burden.

The Institute of Medicine of the National Academy of Sciences pointed out the threat from emerging infectious diseases and emerging pathogens in 1992 and demanded appropriate measures. The factors that justify a new evaluation of communicable diseases are multidimensional (Haggett, 1994; Olshansky et al., 1997). On the one hand, the pathogens themselves or new findings about them can be responsible for a reassessment of infection risks. The five categories listed in Table 5.1 have been suggested by Kistemann and Exner (2000) to be distinguished. On the other hand, environmental changes including physical, social, and psychological aspects, mainly induced by human activities, can favor the spread of pathogens to a considerable extent. Based on the opinion that these factors have their own additional importance for the epidemiology of communicable diseases, they have been

TABLE 5.1
Types of Newly Emerging Pathogens

Type	Characterization	Example (microorganism/disease)
A	Newly discovered pathogens	*Borrelia burgdorferi*/Lyme disease (1982)
B	Newly discovered mutants of pathogens	*Vibrio cholerae* 0 139/cholera (1992)
C	Discovery of new human pathogenic aspects of a well-known microorganism	*Campylobacter* sp./gastroenteritis (1977)
D	Discovery of the pathogen of an infectious disease which has been known for some time	Hepatitis C virus/hepatitis non-A, non-B (1989)
E	Discovery of the association of a microorganism to a well-known malignant or chronic-degenerative disease	*Helicobacter pylori*/stomach ulcers (1983)

named B-factors, in contrast to microbial agents (A-factors) (Rimpau, 1934). Facing the end of the antibiotic era, however, the underlying ecological concept of communicable disease etiology is experiencing a comeback as it is rediscovered by the medical world. In our context, it is of utmost importance that, just as the links of an infection chain do, most of these B-factors show clear spatial differentiation and spatial interaction. Several categories, each comprising different ecological B-factors, have been distinguished (Figure 5.3) (Haggett, 1994; Kistemann and Exner, 2000; Olshansky et al., 1997).

Regarding sociodemography, general population growth, changes in the age structure of populations, mobility, mass migrations, and unplanned urbanization are of distinct importance for the spread of many infectious diseases. Political and economic crises, armed conflicts, under- and unemployment, material deprivation and poor residential conditions can be summarized as socioeconomic conditions.

Today, there is no doubt that large-scale environmental changes such as global climate change, stratospheric ozone depletion, changes in land-use patterns, soil degradation, and hydraulic engineering severely affect the resurgence of communicable diseases. Water has its own implications, in that access to clean drinking and recreational water, closely related to the quality of water supply structures, the availability of freshwater, and the protection of water resources strongly influence patterns of infectious diseases.

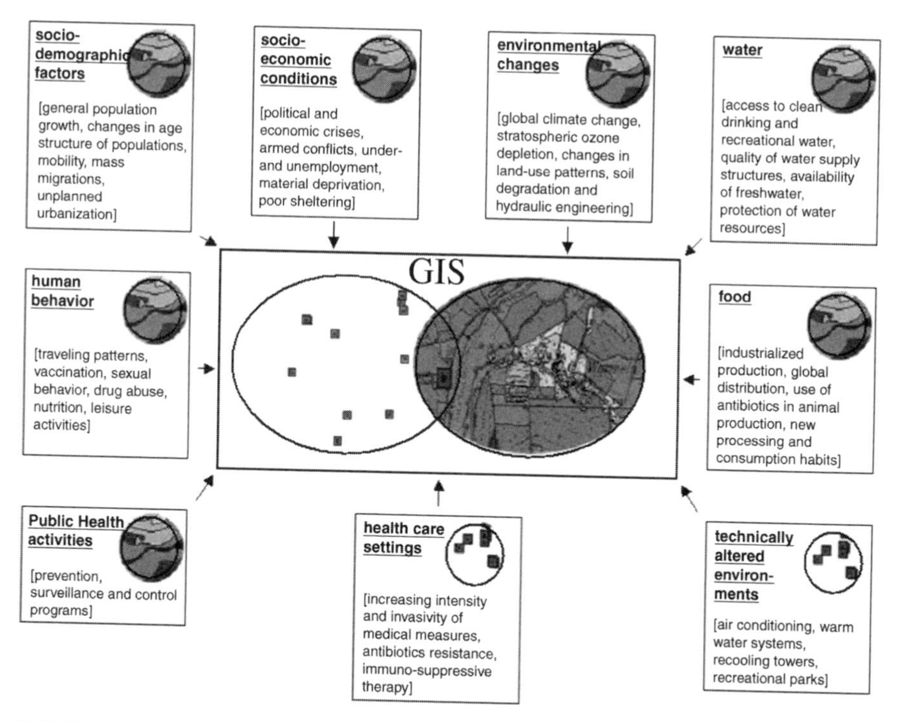

FIGURE 5.3 Different ecological factors (B-factors) affecting the space time patterns of the appearance of communicable diseases. Their spatial features can easily be fitted together using GIS.

Food is another environmental factor that has been subject to dramatic changes during the last few decades, in terms of industrialized production, global distribution, use of antibiotics in animal production, and new processing and consumption habits.

Worldwide, people spend more and more time in technically altered environments. Air conditioning, warm water systems, cooling towers, and recreational parks are examples of water-related techniques with potential impacts on human health and well-being. In particular, healthcare settings are specific environments with an extraordinary high risk. Increasing intensity and invasiveness of medical interventions, resistance to antibiotics, and immunosuppressive therapy contribute to these significant infection risks.

Finally, public health activities such as prevention, surveillance, and control programs, being part of the population's social environment, affect the occurrence of communicable disease.

Many of these environmental factors interact with human behavior, which itself, although individual-based, shows spatial patterns of practices and habits as they are society induced, e.g., traveling patterns, vaccination, sexual behavior, drug abuse, nutrition, and leisure activities.

The discussion about emerging infectious diseases has shown that understanding spatial relations is an important condition for successful prevention, control, and surveillance of communicable disease.

Many factors that influence the occurrence of communicable diseases are determined by their spatial dimensions. GIS provides a broad range of tools to integrate, store, handle, complete, analyze, and display the spatial dimension of these factors and their correlation to the space–time patterns of communicable diseases (Table 5.2).

5.4 USING GIS FOR THE PREVENTION, SURVEILLANCE, AND CONTROL OF COMMUNICABLE DISEASES

There is an incipient change in healthcare strategy from therapeutic medicine, which was very much oriented toward antibiotics, to public health instruments that have been more or less neglected for a long time: prevention, surveillance, and control of communicable diseases.

5.4.1 GIS and Communicable Disease Prevention

Prevention comprises all measures and strategies of health protection and promotion, which ensure that communicable diseases do not occur. This includes a health protecting legal framework, quality assurance of water for human consumption, food hygiene, hospital hygiene, vaccinations, vector abatement, and health promotion. The success of preventive measures depends on identifying the existence and location of a population at risk, spatially allocating preventive actions, and ensuring accessibility to these preventive measures for those at risk.

For example, for the Hlabisa health district, Republic of South Africa, an investigation using GIS demonstrated that there exists a substantial spatial heterogeneity of HIV prevalence among pregnant women and that this heterogeneity closely correlates with the distance of the women's homestead to primary and secondary

TABLE 5.2
Important GIS Analysis Methods

Method	Description	Application for Control of Communicable Diseases (example)
Database query	Identification of objects on the basis of user-defined selection terms	Identification of gastrointestinal disease cases within specific water supply zones (Dangendorf et al., 2001)
Geometric calculations	All functions carrying out calculations on the basis of geometry: distances, longitudes, areas, angles, differences in altitude, etc.	Calculation of distance between the residential address of disease cases and certain risk factors (Tanser et al., 2000)
Overlay, clip, merge	Techniques to calculate new variables by combining different spatial information	Investigation of correlation between anthrax incidence and natural conditions in Russia (Cherkasskiy, 1999)
Buffering	Construction of zones (buffers) of specified dimensions around points, lines, and areas	Determination of amounts of land use in different water protection zones (Kistemann et al., 2001)
Density estimation	Estimation of spatial density of geometric objects on the basis of user-defined conditions (e.g., kernel estimation)	Estimation of spatial density of disease cases (Atkinson and Unwin, 1998)
Interpolation	Estimation of missing data on the basis of space-related relations and distribution of known data (e.g., kriging)	Estimation of influenze incidence on the basis of selected GP practice indices (Uphoff et al., forthcoming)
Smoothing methods	Construction of smoothed (generalized) patterns of attribute data (surface) (e.g., surface trend analysis)	Construction of patterns of vector density on the basis of data for selected sites
Analysis of space-related distribution	Examination of space-related data for correlations and clusters using visualization and geostatistical methods	Identification of disease clusters (McKee et al., 2000)
Modeling and simulation	Development of models and scenarios on the basis of geometric and attribute data, in particular tempospatial distribution and spreading models, etc.	Simulation of the effects of temperature rise on the spread of vectors and vector-borne communicable diseases (Rogers and Randolph, 2000)

roads. This result clearly pointed to the importance of social contacts with road-related populations for women's HIV incidence. It was seen as a starting point for the development of more precise prevention strategies to reduce the spread of HIV infection (Tanser et al., 2000).

5.4.2 GIS and Communicable Disease Surveillance

Surveillance is the continuous and systematic collection, analysis, and interpretation of data on infectious diseases. This is essential for planning, implementing, and evaluating intervention measures and programs for the prevention, identification, and control of infections. It is probably the most popular current application of GIS in the field of communicable disease control, as it covers spatial aspects of infection chains and environmental conditions and changes.

Since the beginning of the 1990s, the Centers for Disease Control and Prevention (CDC) have carried out several GIS-based analyses covering the occurrence of infectious diseases due to environmental factors (Croner et al., 2000). Vector-borne diseases have been the predominant field for GIS application, because the complex interactions between environmental factors and pathogens, vectors (e.g., mosquitoes, ticks), the various host animals and pathogen reservoirs can be recorded in a single system (Mott et al., 1995) and numerous ecological data influencing the appearance of vectors can be included. Recent examples cover, for instance, the surveillance of the following:

- Malaria (Indaratna et al., 1998; Kitron et al., 1994; Martin et al., 2002; Sharma and Srivastava, 1997; Srivastava et al., 1999; Yang et al., 2002)
- Tick-borne diseases (Cortinas et al., 2002; Frank et al., 2002; Glass et al., 1995; Rizzoli et al., 2002)
- Helminth diseases (Abdel-Rahman et al., 2001; Bavia et al., 2001; Brooker and Michael, 2000; Brooker et al., 2000; Kloos et al., 1998; Malone et al., 1992, 2001; Maszle et al., 1998)

For Russia, a national register of historic and contemporary anthrax foci has been assembled to develop contingency plans for different risk locations, a differentiated strategy of vaccination and other control strategies, and preventive recommendations to reduce the risk in high-risk areas. In-depth GIS-based studies of particular clusters compare natural geographic features, such as soil type, climate, etc., with anthrax distributions and aim to identify the factors that are associated with the anthrax outbreaks in Russia (Cherkasskiy, 1999).

The epidemiology of gonorrhea and other sexually transmitted diseases (STDs) is characterized by geographically defined hyperendemic areas (cores). GIS has been used to evaluate the geographic epidemiology of gonorrhea, e.g., on a large military installation in North Carolina (Zenilman et al., 2002) or in Baltimore. There, census tract-specific rates were calculated and the top rate quartile was considered as the core, consisting of 13 geographically contiguous census tracts. As radial distance from the core increased, incidence rates decreased and the male to female ratio increased. This GIS-based study was consistent with previous definitions of the core theory of STDs (Becker et al., 1998).

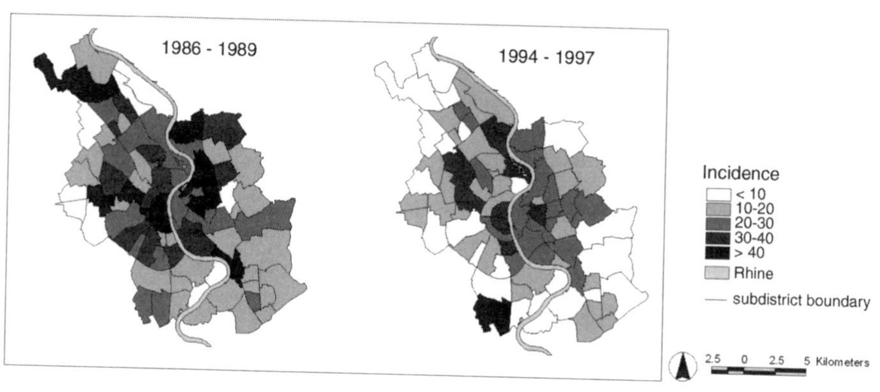

FIGURE 5.4 TB patterns in the city of Cologne, Germany, 1986–1989 in comparison to 1994–1997. From Kistemann, T., Munzinger, A., and Dangendorf, F., 2002, Spatial patterns of tuberculosis incidence in Cologne (Germany), *Social Science & Medicine,* 55, 7–19. With permission.

A small-area, division-based study using GIS was conducted to investigate the inner-urban strength of association between tuberculosis (TB) and 12 independent variables representing contemporary ethnic and economic conditions in Cologne, Germany. Mapping revealed huge inner-urban differences in TB incidence (Figure 5.4). In the statistical analysis for the under-60 age group, a strong positive association was found between TB incidence and percentage of immigrants as well as variables depicting economic conditions. As for the 60-and-older age group, regression analysis failed to model the TB incidence patterns sufficiently. An autonomous, spatially disaggregated TB epidemic of the elderly was assumed echoing the severe postwar epidemic by reactivation. The study contributed to the understanding of TB patterns in Germany, which does not fulfill the WHO definition of a low incidence country yet, and gave cause for inner-urban adjustment of public health TB programs (Kistemann et al., 2002).

Modern software facilitates the development of complex applications for the World Wide Web (Web) in the field of GIS and database technology. These new communication forms can be used for public health purposes as well (Goodchild, 2000).

The novelty of the global networks consists in the fact that space-related data, including the underlying data, can be generated, networked, used, and distributed in a decentralized and simultaneous way (Asche, 2001). Within networked environments, we can distinguish between static, interactive, and dynamic features of geographic data presentation (Asche, 2001; Kraak, 2001; Schröder, 1998).

The Web can be used to generate complete maps interactively. The client does not need separate GIS software. By means of a map server, individual maps are generated and transmitted to the client. Due to these methods, it is possible to generate topical maps via a Web site without having one's own resources (Goodchild, 1998).

Quick data access is of direct benefit to research. Addresses can be geocoded and demographic and socioeconomic data can be downloaded to use them as a basis for a personal GIS application.

The online monitoring of the spatial distribution of infectious diseases is of increasing interest to public health. The Web promotes new strategies for disease surveillance, e.g., the development of early warning systems (Flahault et al., 2000). The Web offers good opportunities to secure efficient healthcare on the national and international level that is accompanied by health policy measures in the field of prevention.

A rather advanced example comes from France. The French National Institute of Health and Medical Research (INSERM) has been developing a national teleinformation system for the electronic monitoring of infectious diseases since 1984 (Flahault et al., 2000; Valleron and Garnerin, 1992). Due to the implementation of GIS technologies on the Internet and to a user-friendly surface, it is possible for every user to scan the current epidemiological situation in the French regions and to display them accordingly. Presently, the spatial distribution of seven communicable diseases can be queried (http://rhone.b3e.jussieu.fr/). FluNet is an advance of this system and monitors the global situation of influenza (http://www.who.int/GlobalAtlas/home.asp).

5.4.3 GIS and Communicable Disease Control

Control comprises all measures that are necessary to identify an increasing number of infections with the same pathogen as well as the specific causes. It includes measures that are directed at the cause and prevent the infection from spreading or recurring (outbreak management).

In North Carolina, a GIS was used in an outbreak of *Shigella sonnei* infection in a single community. A database consisting of demographic, temporal, and home address information was used. Through simultaneous examination of temporal and spatial distribution of the 59 identified cases, a focus of infection in a single housing area was identified. Targeted education among residents of the neighborhood was associated with prompt control of the epidemic (McKee et al., 2000).

Little is currently known about the spatial distribution of parasitic infections other than malaria, trypanosomiasis, and onchocerciasis (Brooker et al., 2000). The construction of the Three Gorges Dam in China, however, prompted a spatial investigation of schistosomiasis, a water-borne parasitic disease, as the dam will increase marshlands and irrigation in areas currently free of schistosomiasis. The potential for the spread of schistosomiasis into these new areas is a major concern. Therefore, a hydrological parasite transport model of water velocity and flow in an irrigation system was developed to provide a means of estimating travel times of the parasites from source sites to water contact/exposure sites for humans and the intermediate vector snail population. It will be part of an overall model of schistosomiasis transmission in the catchment areas. In this context, GIS was used to manage spatial data of the drainage network, land use, infection sources, and population centers (Maszle et al., 1998). It has now become quite common to apply GIS, sometimes combined with remote sensing to provide ecological data, to schistosomiasis control programs (Abdel-Rahman et al., 2001; Bavia et al., 2001; Brooker and Michael, 2000; Kloos et al., 1998; Malone et al., 2001).

Remote sensing has become an important source of ecological data. User-friendly software for remote sensing and GIS are the ideal tools to collect, organize, and use this large quantity of space-related information. In the field of epidemiology, however, this technology has rarely been applied; it is only slowly increasing in use (Goetz et al., 2000; Wood et al., 2000). The potential of remote sensing, however, has in principle been recognized and its wider use is estimated to be very promising (Brooker et al., 2000; Hay, 2000; Hay et al., 2000).

Remote sensing data are increasingly used for disease risk mapping, surveillance or monitoring, particularly of vector-borne diseases (Beck et al., 2000). Since the disease vectors have specific requirements regarding climate, vegetation, soil and other factors, remote sensing can be used to determine their habitat.

As an example, the risk of cholera epidemics in the area of the Ganges delta has been assessed by use of GIS and remote sensing. *Vibrio cholera* is hosted by zooplankton, which reacts like phytoplankton. For this reason, it is possible to correlate cholera incidence and favorable factors for the plankton. This method requires the evaluation of surface temperature and turbidity of the water as well as the sea water level. These factors can be checked by means of remote sensing. Cholera incidence is higher when surface temperature and the seawater level rise (Colwell et al., 2000; Lobitz et al., 2000).

Outbreak situations need urgent public health control measures including risk assessment, outbreak management, cause identification, and risk communication. Much of the relevant information is space related: distribution of cases, patterns of risk factors, health services, infrastructure, and emergency medical services.

Within a small German municipality, an outbreak of diarrheal disease prompted parasitological and epidemiological investigations into the question of whether the cases were related to tap water. Within a retrospective cohort study, 13 asymptomatic cases of giardiasis were identified. The origin of the domestic tap water was traced back for each participant in the study via the place of residence. The drinking water supply structures of the investigation area were recorded in detail. A water supply structure GIS (WSS-GIS) (Kistemann et al., 2001) has been developed to support spatial analysis and communication of results (Figure 5.5). The water supply zone of the residence place turned out to be a significant risk factor for acquiring giardia infection. GIS helped the understanding of complex drinking water supply structures and related epidemiological data to this environmental risk factor (Kistemann et al., 2004, in press).

Hospital environments are high-risk areas, due to immunocompromised hosts, breached host barriers, intensive contact patterns, and multiresistant strains. The costs of sufficient control measures are substantial. Therefore, hospital infection control is an important task. Again, much of the relevant information is space related: localization of patients, diagnostic and therapeutic activities, hospital infrastructure, contact patterns, working areas of personnel. GIS could be the ideal tool to organize and use the data.

Within a hospital salmonellosis outbreak, all case-specific information was transferred to a Hospital-GIS. To investigate the outbreak, the layers — "placement of institutions" and "providing logistics" — were used and a specific "salmonella outbreak layer" was composed, which comprised the database of the cases. The

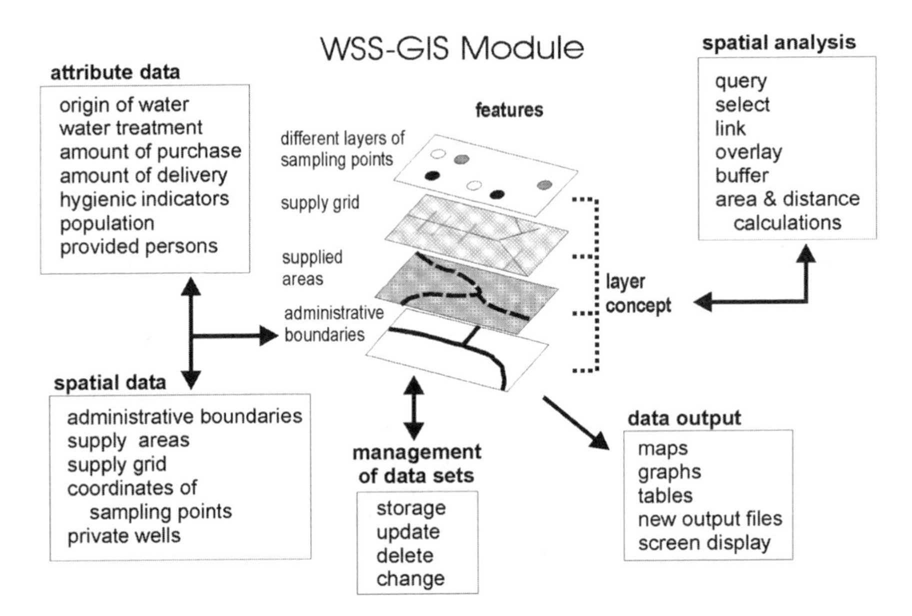

FIGURE 5.5 Principles of WSS-GIS as a basic tool for the surveillance and control of water-related communicable diseases. From Kistemann, T., Munzinger, A., and Dangendorf, F., 2002, Spatial patterns of tuberculosis incidence in Cologne (Germany), *Social Science & Medicine,* 55, 7–19. With permission.

cases were georeferenced, referring to their probable place of infection. With the help of the Hospital-GIS, space-related, continuous updating and interactive management of all case-specific information was feasible. Epidemiological queries for every case as well as for single functional units could be done to get current and precise spatiotemporal information concerning the outbreak. As an output, an epidemic map pointed out the widespread character of the outbreak throughout the clinical area. The "providing logistics" layer was applied to analyze the functional relations between the identified places of infection. The central kitchen was identified as the source of infection. The Hospital-GIS helped to confirm and display the clinicwide extent of the outbreak, to identify several spatially separated sites with high rates of infection, and to uncover their relevant functional relation. Communication of the findings was facilitated (Kistemann et al., 2000).

GIS applications within the fields of hospital hygiene and hospital infection control have not been reported before and are not mentioned as a tool of computerized systems in hospital epidemiology (Freeman, 1998). To use GIS for hospital hygiene purposes requires time and cost-intensive implementation. All relevant functional facilities have to be digitized systematically. Organized within a layer system, this information serves as a base to uncover, analyze, and display spatial, temporal, and functional interrelationships of patients and personnel, which may be important for infection routes. Geographic information scientists should not omit this field when demonstrating the benefits of GIS-supported communicable disease control.

5.5 PROBLEMS OF USING GIS FOR COMMUNICABLE DISEASE CONTROL

5.5.1 The Gee Whiz Effect

As for any disease map, the visual impression of communicable disease maps is open to the influence of cartographical and statistical issues. Projection, size of the areal units, number and limits of categories as well as selection of colors influence the perception of the map by the reader. The results may be affected considerably (Openshaw, 1984) by the modifiable areal unit problem (MAUP). The precision of the data depends on type of map and population size: incidence maps may show rather extreme values in areal units with small populations, probability maps may reveal the opposite (Smans and Estève, 1992). Considering these problems, it is critical to draft a hypothesis on the basis of an impressive map to explain a pattern, the existence of which is quite uncertain (the so-called "gee whiz" effect; Jaquez, 1998). GIS can contribute to overcoming some of these problems, since they permit a more flexible and problem-oriented analysis of the areal units when generating choropleth maps (Dunn, 1992). On the other hand, there is a risk that the easy and quick production of numerous maps may promote the distribution of incorrect conclusions if the underlying theory and methodological restrictions are not sufficiently considered (Briggs and Elliott, 1995).

5.5.2 Ecological Fallacy

Ecological studies are based on the principle of the spatial linkage of health data and risk factors. The current place of residence is frequently taken as point of reference. The exposure of a population to a risk factor is assessed by means of some risk factor level at the place of residence. For communicable diseases, these risk factors include the A- and B-factors mentioned previously. In many cases, this procedure proves to be more reliable than the collection of individual exposure data (English, 1992; Morgenstern, 1998). It implies the differentiated mapping of environmental risk factors in terms of the area to be covered, a task for which GIS is highly suitable. It is obvious that GIS has contributed to the spread of ecological studies.

However, since ecological studies are not based on individual but on aggregated disease and exposure data, the results achieved may be subject to the so-called ecological fallacy, which can only be excluded by a subsequent epidemiological study at the individual level (Morgenstern, 1998; Robinson, 1950; Selvin, 1958). Several techniques are available to reduce the risk of ecological confounding. Important methods are stratifying with regard to time lags due to latent periods, and statistical adjustment for potential confounders. Furthermore, as much data as possible should be sampled at the individual level to avoid the ecological fallacy.

5.5.3 Lack of Spatial Statistical Capabilities

GIS has the prerequisites for the automated implementation of spatial-statistical methods such as autocorrelation and cluster analyses. Commercial GIS does not always include the corresponding analytical tools, yet. While Chapter 2 and Chapter 3 discuss a range of available techniques and specifically designed software tools (e.g., WinBUGS) these specific advances are not yet widespread in the public health sector (Scholten and de Lepper, 1991; Jaquez, 1994; van den Berg and von der Ahé, 1997; Zhang and Griffith, 1997; Wellie et al., 2000).

5.5.4 GIS and the Time Dimension

All human activities have not only a spatial, but also a time dimension. In everyday life, individual, family-related, cultural, economic and environmental issues determine the duration and direction of movements comprising both commuters' behavior as well as long-term and permanent changes of location.

Human activity influences communicable disease processes. A certain period of exposure and latency precedes each outbreak of disease. This inevitably leads to the fact that the place of diagnosis of the disease does not necessarily coincide with the place where the disease was acquired or caused.

For this reason, local risk factors can often not directly be associated with the space-related distribution of diseases. Therefore, a corresponding analysis has to consider the migration of individuals (Schærström, 1996). An aggravating factor in this respect is the fact that risk factors may also vary with regard to time and space. To obtain a meaningful analysis, tempospatial models have to be developed and clipped to cover both the migration of the individuals examined and the considered risk factors. This type of analysis is hard to realize by means of the GIS functionalities currently available.

Since the beginning of the 1990s, efforts to integrate the time dimension into geographical-epidemiological GIS models have been intensified. Peuquet and Duan (1995) presented the first workable GIS model comprising the time dimension by means of an "event-based spatiotemporal data model" (Löytönen, 1998). It is a major task to understand the correlation between the time- and space-related processes of disease development and the resulting space-related patterns. GIS technology ought to have the potential to ameliorate the integration of the time dimension. (See Chapter 4 for a discussion of current research that addresses both space and time issues.)

5.5.5 Lack of Systematically Trained Staff

The WHO explicitly defines trained personnel as a constituent part of GIS (WHO, 1999). Regarding communicable disease control applications, lack of trained staff is probably the most serious deficiency in the field. In Germany, for instance, most local public health officers have little knowledge of GIS. Many do not realize the opportunities provided by GIS. To improve this situation, GIS should become an integral part of public health training courses and the financial resources for GIS hardware and software, as well as the number of GIS professionals within the public health authorities, should be increased.

5.6 CONCLUSIONS

The discussions about emerging infectious diseases during the last decade have unquestionably drawn renewed attention to prevention, surveillance, and control measures. Ecological B-factors, public health, the spatial dimension of communicable diseases, and the ecological approach have been strengthened in this framework. This opens huge opportunities for GIS applications within communicable disease control programs. GIS has meanwhile proved to be a useful tool for prevention, control, and surveillance measures. However, some infectious disease epidemiologists still doubt whether a spatial approach and GIS have a broad application to their work (Giesecke, 2001).

It seems reasonable to adopt additional techniques like remote sensing and the Internet and to be open to specific tasks for GIS like outbreak management and solutions for specific environments (e.g., hospitals).

Some old problems, well known from disease mapping and ecological studies, should be kept in mind: the gee whiz effect, ecological fallacy, the problem of the time dimension. Some new, more GIS-specific problems should be addressed: the lack of spatial statistical capabilities of standard GIS packages and, perhaps most important, the lack of GIS-skilled personnel within the local public health authorities, which play the key role in the prevention, surveillance, and control of communicable diseases.

References

Abdel-Rahman, M.S. et al., 2001, Geographic information systems as a tool for control program management for schistosomiasis in Egypt, *Acta Tropica,* 79, 49–57.

Asche, H., 2001, Kartographische Informationsverarbeitung in Datennetzen – Prinzipien, Produkte, Perspektiven, in Herrmann, C. and Asche, H., Eds., *Web Mapping 1. Raumbezogene Information und Kommunikation im Internet,* Heidelberg: Wichmann.

Atkinson, P.J. and Unwin, D.J., 1998, The use of density estimation techniques in mapping the distribution of hepatitis A, in Gierl, L. et al., Eds., *Geomed '97, International Workshop on Geomedical Systems, Rockstock September 1997,* Leipzig, Stuttgart: Teubner.

Barrett, F.A., 2000, Finke's 1792 map of human diseases: The first world disease map? *Social Science & Medicine,* 50, 915–921.

Bavia, M.E. et al., 2001, Use of thermal and vegetation index data from Earth observing satellites to evaluate the risk of schistosomiasis in Bahia, Brazil, *Acta Tropica,* 79, 1, 79–85.

Beck, L.R., Lobitz, B.M., and Wood, B.L., 2000, Remote sensing and human health: New sensors and new opportunities, *Emerging Infectious Diseases,* 6, 3, 217–227.

Becker, K.M. et al., 1998, Geographic epidemiology of gonorrhea in Baltimore, Maryland, using a geographic information system, *American Journal of Epidemiology,* 147, 7, 709–716.

Briggs, D.J. and Elliott, P., 1995, The use of geographical information systems in studies on environment and health, *World Health Statistics Quarterly,* 48, 85–94.

Brooker, S. and Michael E., 2000, The potential of geographical information systems and remote sensing in the epidemiology and control of human helminth infections, *Advances in Parasitology,* 47, 245–288.

Brooker, S. et al., 2000, Toward an atlas of human helminth infection in sub-Saharan Africa: The use of geographical information systems (GIS), *Parasitology Today,* 16, 7, 303–307.

Cherkasskiy, B.L., 1999, A national register of historic and contemporary anthrax foci, *Journal of Applied Microbiology,* 87, 2, 192–195.

Colwell, R. et al., 2000, Remote sensing of cholera outbreaks: First year report, geo.arc.nasa.gov/sge/health/projects/cholera/cholera.html.

Cortinas, M.R. et al., 2002, Detection, characterization, and prediction of tick-borne disease foci, *International Journal of Medical Microbiology,* 291, Suppl. 33, 11–20.

Croner, C.M., Sperling, J., and Broome, F.R., 2000, Geographic information systems (GIS): New perspectives in understanding human health and environmental relationships, *Statistics in Medicine,* 15, 1961–1977.

Dangendorf, F. et al., 2002, Spatial patterns of diarrhoeal illnesses with regard to water supply structures — a GIS analysis, *Int. J. hyg. Environ. Health*, 205, 183–191.

Diesfeld, H.J., 1995, Geomedicine, in Doerr, W., and Seifert, G., Eds., *Spezielle Pathologische Anatomie* (*Tropical Pathology*), Vol. 8, Heidelberg: Springer.

Dunn, C., 1992, GIS and epidemiology, AGI publication number 5/92, London: Association for Geographic Information.

English, D., 1992, Geographical epidemiology and ecological studies, in Elliott, P. et al., Eds., *Geographical and Environmental Epidemiology,* Oxford: Oxford University Press.

Flahault, A. et al., 2000, Electronic monitoring of diseases, in Flahault, A., Toubiana, L., and Valleron, A.J., Eds., *Geography and Medicine. Geomed'99. Proceedings of the Second International Workshop on Geomedical Systems, Paris, 22–23 November 1999,* Amsterdam: Elsevier.

Frank, C. et al., 2002, Mapping Lyme disease incidence for diagnostic and preventive decisions, Maryland, *Emerging Infectious Diseases,* 8, 427–429.

Frank, J.P., 1779, *System Einer Vollständigen Medizinischen Polizey, Band 1,* Mannheim.

Freeman, J., 1998, The use of computerized systems in hospital epidemiology, in Bennett, V. and Brachman, P.S., Eds., *Hospital Infection,* 4th ed., Philadelphia: Lippincott-Raven Publishers.

Giesecke, J., 2001, *Modern Infectious Disease Epidemiology,* London: Arnold.

Glass, G.E. et al., 1995, Environmental risk factors for Lyme disease identified with geographic information systems, *American Journal of Public Health*, 85, 944–948.

Goetz, S.J., Prince, S.D., and Small, J., 2000, Advances in satellite remote sensing of environmental variables for epidemiological applications, *Advances in Parasitology,* 47, 289–307.

Goodchild, M.F., 1998, Strategies for GIS and public health, in Williams, R.C. et al., Eds., *Geographic Information Systems in Public Health: Proceedings of the Third National Conference,* 63–72, www.atsdr.cdc.gov/GIS/conference98.

Goodchild, M.F., 2000, Communicating geographic information in a digital age, *Annals of the Association of American Geographers,* 90, 344–355.

Haggett, P., 1994, Geographical aspects of the emergence of infectious diseases, *Geografiska Annaler,* 76B, 91–104.

Hay, S.I., 2000, An overview of remote sensing and geodesy for epidemiology and public health application, *Advances in Parasitology,* 47, 1–35.

Hay, S.I. et al., 2000, Earth observation, geographic information systems and *Plasmodium falciparum* malaria in sub-Saharan Africa, *Advances in Parasitology,* 47, 173–215.
Indaratna, K. et al., 1998, Application of geographical information systems to co-analysis of disease and economic resources: Dengue and malaria in Thailand, *Southeast Asian Journal of Tropical Medicine and Public Health,* 29, 4, 669–684.
Jaquez, G.M., 1994, *STAT! Statistical Software for the Clustering of Health Events, User Manual,* Ann Arbor: Biomedware.
Jaquez, G.M., 1998, GIS as an enabling technology, in Gatrell, A. and Löytönen, M., Eds., *GIS and Health,* London: Taylor and Francis.
Kistemann, T. and Exner, M., 2000, Bedrohung Durch Infektionskrankheiten? *Risikoeinschätzung und Kontrollstrategien. Deutsches Ärzteblatt,* 97, A 251–255.
Kistemann, T., Munzinger, A., and Dangendorf, F., 2002, Spatial patterns of tuberculosis incidence in Cologne (Germany), *Social Science & Medicine,* 55, 7–19.
Kistemann, T. et al., 2000, GIS-supported investigation of a nosocomial *Salmonella* outbreak, *International Journal of Hygiene and Environmental Health,* 203, 117–126.
Kistemann, T. et al., 2001, GIS-based analysis of drinking-water supply structures: A module for microbial risk assessment, *International Journal of Hygiene and Environmental Health,* 203, 301–310.
Kistemann, T. et al., 2004, in press, A waterborne giardiasis outbreak in a small German community, *International Journal of Hygiene and Environmental Health,* 206.
Kitron, U. et al., 1994, Geographic information system in malaria surveillance: Mosquito breeding and imported cases in Israel, *American Journal of Tropical Medicine,* 50, 5, 550–556.
Kloos, H., Gazzinelli, A., and Van Zuyle, P., 1998, Microgeographical patterns of schistosomiasis and water contact behavior: Examples from Africa and Brazil, *Memorias do Instituto Oswaldo Cruz,* 93, Suppl. 1, 37–50.
Kraak, M.J., 2001, Webmapping: Webdesign, in Herrmann, C. and Asche, H., Eds., *Web.Mapping 1. Raumbezogene Information und Kommunikation im Internet,* Heidelberg: Wichmann.
Krabbe, H., 2001, Experiences with the conversion of legal regulations in practice, *Deutsche Tierärztliche Wochenschrift,* 108, 8, 353–357.
Lobitz, B. et al., 2000, Climate and infectious disease: Use of remote sensing for detection of *Vibrio cholerae* by indirect measurement, *Proceedings of the National Academy of Sciences of the United States of America,* 97, 1438–1443.
Löytönen, M., 1998, GIS, Time geography and health, in Gatrell, A. and Löytönen, M., Eds., *GIS and Health,* London: Taylor and Francis.
Malone, J.B. et al., 1992, Use of LANDSAT MSS imagery and soil type in a geographic information system to assess site-specific risk of fascioliasis on Red River Basin farms in Louisiana, *Annals of the New York Academy of Sciences,* 653, 389–397.
Malone, J.B. et al., 2001, Satellite climatology and the environmental risk of *Schistosoma mansoni* in Ethiopia and East Africa, *Acta Tropica,* 79, 1, 59–72.
Martin, C. et al., 2002, The Use of a GIS-based malaria information system for malaria research and control in South Africa, *Health and Place,* 8, 4, 227–236.
Maszle, D.R. et al., 1998, Hydrological studies of schistosomiasis transport in Sichuan Province, China, *Science of the Total Environment,* 216, 3, 193–203.
McKee, K.T. Jr. et al., 2000, Application of a geographic information system to the tracking and control of an outbreak of shigellosis, *Clinical Infectious Diseases,* 31, 3, 728–733.

Molyneux, D.H., 2001, Vector-borne infections in the tropics and health policy issues in the twenty-first century, *Transactions of the Royal Society of Tropical Medicine and Hygiene,* 95, 3, 233–238.

Morgenstern, H., 1998, Ecologic studies, in Rothman, K.J. and Greenland, S., Eds., *Modern Epidemiology,* Philadelphia: Lippincott-Raven.

Mott, K. E. et al., 1995, New geographical approaches to control of some parasitic zoonoses, *Bulletin of the World Health Organization,* 73, 247–257.

National Academy of Sciences, 1992, Emerging infections: Microbial threats to health in the United States, Washington, D.C.: National Academy Press.

Nyamogoba, H.D., Obala, A.A., and Kakai, R., 2002, Combating cholera epidemics by targeting reservoirs of infection and transmission routes: A review, *East African Medical Journal,* 79, 3, 150–155.

O'Dwyer, L.A., 1998, Potential meets reality: GIS and public health research in Australia, *Australian and New Zealand Journal of Public Health,* 22, 819–823.

Olshansky, J.S., Carnes, B., and Rogers, R.G., 1997, Infectious diseases — New and ancient threats to world health, *Population Bulletin 1997,* 52, 2, 1–52.

Openshaw, S., 1984, *The Modifiable Areal Unit Problem,* CATMOG No 38, Norwich, U.K.: Geo Books.

Petermann, A., 1852, *Cholera Map of the British Isles Showing the Districts Affected in 1831, 1832, 1833,* London.

Peuquet, D.J. and Duan, N., 1995, An event-based spatiotemporal data model: ESTDM for temporal analysis of geographical data, *International Journal of Geographical Information Systems,* 9, 7–24.

Rimpau, w., 1934, Geomedizin als Wissenschaft (geomedicine as science), *Münchner Medizinische Wochenschrift,* 81, 940–943.

Rizzoli, A. et al., 2002, Geographical information systems and bootstrap aggregation (bagging) of tree-based classifiers for Lyme disease risk prediction in Trentino, Italian Alps, *Journal of Medical Entomology,* 39, 3, 485–492.

Robinson, W.S., 1950, Ecological correlations and the behavior of individuals, *American Sociological Review,* 15, 351–357.

Rodenwaldt, E. and Jusatz, H., 1952–1961, *World Atlas of Epidemic Diseases,* Vols. 1–3, Hamburg: Falk-Verlag.

Rogers, D.J. and Randolph, S.E., 2000, The global spread of malaria in a future, warmer world, *Science,* 289, 5485, 1763–1766.

Schærström, A., 1996, *Pathogenic Path? A Time Geographical Approach in Medical Geography.* Meddelanden från Lunds Universitets Geografiska Institutioner, Avhandlingar 125, Lund: Lund University Press.

Scholten, H.J. and de Lepper, M.J.C., 1991, The benefits of the application of geographical information systems in public and environmental health, *World Health Statistics Quarterly,* 44, 160–170.

Schröder, K., 1998, Thematische Karten im Internet: Neue Möglichkeiten der Karten- und Legendengestaltung, Berlin: Berliner Manuskripte zur Kartographie.

Schweikart, J., 1999, Daten zur Gesundheit in der Karte. Möglichkeiten und Perspektiven. geoinformatik_online 1/99, gio.uni-muenster.de.

Selvin, H.C., 1958, Durkheim's "suicide" and problems of empirical research, *American Journal of Sociology,* 63, 607–619.

Sharma, V.P. and Srivastava, A., 1997, Role of geographic information systems in malaria Control, *Indian Journal of Medical Research,* 106, 198–204.

Smallman-Raynor, M.R., Cliff, A.D., and Haggett, P., 1992, *London International Atlas of AIDS,* Oxford: Blackwell Scientific.

Smans, M. and Estève, J., 1992, Practical approaches to disease mapping, in Elliott, P. et al., Eds., *Geographical and Environmental Epidemiology,* Oxford: Oxford University Press.

Snow, J., 1855, *On the Mode of Communication of Cholera,* 2nd ed., London: John Churchill.

Srivastava, A. et al., 1999, Geographic information system as a tool to study malaria receptivity in Nadiad Taluka, Kheda District, Gujarat, India, *Southeast Asian Journal of Tropical Medicine and Public Health,* 30, 4, 650–656.

Stevenson, L., 1965, Putting disease on the map: The early use of spot maps in the study of yellow fever, *Journal of the History of Medicine and Allied Sciences*, 20, 226–261.

Tanser, F. et al., 2000, HIV heterogeneity and proximity of homestead to roads in rural South Africa: An exploration using a geographical information system, *Tropical Medicine and International Health,* 5, 1, 40–46.

Uphoff, M. et al., 2002, Are influenza surveillance data useful for detailed mapping presentations? Tagungsberichte der als Raümliche Statistik, 5, 105–112.

Valleron, A.J. and Garnerin, P., 1992, Computer networking as a tool for public health surveillance: The French experiment, *Morbidity and Mortality Weekly Report,* 41, 101–110.

van den Berg, N. and von der Ahé, K.-R., 1997, Geoinformationssysteme in der Epidemiologie, *Kartographische Nachrichten,* 2, 52–58.

Wellie, O. et al., 2000, Der Einsatz von Geoinformationssystemen (GIS) in Epidemiologischen Studien Dargestellt am Beispiel der ISAAC — Studie München, *Das Gesundheitswesen,* 62, 423–430.

Wood, B.L. et al., 2000, Education, outreach and the future of remote sensing in human health, *Advances in Parasitology,* 47, 331–344.

World Health Organization, 1999, Geographical information systems (GIS), *Weekly Epidemiological Record*, 74, 281–285.

Yang, G. et al., 2002, GIS Prediction model of malaria transmission in Jiangsu Province, *Zhonghua Yu Fang Yi Xue Za Zhi,* 36, 2, 103–105.

Zenilman, J.M. et al., 2002, Geographic epidemiology of gonorrhoea and chlamydia on a large military installation: Application of a GIS system, *Sexually Transmitted Infections,* 78, 1, 40–44.

Zhang, Z. and Griffith, D.A., 1997, Developing user-friendly spatial statistical analysis modules for GIS: An example using ArcView, *Computing, Environmental and Urban Systems*, 21, 5–29.

6 New Zealand Experience of *Salmonella* Brandenburg Infection in Humans and Animals

John Holmes

CONTENTS

6.1 INTRODUCTION

GIS is a useful tool in the investigation and management of communicable disease outbreaks, as described in Chapter 5. *Salmonella* Brandenburg infection has been

0-415-30655-8/04/$0.00+$1.50

of increasing concern in South Island, New Zealand since 1996. A descriptive study of the pattern of *Salmonella* Brandenburg infection in southern South Island between 1996 and 2001 was carried out. GIS-based tools were useful in highlighting the changing interrelationship between infections in sheep and humans during the course of this outbreak. This chapter describes the New Zealand experience of this infection in South Island.

6.2 INFECTIOUS DISEASE SURVEILLANCE IN NEW ZEALAND

The New Zealand Health Act of 1872 required the notification of all cases of certain infectious diseases to public health authorities. The list of notifiable conditions has changed over time. Since June 1952, all proven and suspected cases of human salmonella infections have been included in the notifiable disease schedule. The attending medical practitioner must give details of cases of notifiable disease to the local medical officer of health. The country is divided into 21 health districts each with a medical officer of health, a public health medicine specialist providing epidemiological oversight of the district. Health protection officers, employed by the local Public Health Service, or environmental health officers, employed by the local authority, undertake investigations into possible causes of notified diseases. Diseases, such as salmonella, that may spread through contaminated food and water are normally investigated by territorial local authorities because the infections may be caused by poor sanitation.

6.3 METHODS

Details of completed investigations of human cases are recorded on EpiSurv, an electronic database maintained by the Institute of Environmental Science and Research (ESR) on behalf of the Ministry of Health. Each Public Health Service office maintains a local electronic EpiSurv register and supplies weekly updates to the national register. The district office can analyze the local pattern of infectious disease morbidity and report to the local community. ESR produces monthly surveillance reports as well as an Annual Summary of Notifiable Diseases.

Since mid-2000, all cases registered on EpiSurv have been automatically geocoded on entry and a retrospective coding of previous cases has been undertaken. Initially there were problems coding rural addresses because many people quote a rural postal delivery zone when asked for their address. The accuracy of geocoding has been improved by the introduction of "Rapid Numbers," which were developed for the location of dwellings by emergency services and are related to distances from road junctions.

Microbiological testing for human isolates is taxpayer funded through health benefits, so the tests are at no direct charge to the patient. The general practitioner may submit fecal specimens to a local pathology laboratory for initial culture, although such testing is of limited value when treating the individual patient. However, the results are of great importance to public health physicians studying the epidemiology of diseases.

Veterinary surgeons working with infected animals may send specimens for analysis to one of the specialist animal health laboratories. Invermay Animal Health Laboratory processed specimens from the Otago and Southland districts. The Lincoln Laboratory processed specimens from South Canterbury and Canterbury. There is no notification of salmonella infections in animals. Funding for veterinary public health specimens is on a user-pays basis. Hence, it is not always possible to relate the extent of concomitant human and animal outbreaks.

ESR's Enteric Reference Laboratory in Wellington carried out the formal identification and typing of all salmonella isolates (human and animal). Data from the local EpiSurv database were combined with similar data from the adjacent health districts (South Canterbury and Canterbury) for this study of the pattern of human cases of *Salmonella* Brandenburg in the southern part of South Island.

AgriQuality is a crown research institute, which among other activities maintains AgriBase, a geographic information system for plotting the location and stocking type of all farms in New Zealand. Plotting of animal isolates of *Salmonella* Brandenburg to the farm of origin was undertaken for data from Otago and Southland for the period of 1997 to 2000. The combination of animal and human data has enabled the detailed study and description of the development of the epidemic. The geocoding of animal cases from South Canterbury and Canterbury has not been possible but data about the date of isolation was available for all the animal isolates.

6.4 THE PATTERN OF *SALMONELLA* INFECTIONS IN NEW ZEALAND

As in many other comparable countries, there has been a gradual increase in the rate of notifications of salmonella infections in New Zealand over the past 50 years (Thornley et al., 2002). On several occasions, the rate of infection in the Otago and Southland districts has exceed the national average. Some of these peaks were associated with single source outbreaks, but in the majority of cases, no apparent source of infection has been noted. The age-specific incidence of all salmonella infections shows a peak in the under-1-year-old age group with a second peak in the early 20s.

Salmonella Brandenburg is one of over 1800 serotypes, originally described by Kauffmann and Mitsui in 1930. It was first identified in humans in New Zealand in 1985 and was a relatively infrequent isolate between 1985 and 1994, accounting for 1 percent of the isolates during the period (Wright et al., 1998). Until 1996, *Salmonella* Brandenburg had rarely been isolated from animals.

6.4.1 Pattern of *Salmonella* Brandenburg Isolates in Southern New Zealand: 1996

The first documented isolate of *Salmonella* Brandenburg infection from a sheep was on a farm in mid-Canterbury during mid-1996. The disease in sheep usually presents as septic abortion of a near term fetus or a uterine infection in the pregnant ewe. It can also infect other animals such as cattle, pigs, and deer.

6.4.2 Pattern of *Salmonella* Brandenburg Isolates in Southern New Zealand: 1997

During the 1997 lambing season (July to September) *Salmonella* Brandenburg infection was found on 17 farms in the mid-Canterbury region (Figure 6.1). It was also reported from one sheep farm and found in one cow in Southland. Ten human cases of *Salmonella* Brandenburg infection were reported from the region. The usual presenting symptoms of human disease are abdominal pains, diarrhea, and vomiting. These symptoms are no different from those found in infections caused by other types of salmonella. The first two people from South Canterbury were hospitalized with a generalized blood stream infection due to *Salmonella* Brandenburg. Fortunately, both patients soon recovered and returned home. Subsequent case investigation showed that although they were from farms, they did not have any evidence of infection in their sheep flocks.

6.4.3 Pattern of *Salmonella* Brandenburg Isolates in Southern New Zealand: 1998

In total, there were 153 infected farms during 1998 and 118 human isolates from the southern half of South Island (Figure 6.2). The epidemic curve shows a peak in late August, which coincides with lambing in the southern part of the country. The number of human cases increased and the epidemic curve shows a similar peak to the animal curve, but there is a delay of about three weeks. Some of this lag may result from the delay between the patient presenting to the general practitioner and a positive fecal specimen being reported to the medical officer of health. The median interval between onset of symptoms and reporting the case to the medical officer of health was 10 days with a range of 2 days to 141 days. Part of this variation may

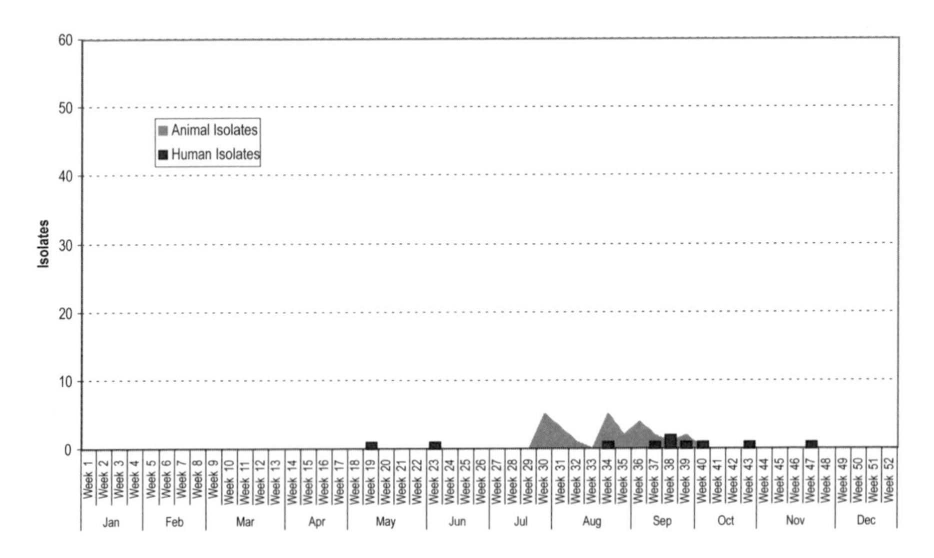

FIGURE 6.1 *Salmonella* Brandenburg isolates in 1997.

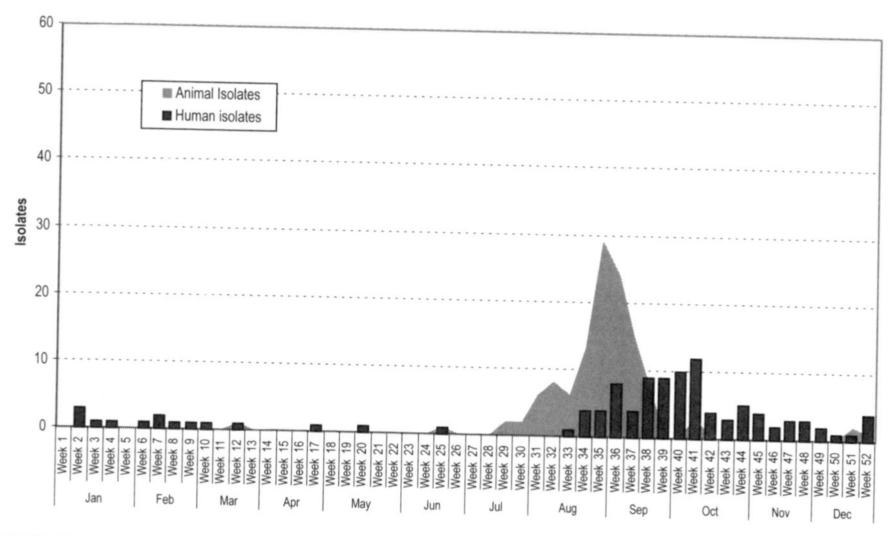

FIGURE 6.2 *Salmonella* Brandenburg isolates in 1998.

reflect reluctance by many rural people to consult a doctor, but it may also reflect a varying awareness by doctors of the need to notify on suspicion all cases of a disease of potential public health importance, such as salmonella infection.

A large number of the human cases were farm workers who had been in close contact with infected sheep. A human case control study was carried out between August and September 1998. This compared the clinical pattern of *Salmonella* Brandenburg infections with other salmonella infections and found no significant differences in the severity or duration of the disease between the different types of bacteria. Local veterinarians sent a detailed questionnaire on management practices and personal hygiene to known infected farms from which there were no human cases. This information was compared with a similar questionnaire from farmers who were identified as suffering from *Salmonella* Brandenburg. No significant differences in personal hygiene or farming practice were noted between any of the groups. Good personal hygiene and changing from work clothes before going indoors were seen as offering the best possibility for controlling the spread of the human disease.

6.4.4 Pattern of *Salmonella* Brandenburg Isolates in Southern New Zealand: 1999

There was again a rapid increase in the number of infected farms at the beginning of August and this prompted joint publicity from the local veterinarians and public health staff (Figure 6.3). The farming media were supportive and ran frequent items about the need for personal protection. The animal epidemic curve was steeper than in 1998, but the number of human cases did not rise to the same extent, suggesting that farmers were taking some precautions. It was of concern that there were more children and other adults affected in 1999.

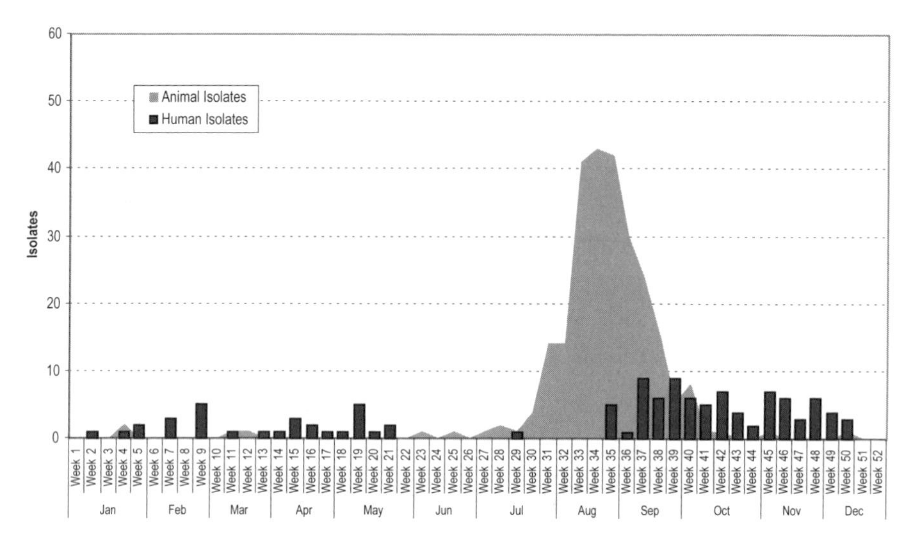

FIGURE 6.3 *Salmonella* Brandenburg isolates in 1999.

In 1999, there were 196 infected farms (178 ovine isolates and 18 bovine isolates) and the human notifications increased to 112.

6.4.5 Pattern of *Salmonella* Brandenburg Isolates in Southern New Zealand: 2000

In 2000, there were 401 infected farms (331 ovine isolates and 70 bovine) and 152 human cases (Figure 6.4). During the year, many groups undertook research into the possible pattern of spread of the bacteria. This work looked at farming practices, livestock handling, meat processing, and general environmental sampling of the farm as a workplace. The organism was found in sheep yard dust from farms that had been infected as well as farms that had not shown any overt infection during the previous year. Sampling of black back gulls (*Larus dominicanus*), which are frequent scavengers of dead sheep and lambs, also showed high levels of *Salmonella* Brandenburg.

6.4.6 Pattern of *Salmonella* Brandenburg Isolates in Southern New Zealand: 2001

In 2001, there were 289 infected farms (216 ovine and 73 bovine) and 91 human cases (Figure 6.5). The isolation dates of animal and human data have been combined to give an epidemic curve for the outbreak since 1997 (Figure 6.6). This shows three important features. First, a marked seasonal peak in animal isolates coincides with lambing in spring. Second, there is a delay of two to three weeks between the peak in animal isolates and the peak in human cases. This may be explained by people delaying in seeking medical attention and the time taken for laboratory confirmed cases to be notified by the general practitioner. Although there is a legal requirement to notify cases, this does not always happen. Not all people with diarrhea will present

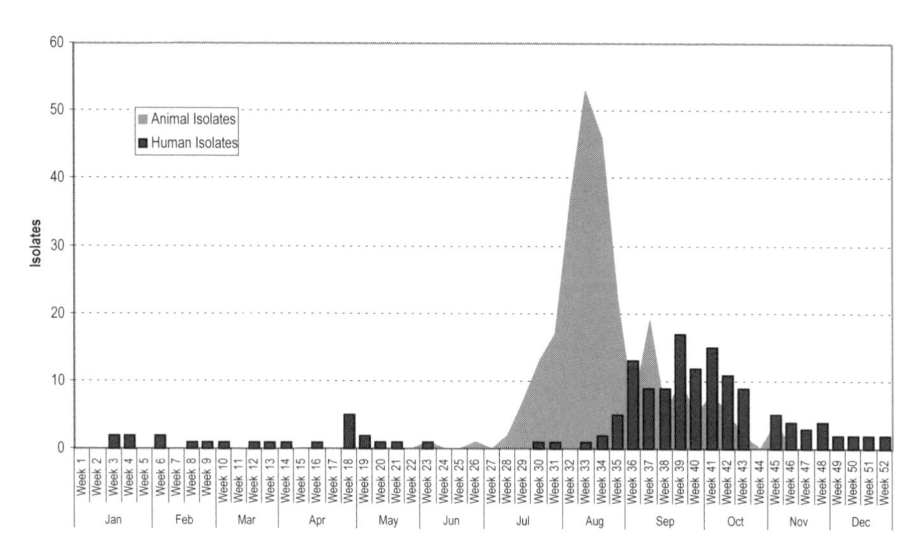

FIGURE 6.4 *Salmonella* Brandenburg isolates in 2000.

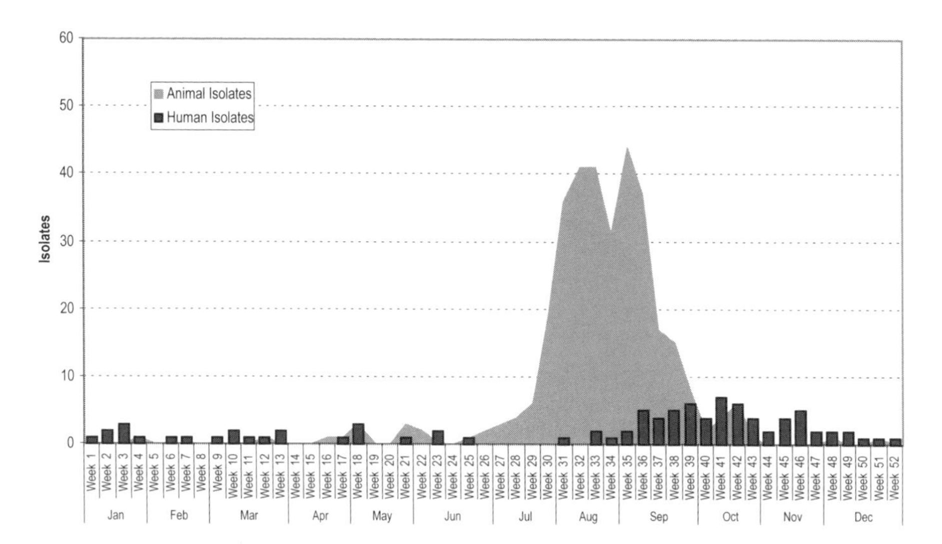

FIGURE 6.5 *Salmonella* Brandenburg isolates in 2001.

themselves to a general practitioner. Not everybody who presents themselves to a general practitioner will be offered a fecal test and, furthermore, not all people from whom a test is requested, actually provide a specimen (Wright, 1996). Hence, notifications of gastrointestinal disease represent the tip of an iceberg of disease.

The human cases are listed from the date of notification. The date of onset of the symptoms was specified in only about 60 percent of the cases in this study. The reported interval between the onset of symptoms and the date of notification ranged from 2 days to 141 days with a mean of 10 days.

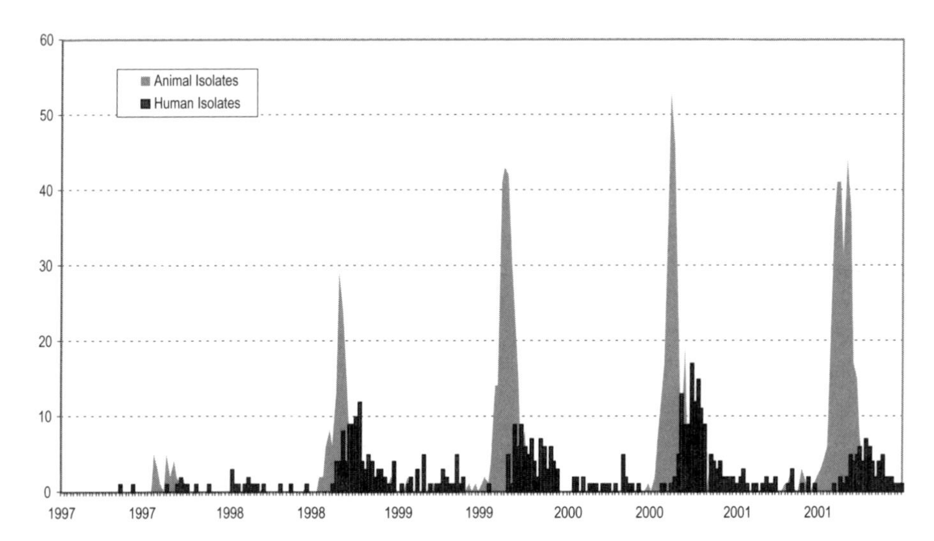

FIGURE 6.6 *Salmonella* Brandenburg isolates, 1997 to 2001.

The third feature is that there now appears to be a year-round incidence of the disease with one or two cases being reported almost every month of the year instead of in seasonal clusters. The disease has passed from being an epidemic to that of low-level endemicity.

This gives a brief summary of the epidemiological knowledge gained from traditional case report forms that can be analyzed by EpiSurv. It was difficult to put the "pins in the map" when dealing with an outbreak lasting five years and spread over an area of several thousand kilometers.

The combined human and animal epidemic curve demonstrated a temporal relationship, but it was difficult to find any relationship between the place of residence and the illness.

6.5 SPATIAL DISTRIBUTION OF CASES

The Public Health Unit acquired a license for a desktop GIS (ArcView® 3.2) in late 1999. Once staff became familiar with the system and were able to use it for the analysis of disease information, it enabled a greater understanding of the spatial and temporal relationship between the human and animal cases. Access to a computer-based GIS has greatly assisted the investigation of links between the human cases of *Salmonella* Brandenburg and the animal isolates. The location of farm isolates of *Salmonella* Brandenburg for the southern part of the country for the period of 1997 to 2000 was geocoded by AgriQuality and these results have been plotted against the location of the human cases. The spatial location of human cases has enabled them to be attributed to a census area unit (AU), which has a denominator population, so data can be analyzed on a population basis.

Statistics New Zealand classifies population areas as rural, rural centers, or urban, based on the population size of AUs. A rural AU normally contains less than 300 people, a rural center usually contains between 300 and 999 people, and all AUs containing more than 1,000 people are classed as urban. Every five years there is a New Zealand Census of Population. There was one in March 1996 and the most recent was taken in March 2001. Data from the most recent census has been used as the denominator population for this study, even though this might introduce a degree of bias. The population of South Island grew by 0.16 percent annually between 1996 and 2001 compared with a 0.81 percent annual growth in North Island. The usual resident population of the study area at Census 2001 was 753,333 people with 104,859 people in rural AUs, 26,442 people in rural centers, and 662,032 people in urban AUs.

A residential classification for the human cases of *Salmonella* Brandenburg infection was derived by mapping the incident points and carrying out a spatial join using ArcView 3.2. This showed that 143 cases lived in AUs classed as rural, 52 lived in rural centers, and 275 cases lived in urban AUs. The annual infection rates for the three areas were calculated (Table 6.1).

Thus, the risk of infection appeared much greater for rural residents and those who lived in rural centers than for urban dwellers.

The occupations were grouped into five major categories:

1. Farmers, including all occupational groups associated with animals such as freezing workers, veterinarians, stock agents as well as sheep and dairy farmers
2. Other workers, including unemployed
3. Retired, reclassified as farmers if there was a mention of farming in their previous occupation
4. Students, from five years of age to tertiary level
5. Preschoolers

Analysis of the distribution of cases by these occupation groups showed the proportion of cases in farmers decreased since 1998 (Figure 6.7). However, the proportion of cases in younger people increased over time suggesting the need for education programs aimed at parents and schools.

The patterns for the three location types differ and this information was valuable in targeting health promotion interventions (Figure 6.8 to Figure 6.10).

TABLE 6.1
***Salmonella* Brandenburg Infection Rates by Residential Location, 1997 to 2001**

Location	Population	Average Cases per Year	Annual Infection Rate per 100,000
Rural area units	104,859	29	27.3
Rural centers	26,442	10	39.3
Urban area units	662,032	55	8.8
Total population	753,333	94	12.5

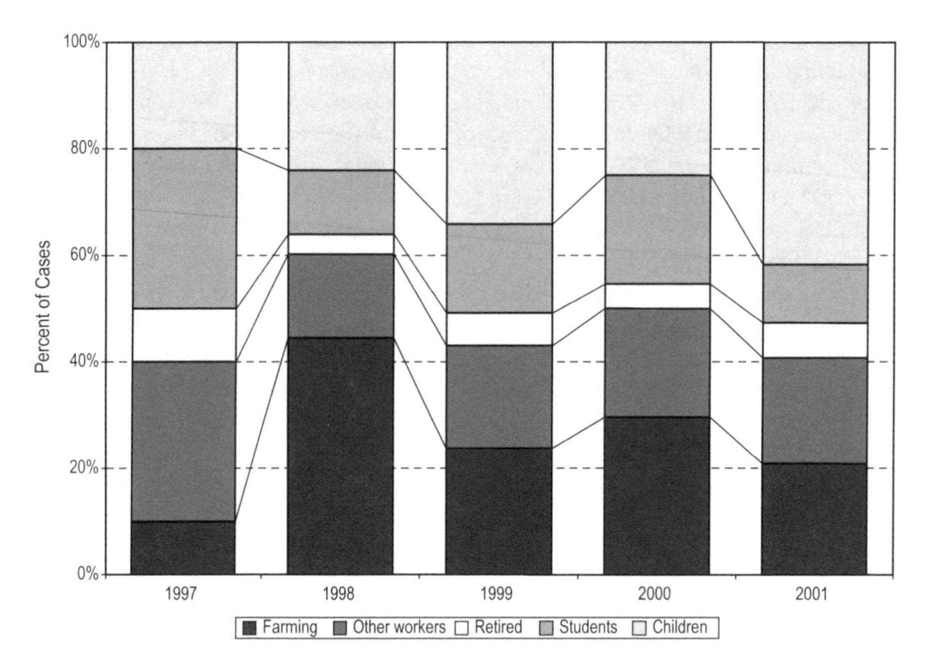

FIGURE 6.7 Notifications for the total population, 1997 to 2001.

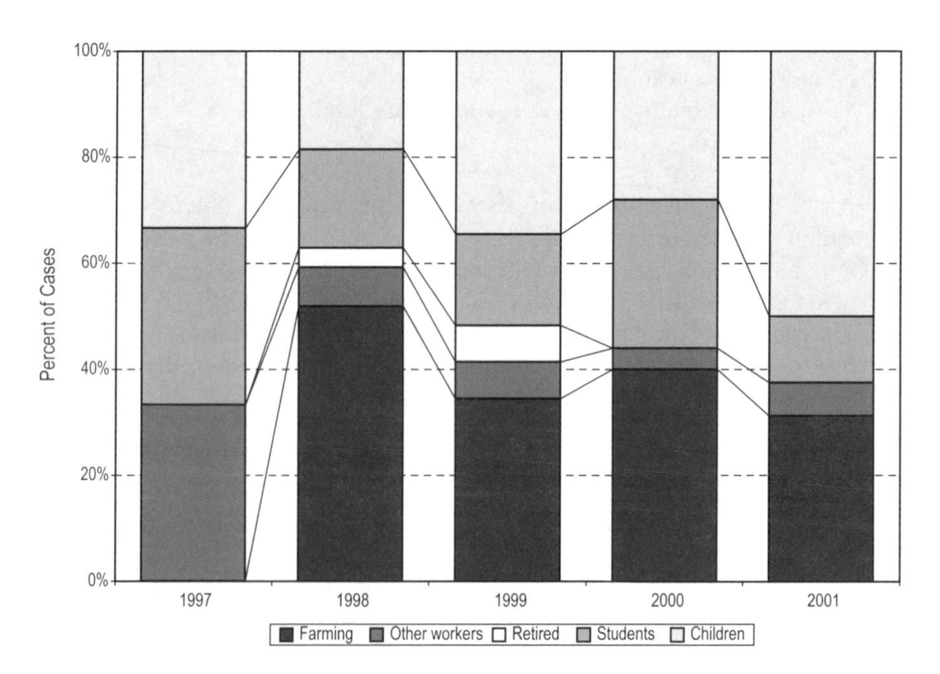

FIGURE 6.8 Notifications for the rural population, 1997 to 2001.

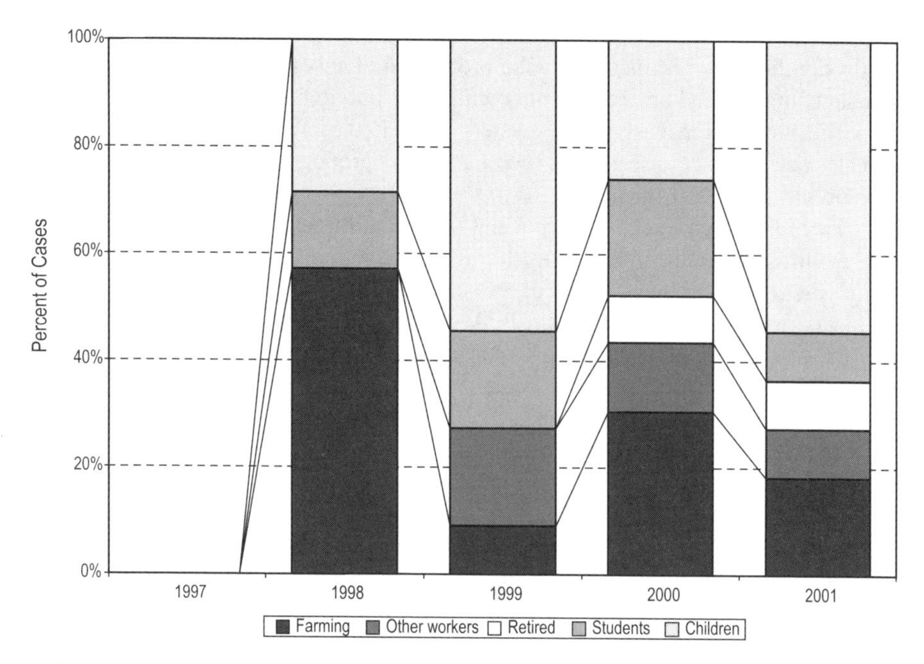

FIGURE 6.9 Notifications for rural centers, 1997 to 2001.

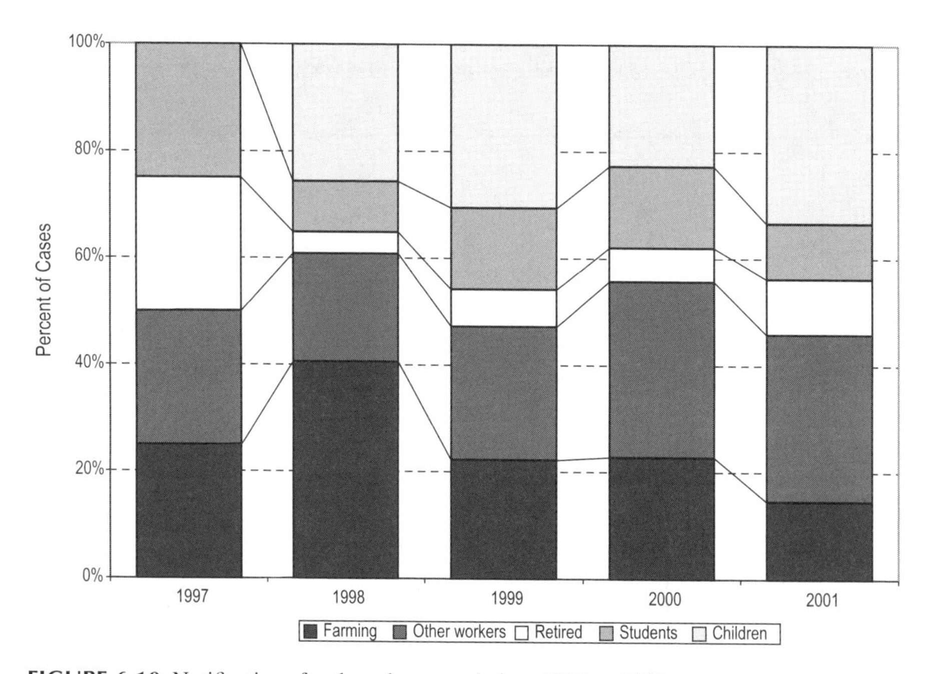

FIGURE 6.10 Notifications for the urban population, 1997 to 2001.

There were only 10 cases identified in 1997, so the relative proportions have little significance. The increase in the proportion of cases in preschool children and students highlighted an area for intervention by public health staff.

The notifications from rural centers also showed that young people were at greater risk from the disease, but it was noted the proportion of cases in the farming sector had decreased since 1998.

There has been a relatively constant pattern of disease in the urban population.

A different pattern is seen in the age distribution of cases of infection with *Salmonella* Brandenburg. The proportion of cases in children (under 5 years) and students (up to 18 years) has increased, especially in those living in rural centers. As the urban population appears to have had a relatively constant distribution of cases, it has been used as the baseline category for calculating the relative risk of infection for the residential groups.

The relative risk of disease was calculated by comparing the rate of disease in people from rural areas and rural centers with that found in urban cases (Figure 6.11). Thus, the relative risk is taken as one for the urban population, so the excess infections in the other groups can be seen. The high relative risk of disease found in young people living in rural centers was surprising, but not unexpected. Many agricultural workers live in these centers and travel to work on nearby farms. Their children will go to school with children from the rural AUs and will often travel together on the rural school bus. In general, there will be closer contact with animals than found in children from urban AUs. The information provided the basis for further education to schools in the rural areas stressing the importance of good personal hygiene as a means of preventing infection with *Salmonella* Brandenburg.

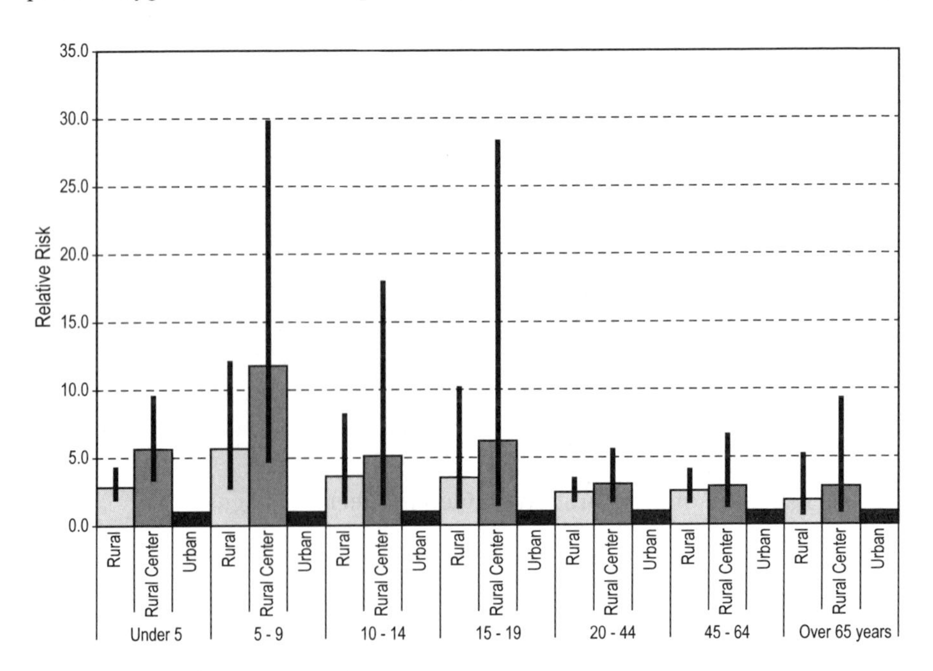

FIGURE 6.11 Relative risk of infection by residence.

6.6 PLOTTING SPATIAL DATA

Information about the number of sheep in the various AUs from AgriBase has enabled calculation of an approximate stocking density. The density of sheep by AU suggested the areas of highest sheep density. Land use data indicates the areas of high pastoral activity compared with the areas of forest and scrub. Sheep farming is mainly restricted to pastoral land and hence the animal isolates of *Salmonella* Brandenburg tend to be confined to areas of pastoral land. The density of sheep in AUs was recalculated on the basis of available pastoral grazing land to recognize that the whole of the AU was not available for grazing. The area of land suitable for pastoral use was reduced by 58 percent. The areas of the AUs were adjusted using the geoprocessing function of ArcView 3.2 and a revised map of the stocking densities was drawn. This increased the density of stocking levels. The overall reduction in land area and consequent increase in stock density is shown in Table 6.2. The map clearly demonstrates the location of the actual pastoral areas and compares the stocking density before and after recalculation (Figure 6.12).

A combined map of sheep and human cases of *Salmonella* Brandenburg infection (Figure 6.13), the high stocking rates of sheep, and a high rate of infection in sheep suggests a relationship. However, the overall numbers of human cases in the four year period for which geocoded sheep infections are available are small and the relationships do not reach statistical significance.

Environmental water samples from two of the major rivers in the south both showed detectable levels of the endemic strain of *Salmonella* Brandenburg.

One feature of the outbreak, which became apparent from a survey of farming practices, was the correlation between lowland sheep pastures and isolates of *Salmonella* Brandenburg. Most infected farms were below 300 meters above sea level. These areas provide good sheep grazing and hence have high stock numbers. An estimated 20 percent of New Zealand's sheep are located within the endemic area, which accounts for about 5 percent of the total land area. GIS software can easily demonstrate the relationship between pastoral land and contour.

The outbreak of *Salmonella* Brandenburg infection has been limited to the southern half of South Island (Figure 6.14). Pulse Field Gel Electrophoresis (PFGE) of the animal and human isolates shows that all those tested have been from an identical type, which is one of 14 variants known in New Zealand. This particular type has not been isolated from cases of *Salmonella* Brandenburg infection reported from other parts of the country or other parts of the world. The reason for the

TABLE 6.2
Revision of Land Area Available for Sheep Stocking

	Calculated Area of Census Units (ha)	Area of Pastoral Land (ha)
Area	5,554,628	2,327,047
Stocking density	2.4	5.7

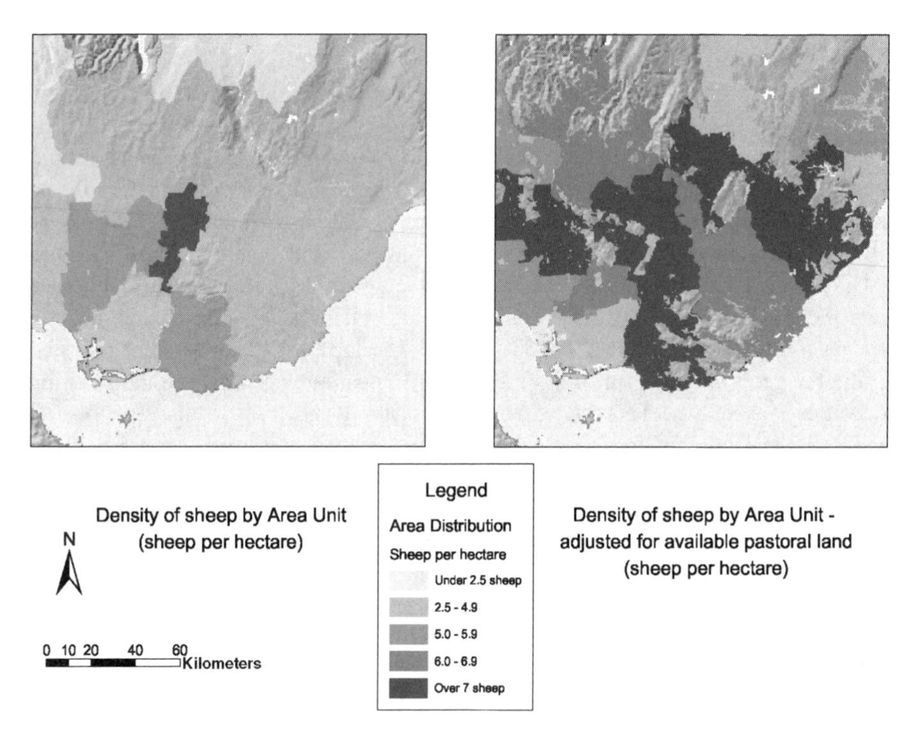

FIGURE 6.12 Distribution of sheep in southern New Zealand in 2000.

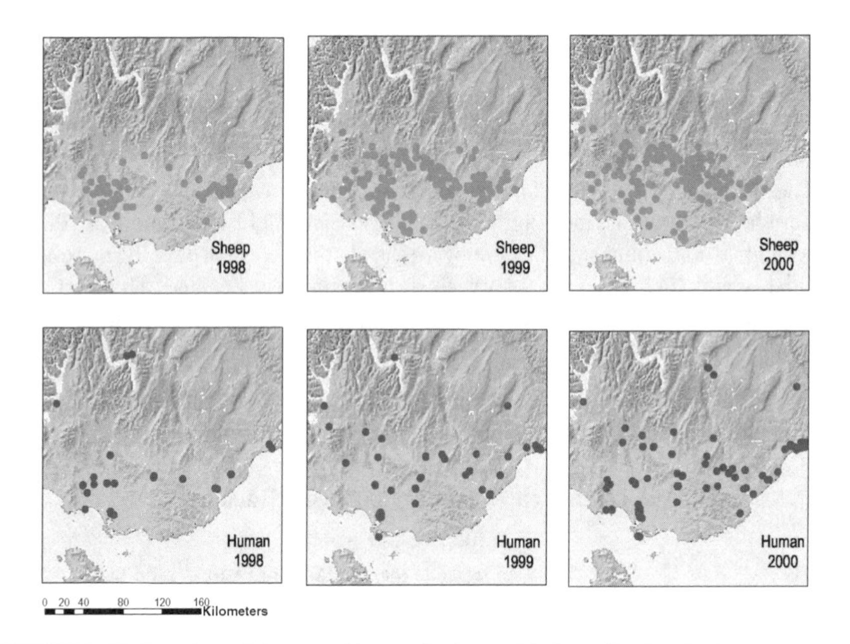

FIGURE 6.13 Location of sheep and human isolates of *Salmonella* Brandenburg.

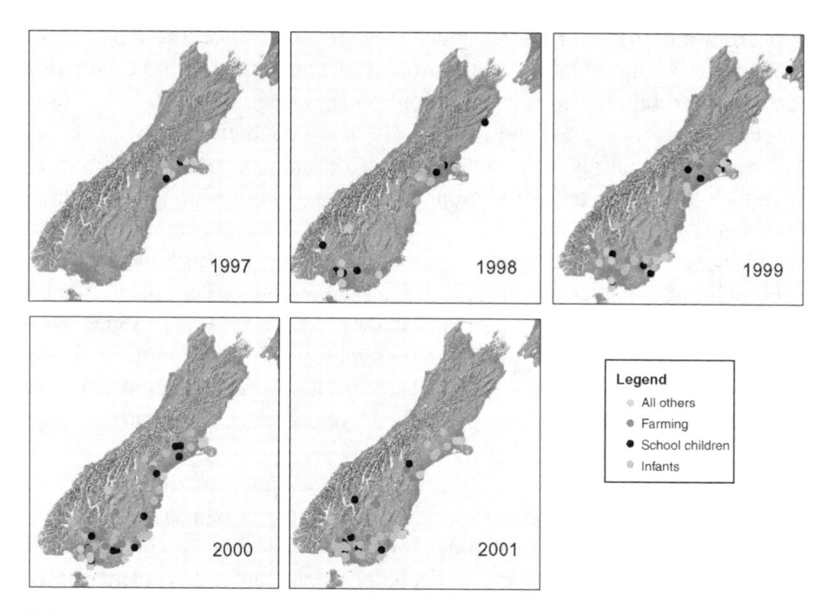

FIGURE 6.14 Human isolates of *Salmonella* Brandenburg in South Island, 1997 to 2001.

restriction to the southern part of South Island is unknown, but this study has shown that the area is characterized by particularly high stock densities, which are associated with intensive farming practices.

In 1998, *Salmonella* Brandenburg infection was considered an occupational disease of farm workers. They appear to have responded to the educational messages and instituted safe working practices, which have reduced the number of farm-related infections. The same cannot be said for cases in children and students.

6.7 CONCLUSION

Cooperation and sharing of GIS information between animal health and human public health services has given a greater understanding of the epidemiology of this epidemic. The ability to share and integrate spatial data from a variety of sources, including veterinarians and the Ministry of Agriculture, with routine health surveillance data has been an important tool in these investigations. There have been problems over the confidentiality of some data, especially the geocoding of the location of farm isolates. Hence, this study has only looked at the geocoded animal data collected from the Otago and Southland regions. Noncoded data for all isolates has been provided and incorporated into the epidemic curve. Human data for the whole of the greater Canterbury, Otago, and Southland regions has been geocoded and plotted to reveal the extent of the human outbreak. It appears to have spread southward from the initial ten cases reported in Canterbury in 1997.

Disease prevention strategies have targeted farm workers and farming practices in an attempt to control the human and animal outbreaks. They appear to have had a degree of success within the farming community, but they have not prevented the infection from moving out into the wider population. To date, there have been no outbreaks directly attributable to consumption of contaminated food, but we have been unable to explain the wide distribution of cases. Many New Zealand residents have contact with farming families, especially in the southern part of the country.

It is of concern that residents of the two major cities, Dunedin and Invercargill, appear to have been infected without apparent farm or animal contact. Some urban residents who work in farming-related occupations may have been exposed to the organism in the course of their work. In other cases, domestic pets have been infected either through rural contacts or through eating infected meat. The role of black back gulls as a vector has not been studied, but they are known to scavenge on dead lambs. They may become infected and spread the organisms to uninfected flocks.

Education of the rural communities has been the prime target for action and it will be interesting to see how the epidemic develops during the current lambing season.

This study has only been possible through close and continuing cooperation between veterinary staff, public health staff, and farming organizations. We have all learned to value each other's contributions toward solving an emergent disease within our community. The tools offered by GIS helped delineate the problem and added a graphic dimension to the epidemiological analysis of the disease in terms of time and place. The study has reintroduced the public health unit to the topographic map as one of the basic tools of epidemiology.

In 1854, John Snow demonstrated this and was able to control the outbreak of cholera associated with use of the Broad Street pump. Over 160 years later, we have been able to demonstrate an interrelationship between sheep farming practice and human disease caused by a new variant of *Salmonella* Brandenburg. Now that some of the causative factors and features of the outbreak have been ascertained, it has proved possible to control it through a variety of means. The introduction of simple techniques, such as good personal hygiene coupled with changing agricultural practices has seen a marked reduction in the scale of the disease since it was first found in sheep in 1996.

ACKNOWLEDGMENTS

This study is the result of help from many people including Gary Clark, Labnet, Invermay; Quenten Higgan, AgriQuality, Invermay; Chris Ambrose, Crown Public Health, Christchurch; David Peacock, previously Public Health Medicine Registrar, Dunedin; and many others. My greatest thanks go to Carolyn Nicol, scientist, ESR Porirua and her team who have typed all the isolates and who have infinite patience when asked for additional information about the pattern of disease. Dr. Chris Scally, Ministry of Health, Wellington has facilitated the introduction of GIS into public health units and supplied basic information about population and area mapping. He has encouraged staff to get additional training to use this resource.

References

Thornley, C., Baker, M. and Nicol, C., 2002, The rising incidence of Salmonella infection in New Zealand, 1995–2001, *New Zealand Public Health Report*, 9, 25–28.

Wright, J., 1996, Gastrointestinal illness: What are the causative organisms? *New Zealand Public Health Report*, 3, 9–11.

Wright, J.M., Brett, M. and Bennett, J., 1998, Laboratory investigation and comparison of *Salmonella* Brandenburg cases in New Zealand, *Epidemiology and Infection*, 121, 49–55.

7 Using GIS for Environmental Exposure Assessment: Experiences from the Small Area Health Statistics Unit

Kees de Hoogh, David Briggs, Samantha Cockings, and Alex Bottle

CONTENTS

7.1 INTRODUCTION

Relationships between the environment and health are intrinsically geographical. They involve the intersection of two geographies: that of the agents of risk (the environmental hazards) and that of the population at risk. GIS clearly has much to offer in this respect, for they provide the means both to map and model these two geographies, and to bring them together and link them for the purpose of exposure and health risk assessment. In recent years, this potential has begun to be exploited. Gradually, GIS is gaining a foothold in epidemiology and is becoming a standard tool for visualization and exploration of health outcomes and for exposure modeling.

0-415-30655-8/04/$0.00+$1.50

Among the small but increasing body of research groups using GIS for epidemiological enquiries, the Small Area Health Statistics Unit (SAHSU) at Imperial College, London, has an important place. Since its establishment in 1987, SAHSU has undertaken a large number of geographical studies, focusing on a wide range of health outcomes and exposure pathways. This chapter outlines some of the methods devised and used. It presents examples from a series of studies, differing in terms of the environment–health relationship of interest, the scale of analysis, and the modeling methods used. In each case, the methods used for exposure assessment are described and results of the exposure assessment presented. In each case, also, the problems posed by inadequacies in the available data, differences in spatial structures and zone systems, scale limitations, and time–space interactions are discussed. The ways in which these problems have been addressed are illustrated.

7.2 BUFFERING: HEALTH RISKS IN POPULATIONS LIVING AROUND LANDFILL SITES

Buffering is certainly one of the most widely used techniques for exposure assessment in epidemiological studies. It has been employed to study health effects in populations living both around point sources, such as incinerators (Elliott et al., 1996) and coke works (Aylin et al., 2001), and near to line-sources, such as roadways (Briggs et al., 1997, 2000; English et al., 1999).

It is based on the simple principle that exposures decline with distance from source to a threshold beyond which the population can be considered unexposed. Buffer zones of a suitable radius may be defined around any source — a point, line, or area — to identify supposedly exposed and unexposed groups. A single buffer might be used to divide populations into exposed and unexposed groups or multiple buffers can be created to define degrees of exposure. Standard epidemiological techniques can then be used to compare disease rates in the various groups with control, if appropriate, for confounding by other factors.

The technique is straightforward, data and processing requirements are relatively limited, and therefore it can be applied to large numbers of points with comparative ease. Several issues nevertheless arise in using buffering, as exemplified in a recent SAHSU study to investigate congenital malformations, low birth weight, and cancers in children born to mothers living near landfill sites (Elliott et al., 2001; Jarup et al., 2002).

This study was a national investigation and was instigated in response to suggestions from a number of previous studies that populations living close to hazardous waste sites were at increased risk of congenital malformations and cancers (Dolk et al., 1998; Fielder et al., 2000; Marshall et al., 1997). Data on all known landfill sites (some 19,196 in total) in Great Britain were provided by the regulatory agencies (the Environment Agency in England and Wales and the Scottish Environment Protection Agency in Scotland). Health effects reported during the study period of 1986 to 1997 were analyzed in relation to the status, licensed waste types, and proximity of landfills during the preceding year (for birth defects, birth weight, and childhood leukemia) and five years previously (for childhood cancers). All health data were available by postcode of place of residence at time of diagnosis.

Exposure assessment posed several problems. One of these was the lack of any clear etiological hypothesis indicating either the key agent of concern or its exposure pathway. Many different pollutants might be generated from wastes during either disposal or subsequent decomposition. These pollutants might be dispersed into the surrounding environment via the air, groundwater, surface water, soil, or animals (including birds). Although data on actual exposures around landfill sites are sparse, what evidence there is suggests that they usually are limited to no more than a few hundred meters — and at most a kilometer or two — from the site.

Another problem was the possibility that exposures might occur either while sites were operational or long after they had been closed. Indeed, opinions from those working in the industry were that the older sites, which had been closed before modern management practices and licensing arrangements came into force, were more likely to pose hazards than newer sites. A further, serious constraint was the relatively poor quality of the available data on landfill sites: exact boundaries of these were rarely known and most were identified only by a point location (usually the gateway), in some cases with a large degree of error (e.g., due to rounding of geographic coordinates to the nearest kilometer). The status (e.g., whether open or closed) of landfill sites and their spatial extent also change over time, so that the probabilities, pathways, and levels of exposure may also be expected to vary from year to year. The types of waste handled by different sites also vary, so that sites cannot be regarded as of equal hazardousness. At the same time, the large number of sites that had to be considered and their often close clustering meant that many people lived within a few kilometers of one or more landfill sites. In addition, the accuracy of postcodes is questionable. Testing of the available postcode files showed that the geographic coordinates provided tended to migrate from year to year (sometimes by several hundred meters or more), while some postcodes were clearly located incorrectly (e.g., in the sea or in the wrong postcode district) or were missing. Over the years, postcodes may also be closed and reused in a different location, creating possible ambiguities in the georeferencing of the health data (these issues are discussed further in Section 7.3).

For all these reasons, the use of sophisticated models to estimate exposures was not considered worthwhile, nor was it possible to formulate a single, integrated measure of hazardousness that could be aggregated across several sites. Instead, exposure classification was conducted using a rule-based approach, based on distance of place of residence from nearby landfill sites (Figure 7.1). A distance of two kilometers was set as the likely limit of exposure and buffers of this radius were constructed around each landfill site for each year. These were then intersected with the postcode locations, allowing each postcode to be assigned an exposure category according to its distance from landfill sites, the operational status of those sites, and the types of waste received or for which they were licensed (Figure 7.2). Unexposed postcodes were defined as those that lay outside the two-kilometer buffers around all known landfill sites, whenever they had been operating (these thus remained fixed for all years). Operational sites were those that were classed as open in that study year. Closed sites were those that had been closed at some earlier date during the

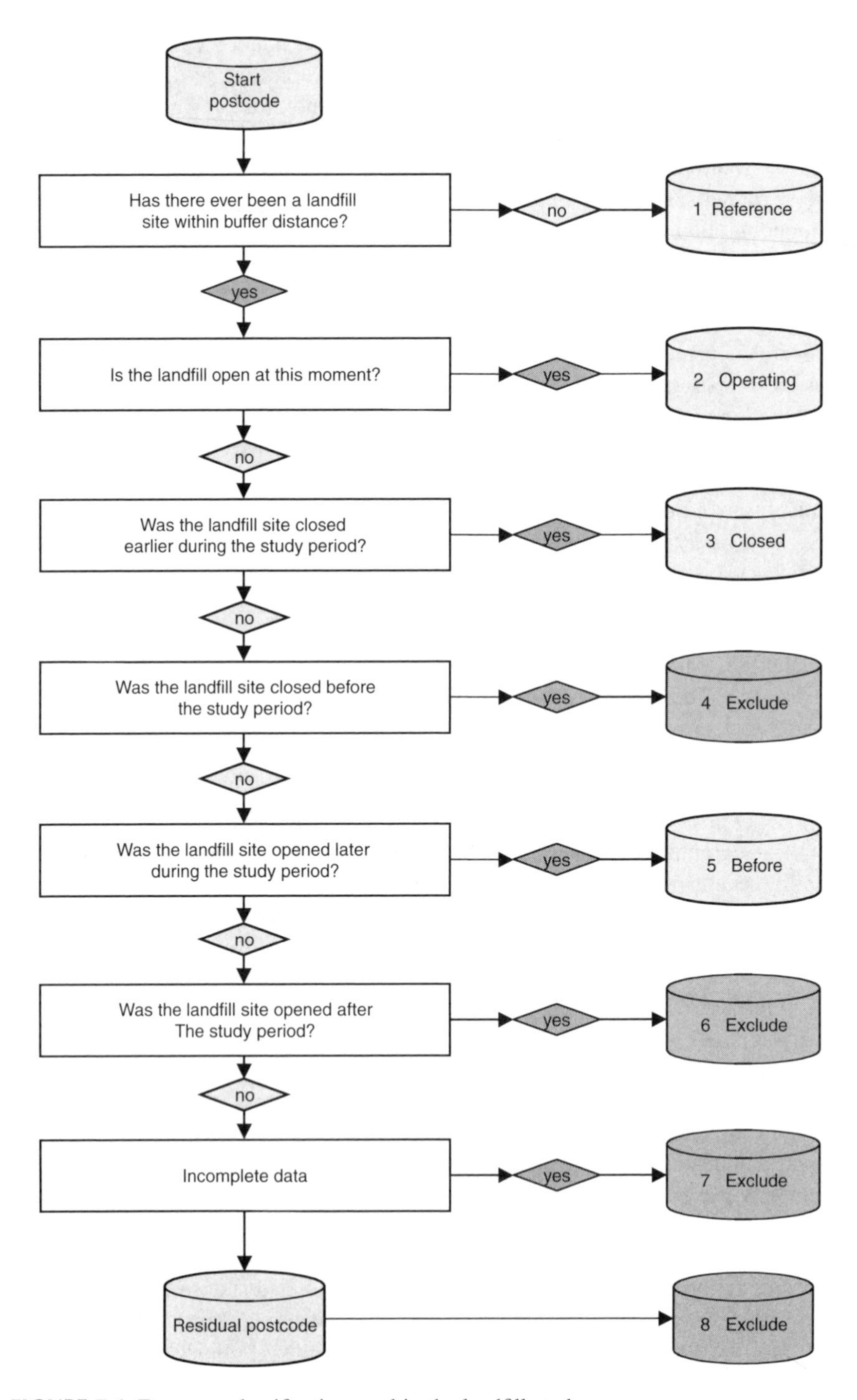

FIGURE 7.1 Exposure classification used in the landfill study.

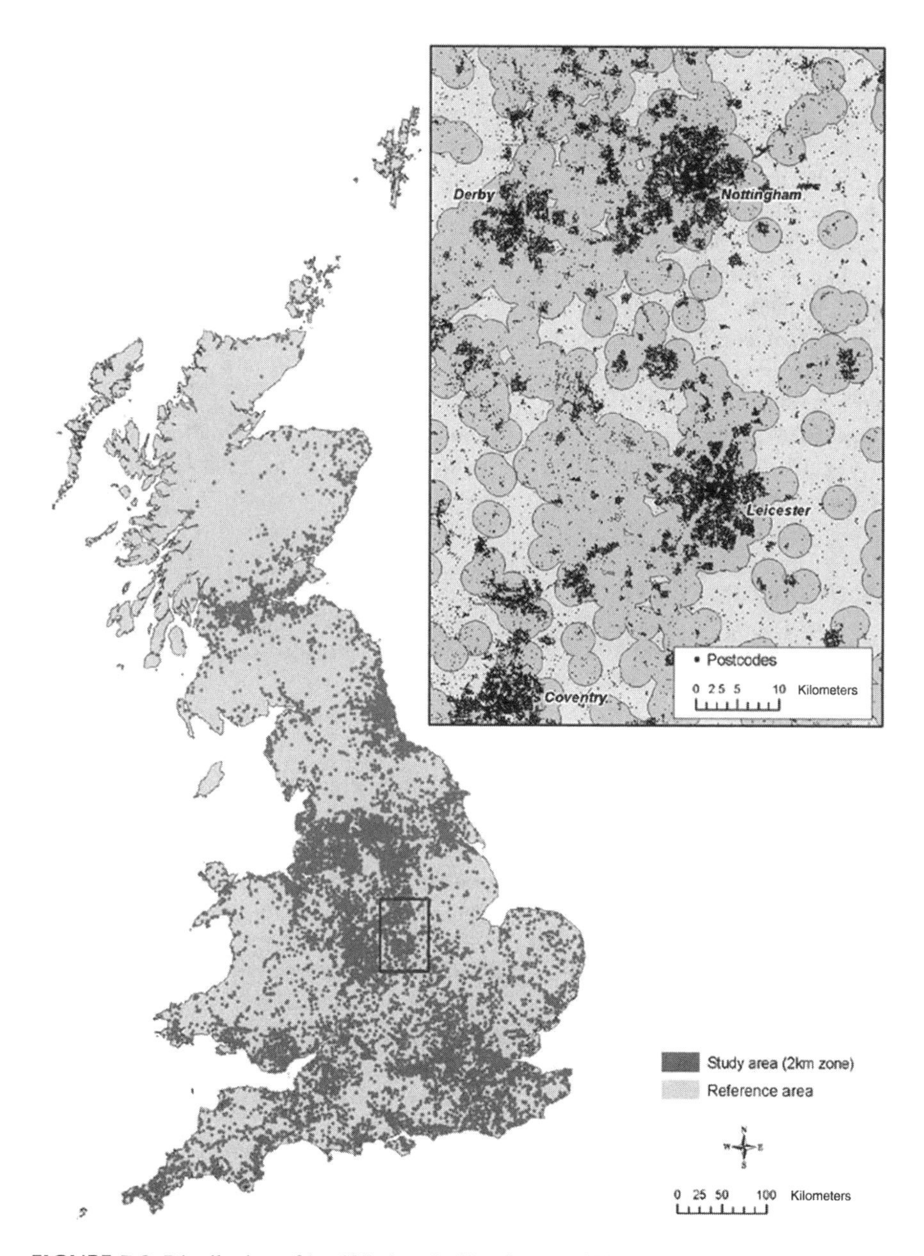

FIGURE 7.2 Distribution of landfill sites, buffered to two kilometers, with an inset showing the character of the buffer zones.

study period (1982 to 1996). Postcodes were classified as before opening if, in that year, they lay within the buffer zone of a site, which opened later in the study period. Postcodes around all other sites, including those for which there were missing opening or closing dates, were masked out (excluded) from the analysis. In total, 9631 sites were excluded, leaving 9565 sites in the analysis.

The scale of the analysis used in this study merits mention. The intersection of some 19,000 buffer zones with around 1.6 million postcodes for 16 years of data and for two groups of health endpoints involved some 10^{11} buffering operations, a process that took several days processing time on a high-powered desktop computer.

Using this exposure measure, the authors found that about 80 percent of the population lived within two kilometers of landfill sites. Exposed populations were found to be slightly less affluent, based on their Carstairs score, than unexposed populations (Table 7.1). People living around landfill sites excluded from the study were intermediate between the two. The authors reported slightly increased risks of a number of congenital malformations among the exposed group, especially for abdominal wall defects and neural tube defects (Elliott et al., 2001), though no significant increases were found for childhood cancers (Jarup et al., 2002). Notably, raised disease rates for some health outcomes were evident even before the landfill sites opened, suggesting that the landfill sites themselves may not be the cause of the increased risk.

7.3 POINT-IN-POLYGON TECHNIQUES: DISINFECTION BY-PRODUCTS IN DRINKING WATER

Point-in-polygon techniques are typically applied in one of two ways in epidemiology:

1. Attribute point measurements of pollution (e.g., at a monitoring site) to a surrounding population
2. Relate health events assigned to a point location (e.g., a postcode) to environmental and social conditions in the surrounding area

TABLE 7.1
Numbers and Percentages of Population by Carstairs Tertile and Exposure Status, 1982 and 1997

Year	Carstairs[a]	Exposed		Unexposed		Excluded	
		No	Percent[a]	No	Percent[a]	No	Percent[a]
1982	1	8,717,580	30.4	4,757,201	43.1	5,342,394	35.2
	2	9,791,927	34.2	3,579,180	32.4	5,036,716	33.2
	3	10,119,173	35.3	2,688,149	24.4	4,771,299	31.5
	N/A	8,333	0.0	10,550	0.1	5,404	0.0
1997	1	10,579,449	32.2	5,262,844	44.4	4,755,429	36.9
	2	11,167,044	34.0	3,847,654	32.4	4,369,923	33.9
	3	11,056,529	33.7	2,739,554	23.1	3,748,996	29.1
	N/A	9,568	0.0	11,719	0.1	4,559	0.0

[a] Carstairs tertile 1 = most affluent; tertile 3 = least affluent.

The methodology is so simple that it does not need sophisticated mapping tools. It is routinely done, for example, in many time series studies of air pollution, merely by assigning populations to the monitoring stations within their city (e.g., Moolgavkar, 2000). Daily concentrations from the monitoring stations are then computed (e.g., by averaging data from all the available sites within a city) and assigned to everyone living within that area. Associations may then be sought between this averaged pollution concentration and health outcome (e.g., mortality or numbers of hospital admissions) from day to day.

One example of the application of this approach within SAHSU has been the study of associations between long-term exposures to air pollution (SO_2 and black smoke) and cardio-respiratory and all-cause mortality in Great Britain (Shaddick, 2002). In this case, point-in-polygon methods were used to assign monitoring sites to the wards within which they fell. Four yearly averaged estimates of exposure were then compiled and geographic associations with health outcome analyzed for different lag periods (from 0 to 16 years). Another example is the ongoing investigation of associations between disinfection by-products in drinking water and low birth weight and stillbirths in three water company areas — Northumbria Water (NW), North West Water (NWW), and Severn Trent Water (STW) — in England.

In this latter study, several aspects of the available data and the study design need to be noted. Drinking water in the United Kingdom is no longer simply a local resource. Instead, most drinking water is the result of the mixing and treatment of water drawn from different sources. Water supply zones (i.e., areas that receive the same water) are also relatively small, covering a population of up to 50,000 people and may change from year to year. The disinfection by-products of concern — trihalomethanes (THMs) — are routinely measured at the tap of sample households by water companies in accordance with regulation. The water companies provided data on THM levels for the study years. The number of measurements taken varies according to the level of risk and may be as few as four measurements per year per supply zone where concentrations are low. Bayesian statistical methods were used to generate modeled quarterly estimates of exposures to THM in each water supply zone, taking account of the sample size, data uncertainty, and the concentrations of individual THMs. Each water supply zone was classified into one of three predefined exposure categories: low (<30 μg/l), medium (30 to 60 μg/l), and high (>60 μg/l). Health data in this study comprised postcode level information on birth weight and birth outcome, for the years 1992 to 1998. The denominator for analysis was the total number of live and still births.

To link the health data to the modeled exposures, postcode locations had to be matched to the water supply zones using point-in-polygon techniques. For this purpose, the postcode of the maternal residence at time of birth was used to identify the water zone of residence to ensure that the appropriate exposure status was assigned to each birth. The exposure estimates were also lagged to the quarter covering the period of 6 to 9 months before the time of birth so that exposures were assessed for the period in which the critical trimester of pregnancy fell.

Although an essentially simple operation, point-in-polygon analysis again faced several important difficulties. For example, digital boundary data for water supply zones were available from only a few companies and for a few, recent years. Hard copy maps were also of variable quality and completeness. Usable data (in either digital or hard copy form) were therefore obtainable only for 1997 for NW, 1992 to 1997 for NWW, and 1993 to 1997 for STW and these were subject to a number of errors and inconsistencies (Figure 7.3). These included zones that lacked THM data, missing or invalid zone identifiers, overlaps between boundaries of adjacent zones, and void areas (i.e., areas not attributed to a water supply zone). To resolve these as far as possible, the digitized maps were returned to the water companies concerned. Where they could not be resolved, the problem zones were excluded from the analysis. Areas were excluded if they were served by private water supplies or by other water companies.

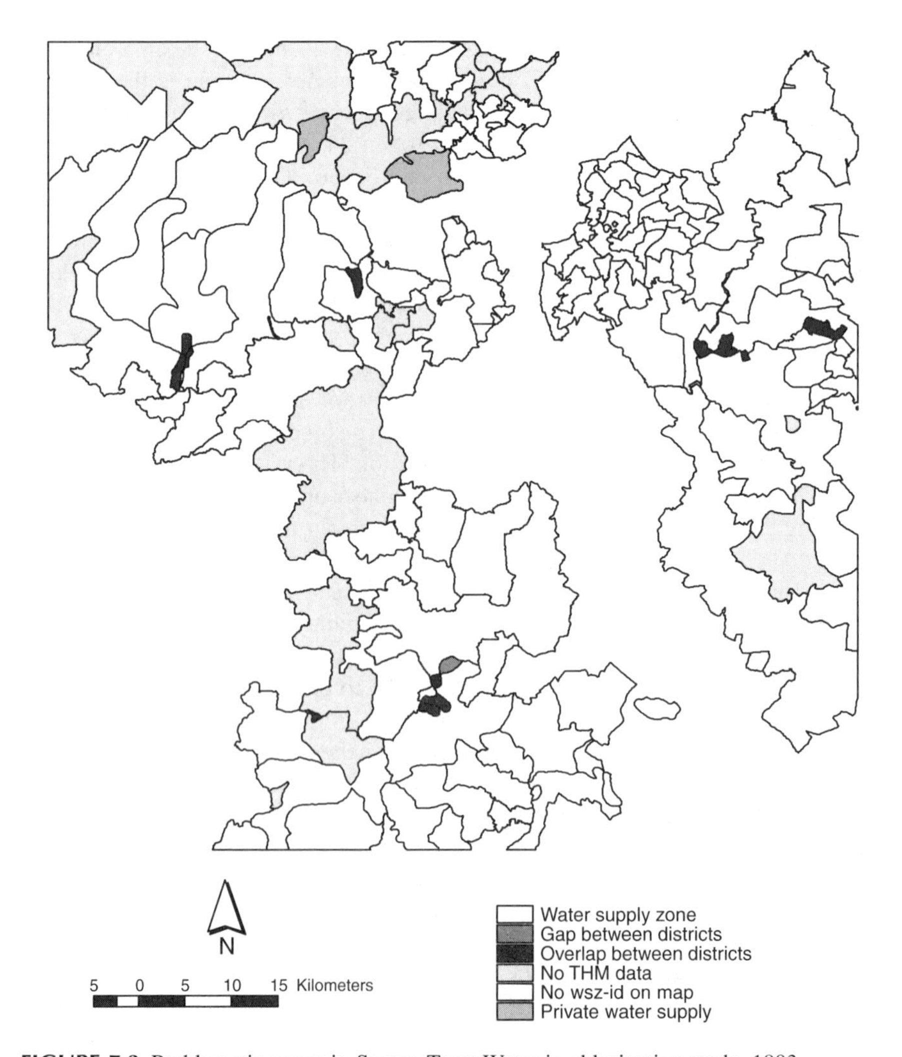

FIGURE 7.3 Problematic zones in Severn Trent Water in chlorination study, 1993.

Problems also arose because of the uncertainties in the All Fields Postcode Directory (AFPD99), which at that stage was the most recently available postcode file. This contained a record for all postcodes operational at that time and all postcodes that were terminated, but not subsequently reused in the United Kingdom. Postcodes that are operational but have never been terminated, reused, or reorganized have a date of introduction, but no date of termination. Terminated postcodes that have not been reused or reorganized are also reported in AFPD99; these have a date of both introduction and termination. Subject only to errors in georeferencing, as noted above, the grid references of both these sets of postcodes could thus be identified and used for each year. More problematic were postcodes that had been closed and reused. Once the postcode is reused, the grid references from the old record are deleted and replaced with the new ones and the termination date is removed from that postcode. Essentially, the postcode's previous attributes are deleted from AFPD99. This means that, using AFPD99, the postcode's previous grid references cannot be obtained and its prior existence cannot be determined. Any births occurring in these postcodes will be matched to the most recent occurrence of the postcode, which may be in a different water supply zone. At best, this may lead to exposure misclassification. If postcode reorganization during the study period preferentially affects specific socioeconomic areas, or areas with a particular level of exposure, it may lead to bias.

Nationally, the number of missing postcodes ranged from about 1.3 percent in 1992 to almost 7 percent in 1997. Several reasons for these missing postcode coordinates exist. The largest proportion (about 70 percent of missing postcodes in 1997) are nongeographic or postboxes, which are mainly business addresses and are thus unlikely to represent populations of interest in this study. However, the remaining postcodes are potentially relevant. As far as possible, locations for these were imputed by taking the average location of all other postcodes within the postal sector. Table 7.2 summarizes the number of postcodes involved in each water zone in each year.

TABLE 7.2
Postcode Status by Water Company Area and Year

	Numbers of Postcodes					
	North West Water		Severn Trent Water		Northumbria Water	
Year	Existing	Imputed	Existing	Imputed	Existing	Imputed
1992	169,639	1,926				
1993	171,480	2,470	181,443	3,216		
1994	192,038	3,642	182,166	5,671		
1995	183,043	6,007	178,991	8,193		
1996	178,983	8,083	181,566	9,728		
1997	179,571	8,931	184,509	7,829	68,598	2,090

7.4 INVERSE DISTANCE WEIGHTING: MODELING FOOD PURCHASES FROM SUPERMARKETS

In the absence of independent data on exposures, many epidemiological studies rely ultimately on the principle of proximity: distance from a source provides a reliable proxy for exposure. In the case of pollutants in the ambient environment, this approach has some merit: most pollutants do show a general decline in intensity away from their source, because of dilution, deposition, and decomposition during dispersion. In these situations, distance-based measures can be powerful tools for exposure assessment. In addition to methods such as buffering (outlined in Section 7.2), a wide range of other distance-based modeling techniques are now becoming standard in proprietary GIS that might serve these needs, including methods such as kriging, inverse distance weighting, and spline interpolation. Somewhat surprisingly, few of these have yet been widely applied for exposure assessment, although kriging has been applied on an exploratory basis (e.g., Cressie, 2000; Liu and Rossini, 1996).

One example of their application is the SAHSU-related study of relationships between socioeconomic conditions, diet, and health. Most food purchases these days are from supermarkets, but the range of food purchases made — and thus the level of nutrition attained — is believed to vary considerably in relation to socioeconomic status. This may be one of the reasons why social deprivation is often so strongly linked to a wide range of health effects. Unfortunately, although data on actual purchases from supermarkets are increasingly being collected — and often (e.g., via loyalty cards) at an individual level — to support marketing, these data are not usually available to the research community for reasons of commercial confidentiality. Modeling procedures thus had to be employed in an attempt to allocate populations to the supermarkets for which they are likely to be customers. The approach taken was to use inverse distance weighting methods to distribute the population in each enumeration district to supermarkets based on their proximity and size.

The supermarket companies provided a database of 5762 supermarkets across Great Britain. This was believed to include about 80 percent of all supermarkets in the country and gave information on the location and size (floor area) of the supermarkets, but contained no information on their customer base. Also collected was population data by enumeration district (ED), classified by age and gender from the 1991 U.K. census data and age- and gender-specific average daily calorie demands for five classes comprising:

1. 0 to 4 year olds
2. 5- to 18-year-old males
3. 5- to 18-year-old females
4. >18-year-old males
5. >18-year-old females

As a basis for modeling, the total calorie demand (CD_i) for each age/gender group (i) was first calculated and used to derive relative weights ($W_i = CD_i/CD_{tot}$)

for each stratum, taking Stratum 5 (adult males over 18) to have weight = 1. The census data on the population (N_{ij}) was obtained for each age/gender group (i) in each ED (j). The calorie-weighted population of each ED was calculated using:

$$CWP_j = \Sigma_i W_i . N_{ij} \quad (7.1)$$

A target customer base (B_k = calorie-weighted population needed to support the supermarket) was derived for each supermarket (k) by:

- Calculating the total calorie-weighted population of Great Britain (Σj CWPj)
- Dividing by total floor area (F) across all types (k) of supermarkets ($\Sigma F_k . n_k$), where:
  - F = 10,000 m^2 for small supermarkets
  - F = 20,000 m^2 for medium-sized supermarkets
  - F = 30,000 m^2 for large supermarkets
  - n_k = the number of supermarkets in each size class
- Multiplying by the area of each supermarket:

$$B_k = F_k . ((\Sigma_j CWP_j)/(\Sigma_k F_k . n_k)) \quad (7.2)$$

Catchment areas were grown around each supermarket by progressively buffering and incorporating calorie-weighted populations from each ED centroid until the target customer base was achieved. The rate of growth (i.e., the power of each supermarket to capture customers) was modeled as a function of the inverse squared distance and unmet capacity. Where catchments interact or overlap, the available population is shared according to this pull variable (Figure 7.4).

The method described above has a number of recognized weaknesses. In particular, it takes no account of the effect of product range, advertising, price, or deliberate social targeting of supermarkets, which may severely distort shopping patterns. Instead, the only pull factors are seen to be the Euclidean distance to the supermarket and its floor space. A further assumption was made that people do not travel further than 50 km to visit a supermarket. The model thus also ignores the effect of natural geographical obstacles such as rivers, estuaries, lakes, and mountains that might act as obstructions to access specific supermarkets. In principle, this weakness could have been overcome by modeling distance along the road network instead of in simple, linear form. However, trials with the ArcInfo™ system indicated computing times of 5 hours for the analysis for one supermarket and a 2.5-kilometer buffer, which would have translated into a total computing time of approximately 1200 days for all 5762 supermarkets! Unfortunately, validation of the model was not possible due to restrictions on access to customer data even for a sample of individual supermarkets.

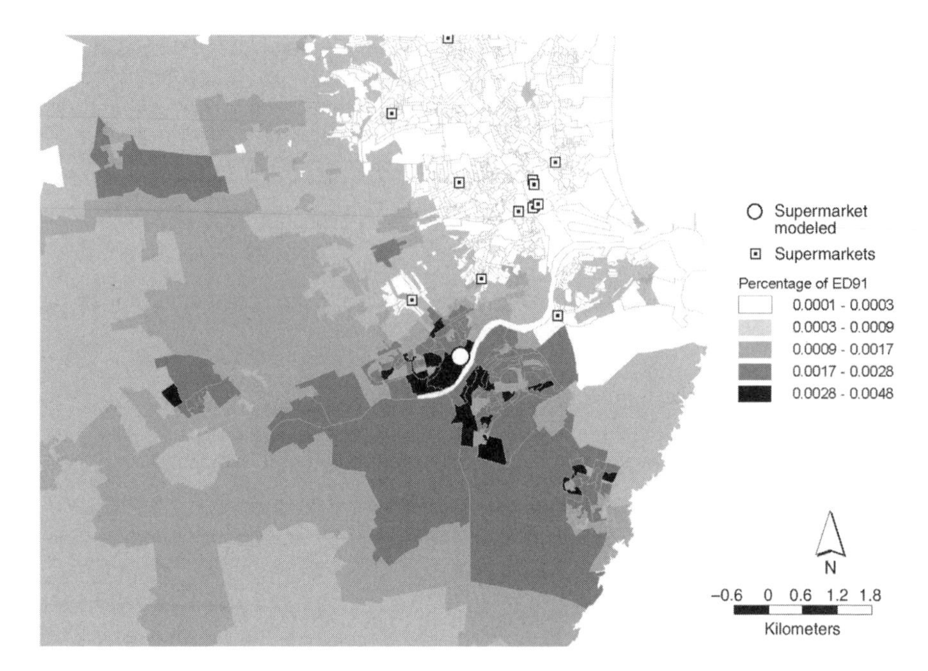

FIGURE 7.4 Modeled percentages of allocations for one supermarket by ED.

7.5 DISPERSION MODELING: EXPOSURES TO AIR POLLUTION FROM COKE WORKS

As hinted earlier, dispersion — rather than simple distance — is often a fundamental process in environmental epidemiology. Exposures to pollution depend not so much on how far away people live from emission sources, but the effects of dispersion on the pollutants within the intervening space. Because dispersion is affected by several factors including environmental conditions, such as the flow speed, flow direction, and degree of turbulence and mixing, simple distance-based measures will almost inevitably provide only approximate estimates of exposure. Enhanced methods of exposure assessment thus rely on the use of dispersion modeling.

Although dispersion models have been developed for a wide range of environmental media and pathways, by far the most extensive applications have been in relation to air pollution. Examples include the use of the Danish Operational Street Pollution Model (OPSM) to assess exposures to nitrogen dioxide (NO_2) in a study of traffic-related air pollution and cancer (Berkowicz et al., 1994) and the Dutch CAR (calculation of air pollution by road traffic) model to estimate exposures to the same pollutant in a case-control study of respiratory illness in Haarlem (Oosterlee et al., 1996). Nyberg et al. (2002) used the Airviro model to map concentrations of NO_2 and SO_2 between the 1960s and 1980s in Stockholm. Exposures were estimated for approximately 1000 cancer cases and 2000 controls by dropping the place of residence onto the pollution maps within GIS. When adjusted for confounding by smoking, the results showed a small, but statistically significant, increased risk of lung cancer for exposures to NO_2, though not to SO_2. Since NO_2 is largely generated by road traffic, while SO_2 tends to come from stationary combustion sources such as domestic heating systems, the implication was that this risk is primarily a function of traffic-related air pollution. Basham and Whitwell (1999) used ISCST3 (Industrial Source Complex Short Term) to estimate ground level concentrations of dioxins emitted from the Avonmouth municipal waste incinerator in Bristol. These were fed into an existing multipathway human exposure model.

In general, dispersion models consist of mathematical representations of the processes that generate pollutants and control their movement, dilution, and fate in the environment. The ability to use dispersion modeling for exposure assessment — and, indeed, the reliability of these models — depends more on the availability of the necessary input data than anything else. These data requirements are often demanding and far beyond the capabilities of many epidemiological studies. In air pollution modeling, detailed data may be needed not only on the characteristics of the emission source (e.g., traffic volume, composition, speed, emission control technologies, percentage of cold starts), but also on meteorological conditions (wind speed, wind direction, mixing height, etc.), surface topography, and building characteristics. Data constraints often limit the use of dispersion modeling, especially for large area or long-term studies. On the other hand, as links between proprietary dispersion models and GIS have been strengthened, opportunities to use these models have improved. GIS increasingly provides the means not only to display the results of dispersion modeling and intersect them with data on the population, but also to capture and provide the necessary input data (e.g., on road networks, traffic flows, emissions, topography, and meteorology).

One example of their use in SAHSU is the study of hospital admissions for respiratory and cardiovascular diseases in areas close to operating coke works in England and Wales (Aylin et al., 2001). Following an initial investigation, using distance from the site as a proxy for exposure, a more detailed study was carried out in which the Atmospheric Dispersion Modeling System (ADMS) was used to model dispersion of SO_2 emissions from one of the sites (Teesside) and the surrounding industrial complex coke work (Bottle, 2000). Figure 7.5 shows the resulting SO_2 pollution map. Exposure estimates were calculated by intersecting the map with ED centroids. Results showed that the coke works accounted for only about 10 percent of the modeled concentrations from the Teesside industrial complex as a whole. Modeled SO_2 concentrations from the entire complex were therefore included in a Poisson regression model for respiratory disease in the under-five age group. After adjusting for sex, Carstairs quintile, and health service provider, risk was found to be nearly twice as high in the highest pollution stratum (6 to 8 $\mu g/m^3$) as the lowest stratum (<2 $\mu g/m^3$).

7.6 CONCLUSIONS

Without doubt, the availability of GIS has greatly enhanced the potential for exposure assessment in studies of associations between the environment and health. As of yet, that potential has been relatively little used: in most cases, studies still tend to rely on relatively simple exposure measures; by doing so, it seems that the studies are

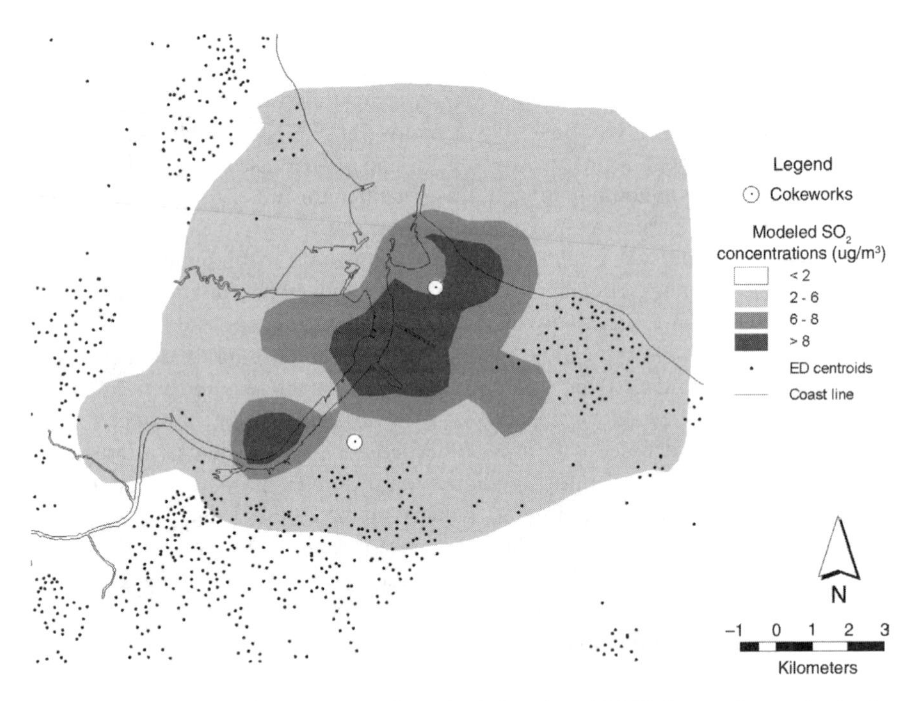

FIGURE 7.5 Modeled SO_2 concentrations (µg/m^3) using ADMS from coke works in the Teesside area.

unnecessarily constraining the quality of the exposure data used in epidemiological investigations. Many of the GIS-based methods that are now beginning to emerge, including those being developed in SAHSU, offer greatly improved estimates of exposure in terms of both their geographical resolution and their accuracy of estimation.

Even so, further improvements to these approaches are possible. Indeed, strictly speaking, few of the methods used so far actually model exposure. Rather, they are measures of pollutant concentrations: they take no direct account either of where people are or of the microenvironments within which exposure occurs. Exposures are usually assessed simply by dropping the place of residence of the individual participants onto the resulting pollution map or by computing some form of population-weighted average across an area. In all these situations, people are seen as fixed to their home. The reality of exposure is very different. In most cases, people are mainly at home during the night. At these times, many of the activities that cause pollution are latent or operating at a reduced rate. Exposures at these times are also likely to be more strongly affected by indoor sources. The combination of exposure estimates relating to ambient conditions with population distributions that reflect places of residence thus provides a relatively poor basis for understanding geographical associations between the environment and health.

The next step in exposure estimation, therefore, is to model people not as static, homebound receptors, but as dynamic and mobile individuals. This poses enormous challenges, not least because of the scarcity of data on human time-activity patterns, both in the long term (e.g., migration) and in the short term (e.g., daily commuting). Techniques that enable this are now emerging. For example, a prototype GIS-based model (Space–Time Exposure Modeling System, STEMS) has been developed that simulates the movement of people through changing pollution fields in different microenvironments and gives estimates of individual-level exposure profiles at averaging times from seconds to days (Gulliver, 2002; Briggs and Gulliver, 2002). Further development as part of SAHSU-related work will not only provide more extensive calibration and validation of this model, but also will see it expanded to provide a stochastic model of exposures across whole population groups. Beale and colleagues (Beale and Briggs, 2002) have developed a network-based system to model route choice and behaviors in urban environments. Though initially devised to simulate access to urban areas by disabled people, this can be integrated into STEMS to provide more-realistic algorithms for defining and simulating route choice.

Use of these new approaches also begins to raise new questions for environmental epidemiology. The ability to model dynamic patterns of exposure, for example, blurs the traditional distinction between ecological and time-series studies. Now we can begin to investigate associations between the environment and health in both time and space together. We can even start to imagine modeling lifetime exposures in a reasonably reliable manner. Whether chronic illness or mortality is a response to repeated, long-term exposures or a delayed response to short-term extreme exposures in the past can then be explored. Similarly, questions arise about the very concepts of exposure, as well as how to characterize it. The choice of exposure measure is no longer constrained so fiercely by data availability and logistics: different measures can be modeled, more or less, according to need. Because these various measures are not always closely correlated and are not strict proxies for each other, which measure we choose is likely to influence our results. The choice must be made on etiological principles. Yet which exposure — where, when, over what averaging period — is the most relevant in terms of disease etiology is often not known. For the future, this question can be less easily ignored.

References

Aylin, P. et al., 2001, Proximity to coke works and hospital admissions for respiratory and cardiovascular disease in England and Wales, *Thorax*, 56, 228–233.

Basham, J.P. and Whitwell, I., 1999, Dispersion modelling of dioxin releases from the waste incinerator at Avonmouth, Bristol, U.K., *Atmospheric Environment*, 33, 3405–3416.

Beale, L. and Briggs, D.J., 2002, A GIS-based route mapping tool for disabled access in urban environments, in Pillman, W. and Tochtermann, K., Eds., *Environmental Communications in the Information Society. Proceedings of the 16th International Conference: Informatics for Environmental Protection*, Vienna, 161–167.

Berkowicz, R. et al., 1994, Modelling air pollution from traffic in urban areas, in *Proceedings of the IMA Conference on Flow and Dispersion through Groups of Obstacles,* Cambridge, U.K.: University of Cambridge.

Bottle, R. A., 2000, Adjustments for the provider effect using hospital data in small area studies, unpublished Ph.D. thesis, Imperial College of Medicine.

Briggs, D.J. and Gulliver, J., 2002, Modelling journey-time exposures to traffic-related air pollution, in Pillmann, W. and Tochtermann, K., Eds., *Environmental Communications in the Information Society. Proceedings of the 16th International Conference: Informatics for Environmental Protection*, Vienna, 151–160.

Briggs, D.J. et al., 1997, Mapping urban air pollution using GIS: A regression-based approach, *International Journal of Geographical Information Science*, 11, 7, 699–718.

Briggs, D.J. et al., 2000, A regression-based method for mapping traffic-related air pollution: Application and testing in four contrasting urban environments, *Science of the Total Environment*, 253, 151–167.

Cressie, N., 2000, Geostatistical methods for mapping environmental exposures, in Elliott, P. et al., Eds., *Spatial Epidemiology: Methods and Applications,* Oxford: Oxford University Press, 185–204.

Dolk, H. et al., 1998, Risk of congenital anomalies near hazardous-waste landfill sites in Europe: The EUROAZCON study, *Lancet*, 352, 423–427.

Elliott, P. et al., 1996, Cancer incidence near municipal solid waste incinerators in Great Britain, *British Journal of Cancer*; 73, 702–710.

Elliott, P. et al., 2001, Risk of adverse birth outcomes in populations living near landfill sites, *British Medical Journal*, 323, 363–368.

English, P. et al., 1999, Examining associations between childhood asthma and traffic flow using a geographic information system, *Environmental Health Perspectives*, 107, 761–767.

Fielder, H.M.P. et al., 2000, Assessment of impact on health of residents living near the Nanrt-y-Gwyddon landfill site: Retrospective analysis, *British Medical Journal*, 320, 19–22.

Gulliver, J., 2002, Space-time modelling of exposure to air pollution using GIS, unpublished Ph.D. thesis, University College Northampton and University of Leicester.

Jarup, L. et al., 2002, Cancer risks in populations living near landfill sites in Great Britain, *British Journal of Cancer*, 86, 11, 1732–1736.

Liu, L.J.S. and Rossini, A.J., 1996, Use of kriging models to predict 12-hour mean ozone concentrations in metropolitan Toronto: A pilot study, *Environment International*, 22, 677–692.

Marshall, E.G. et al., 1997, Maternal residential exposure to hazardous wastes and risk of central nervous system and musculoskeletal birth defects, *Archives of Environmental Health*, 52, 416–425.

Moolgavkar, S.H., 2000, Air pollution and daily mortality in three U.S. counties, *Environmental Health Perspectives*, 108, 777–784.

Nyberg, F. et al., 2000, Urban air pollution and lung cancer in Stockholm, *Epidemiology*, 11, 487–495.

Oosterlee, A. et al., 1996, Chronic respiratory symptoms in children and adults living along streets with high traffic density, *Occupational and Environmental Medicine*, 53, 241–247.

Shadick, G., 2002, Statistical methodological aspects of modelling relationships between air pollution, temperature and health, unpublished Ph.D. thesis, Imperial College of Science, Technology and Medicine.

8 Using Modeled Outdoor Air Pollution Data for Health Surveillance

Paul Brindley, Ravi Maheswaran, Tim Pearson, Stephen Wise, and Robert P. Haining

CONTENTS

8.1 INTRODUCTION

There is substantial evidence linking outdoor air pollution and health. Numerous studies have examined the association between daily mortality and short-term fluctuations in air pollution (Pope, 2000). A smaller number of studies have reported an increase in mortality with long-term exposure to outdoor air pollution (Dockery et al., 1993; Hoek et al., 2002; Pope et al., 1995).

From a public health practitioner's perspective, it would be useful to be able to monitor, on a regular basis, the association between air pollution and health. Although a number of cities monitor air pollution levels, recordings are taken at relatively few sites. However, an increasing number of cities have access to software that may be used to model air pollution. These software programs have the potential to provide information at a much finer spatial resolution than that derived from

0-415-30655-8/04/$0.00+$1.50

monitoring. These data could link to health data within GIS, which could also be used to manipulate the data in a number of ways. This can then provide a local system for monitoring air pollution and health using available data.

In this chapter, we describe our work in Sheffield using modeled air pollution data provided by Sheffield City Council. We discuss the opportunities and pitfalls of using such data in analyzing health outcomes.

8.2 AIR POLLUTION DATA

The actual levels of air pollution are monitored at specific sites. For example, there are 47 automatic sites in the United Kingdom (Bower and Vallance-Plews, 1995) that measure carbon monoxide (CO), nitrogen dioxide (NO_2), nitrogen oxides (NO_x), particulate matter (PM_{10}), ozone (O_3), and sulfur dioxide (SO_2), although not all pollutants are measured at all sites (Collins, 1998). It is then possible to interpolate between the known set of sample points. There are many different methods of spatial interpolation (see, e.g., Haining, 2003). Briggs et al. (1997) suggest that kriging estimates are better suited to national scales, while inverse distance weighting (IDW) is more appropriate for regional mapping. An example of IDW is illustrated in Figure 8.1. The new point's value is proportional to the observed values and distances to the locations of these observed values.

However, due to the financial costs involved in monitoring pollution it is rare that sufficient measuring points are available to reflect accurately the spatial texture and dynamic variability of the pollution surface. Within the urban environment, levels of air pollution exhibit extreme variation over very short distances, frequently no more than a few tens of meters (Briggs et al., 1997; Hewitt, 1991; Leicester City Council, 2000). While coarse resolutions are viable for mapping elevated industrial sources (stacks) of air pollution, much greater pollution gradients are evident for ground-level sources (notably traffic). Small numbers of sampling points could never adequately reflect the space-time variability of air pollution within a city and such methods are better suited to regional or national scales of analysis.

Briggs et al. (1997) (also see Collins, 1996, 1998; Collins et al., 1995) use regression modeling to estimate pollution levels, incorporating the following variables: traffic volume, land cover, and topology. Although the method provides

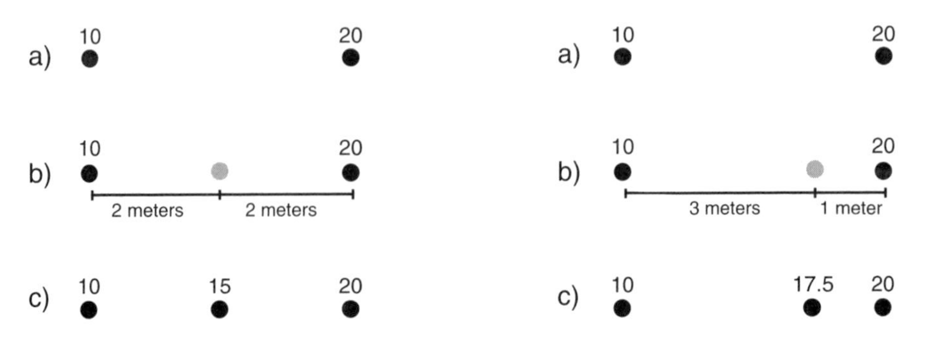

FIGURE 8.1 Examples of IDW interpolation.

generally sound results for pollutants that are influenced heavily by pollution from transportation sources (e.g., NO_x or CO), it is less successful for pollutants that are more reliant upon other sources of pollution (e.g., PM_{10} or SO_2). The model also treats all industrial land use areas as emitting the same levels of pollutants. Such a method is suitable when pollution sources and the levels of emissions are unknown. However, if such additional data are available it seems sensible to endeavor to use them to estimate pollution levels.

Complex dispersion modeling uses information relating to pollution emission sources and the characteristics of dispersal into the environment (Collins, 1998). More simplistic dispersion modeling is appropriate for estimating polluting levels close to emission sources (Collins, 1998) and thus more suited to estimating pollution at a small number of specific points rather than for a whole city (Zannetti, 1990). However, with increasing computer performance it is possible to model very complex phenomena. Such systems include Indic-Airviro (http://www.indic-airviro.smhi.se) and Atmospheric Dispersion Modeling System (ADMS) (http://www.cerc.co.uk/).

8.2.1 The Indic-Airviro System

Indic-Airviro, originally developed by Indic, is distributed and supported by the Swedish Meteorological and Hydrological Institute (SMHI) and is currently one of the most commonly used pollution modeling packages along with ADMS-Urban and the more simplistic Design Manual for Roads and Bridges (DMRB) (Beattie and Longhurst, 1999). The system calculates air pollution given weather conditions and the pollution sources that exist:

- Point sources such as factories
- Line sources such as major roads
- Grid (area) sources to represent background pollution levels such as housing estates and minor roads

The emissions database used for the Sheffield system is illustrated in Figure 8.2.

The system operates within a UNIX environment and the large processing requirement is demonstrated by the fact that each model run for our study area of Sheffield (for a given pollutant and year) took approximately five days to complete due to the inherent complexity and sophistication of the procedure.

As an illustration of the complexity of the model, each major road link is described in terms of estimated hourly traffic flow (derived from daily average flows), road-type, speed limit, proportion of heavy vehicles, and road width. Hourly flows of traffic are available for Monday to Thursday, Friday, Saturday, and Sunday to represent the different types and times of traffic flow on these days (see Veal and Appleby, 1997). Hourly flows are multiplied by a pollution-specific emission factor for the vehicle type to obtain an emission rate at differing speeds (in steps of ten kilometers per hour) (Leicester City Council, 2000).

The system requires the following weather variables (those in italics are critical, those not in italics can be estimated using the critical values):

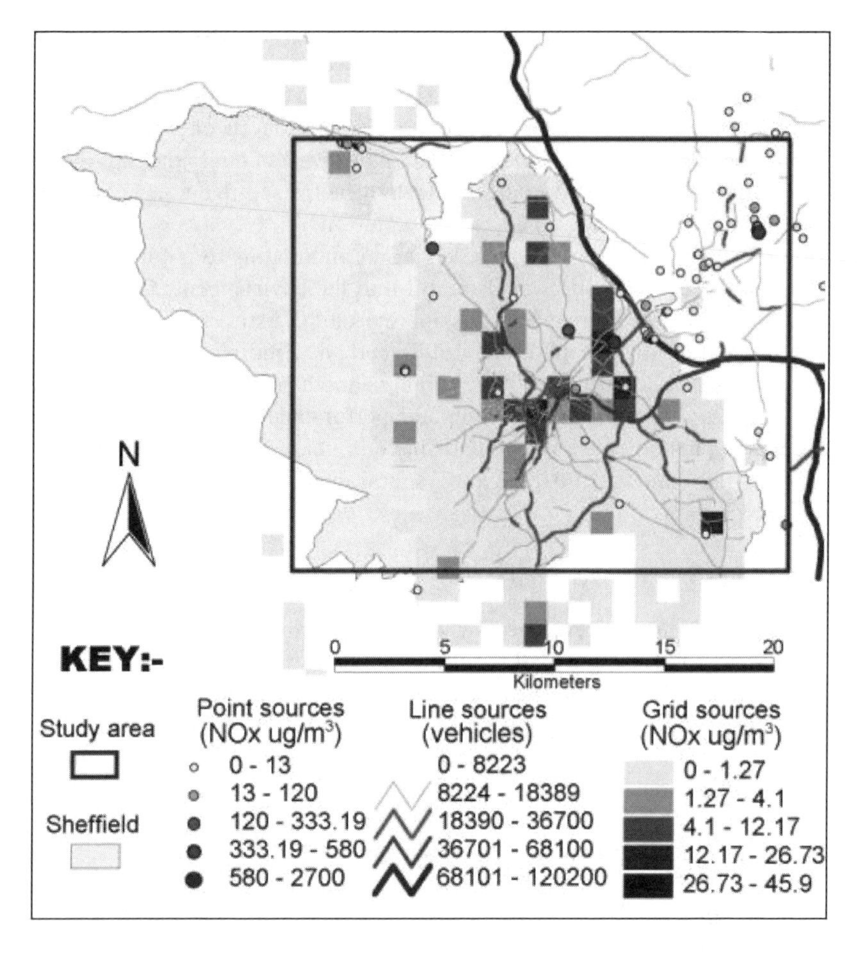

FIGURE 8.2 Example emissions database for NO_x.

- *Wind speed at 10 meters* and 35 meters
- *Wind direction at 10 meters* and 35 meters
- Vertical wind speed at 35 meters
- Absolute temperature at 2 meters
- Temperature difference between 2 meters and 8 meters
- Temperature difference between 2 meters and 20 meters
- Global radiation at 2 meters
- Gamma radiation at 2 meters

8.2.1.1 Modeling Assumptions

Indic-Airviro is heavily reliant on the data input: pollution emissions or weather data. When the weather mast was out of order for 13 weeks starting in September 1998, Indic-Airviro would not output results for that year.

The model used in Sheffield did not have the capacity to handle terrain, which is a severe limitation, as anyone who has ever visited Sheffield (and its "seven hills") will know. Any differences in elevation (also the location and height of buildings) have an impact upon air movements and, hence, pollution concentrations. Unfortunately, at present it is simply not computationally possible to incorporate these elements. Any model by definition is a simplification of reality, which will make generalized assumptions about extremely complex real-life situations. The output of a model can only be as good as its specification and the quality of its input data.

Different pollutants may be suited to differing spatial scales depending upon their emission sources. For example, 91 percent of CO is derived from transport sources (National Atmospheric Emissions Inventory, 1998), which exhibit high variation within short distances. In comparison, 66 percent of SO_2 emissions are from public power sources with a further 24 percent from industry (National Atmospheric Emissions Inventory, 1998) and, hence, levels of SO_2 generally have less spatial variation. Modeling this pollutant is heavily dependent upon power station emissions. However, emissions data collected by Sheffield City Council did not include pollution sources from outside the county (with the exception of nearby Rotherham) and no power stations fall within the county. As such, any modeling of this pollutant would not reflect the true pattern. This clearly demonstrates the importance of interregional cooperation and data sharing for air pollution assessment.

The Sheffield Indic-Airviro system only uses two different vehicle classes (cars and heavy vehicles) whereas in reality even two identical vehicles will probably have different emission patterns due to driving preferences. More significantly, there is no specific class to represent diesel vehicles, which produce very different emission patterns to petrol engines (see Watkins, 1991). Also, average speeds are constant at all hours, being recorded simply as the speed limit, rather than reflecting congestion at peak traffic times. In comparison, Mukherjee et al. (2000) found that off-peak average speeds were 18 percent higher than for peak times.

Traffic counts may be inaccurate (Kühlwein and Friedrich, 2000) and often do not reflect the dynamic behavior of traffic flows (Schmidt and Schäfer, 1998). There is no account taken of the difference in emissions caused by acceleration and deceleration found in congested areas or at traffic lights (DETR, 1998; Schmidt and Schäfer, 1998). It is important to bear in mind that in all situations there will be some pollution component not incorporated within the model: the goal is to make this as small as possible or as is necessary for the application (Peace et al., 1998).

Meteorological data will never be entirely accurate and realistic attempts to model atmospheric diffusion and mixing processes are extremely difficult (Hewitt and Harrison, 1986; Dabberdt and Miller, 2000). The mixing height is an important meteorological input parameter and can lead to large errors in modeled ground-level pollution concentrations (Lena and Desiato, 1999).

The urban environment is so complex that although it is possible to model modest street-level wind patterns, it is impossible to adapt the methods to a whole city area (Johnson and Hunter, 1999; Theurer, 1999). The type of roof, vegetation cover, and even the location of parked cars affect wind patterns and with the added complexity of turbulent flow, it is difficult to extrapolate concentrations from one location to another (Tirabassi, 1999).

8.2.1.2 Model Output

The Eularian Grid (or regional) model within Indic-Airviro calculates hourly pollution levels across each grid by assessing emission sources directly within the grid, emissions that migrate from adjacent grids, and pollution levels remaining in the grid from the previous hour (SMHI, 2000). The resulting grid pollution estimates can be exported as shapefiles (the file format for the GIS ArcView® system) or text-delimited ASCII for further analysis and manipulation within a GIS.

The study area (Figure 8.2) was set up to include as much of the populated area within Sheffield as possible, while maintaining a 200-meter grid resolution. For each of the 10,847 200-meter grids, air pollution was calculated on an hourly basis, as micrograms per square meter ($\mu g/m^3$) and the following statistics were derived: mean annual, minimum, maximum, daily maximum, standard deviation, and 90th percentile. The pollutants for the data collected include CO, NO_x, and PM_{10}. Data were collected on an annual basis for the years 1994 to 1999 (excluding 1998 due to problems with the metrological data, see above).

A background figure of 15 $\mu g/m^3$ was added to all PM_{10} grid cells to represent PM_{10} emissions from external sources outside the study area. This is in accordance with the Department for Environment, Food, and Rural Affairs' (DEFRA) guidelines and supported by the Environmental Protection Service, Sheffield City Council. The data output from Indic-Airviro is illustrated in Figure 8.3A–C.

8.2.2 Model Validation

Model validation is undertaken to check that modeled results are similar to the real world pollution values as measured by monitoring stations. Any differences between modeled and actual results may be due to modeling errors. Errors can take one of two forms. Systematic error (or bias) is where a model persistently over- or under-predicts given certain conditions and requires the model to be calibrated (DETR, 1998). Uncertainty (or random error), on the other hand, can never be eliminated and all predictions should be given with an accuracy assessment (usually incorporated using standard deviations) obtained through assessing model validity (Hedley et al., 1997). There is also the problem that errors may propagate within the model (Benarie, 1987).

The first stage of model validation is a visual check to see if the data appear as we expect it. In the case of air pollution, we expect levels to be high around major road networks, industrial, and city center areas. In the case of the PM_{10} data, there were high concentrations around the city center that were not expected. These proved to be council estates that were still being recorded within the emissions database as nonsmokeless coal burners. This is no longer the case, so areas affected by this problem will be excluded from future analysis. This highlights the need to continually use and check the data to improve it. The more the data are utilized, the greater the incentive to maintain data. Comparisons were made with the original data within the emissions database and previous data runs produced by the Environmental Protection Service, Sheffield City Council.

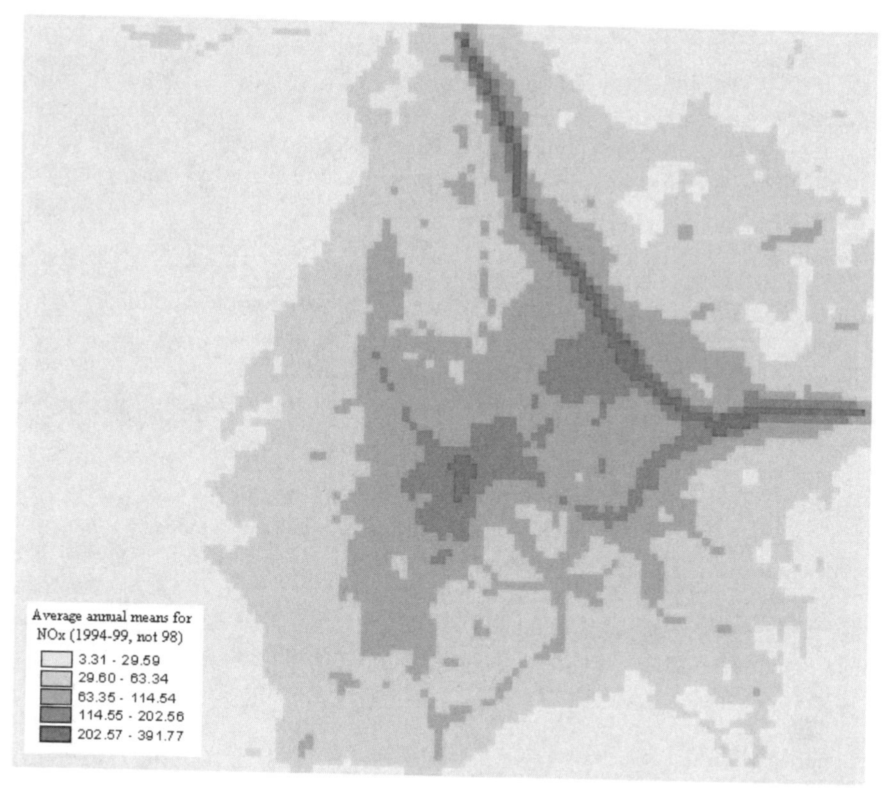

FIGURE 8.3A The average of the annual mean pollution levels, 1994 to 1999 (excluding 1998): NO_x ($\mu g/m^3$).

The second and more rigorous stage of model evaluation compares modeled pollution concentrations at specific points where monitored data are also available. Two suitable validation methods are possible: root mean squared error (RMSE) and the National Society for Clean Air (NSCA) and Environmental Protection regression approach. There are two fixed pollution-monitoring sites within Sheffield, monitored by DEFRA and the Environmental Protection Service (within Sheffield Council) owns three mobile Groundhog monitoring units.

RMSE computes the square root of the average squared difference between each corresponding monitored and modeled pollution value. By taking the square root, the index is scaled back to the original units. The procedure entails first squaring and then summing the difference between the monitored and modeled pollution values, dividing by the sample number, and finally taking the square root. In contrast, the NSCA regression approach creates a best-fit line between the monitored and modeled pollution values and then compares the monitored values to those expected from the best-fit relationship. Each monitored value is multiplied by the slope of the best-fit line and added to the intercept to give the corresponding value of the best-fit line. The standard deviation of the difference between the best-fit line value and modeled values is divided by the mean of the monitored values to give an

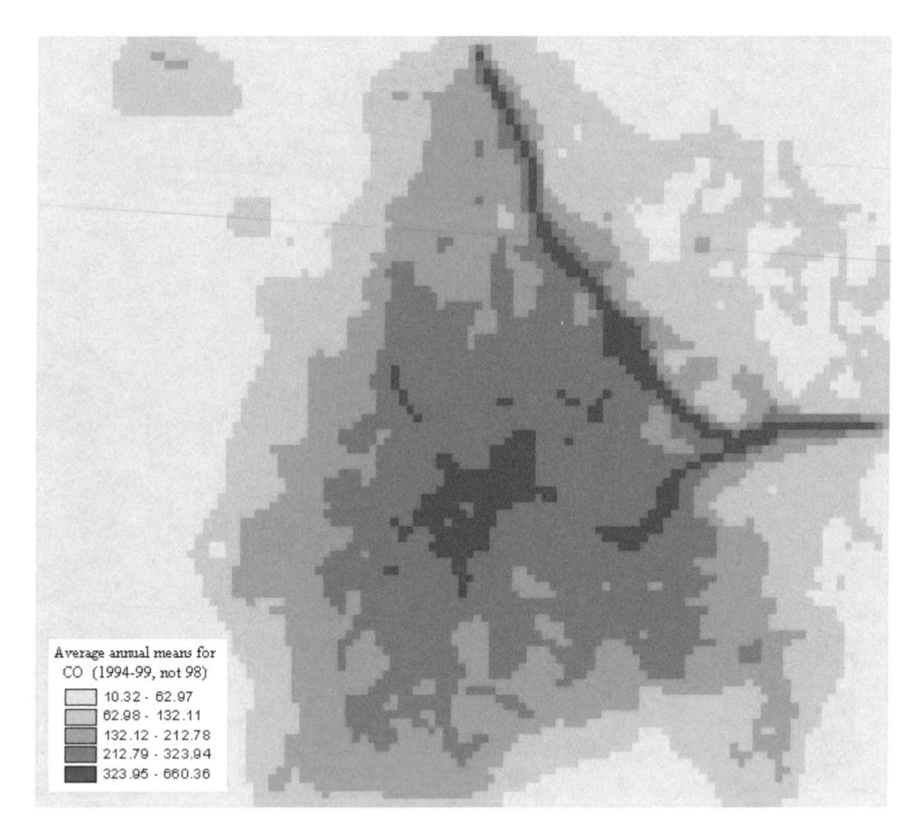

FIGURE 8.3B The average of the annual mean pollution levels, 1994 to 1999 (excluding 1998): CO (μg/m³).

uncertainty factor. The pollution value of interest (e.g., mean annual CO level for 1994) is multiplied by the uncertainty factor to provide an estimate of the level of uncertainty relevant to the level of pollution itself.

The NSCA regression approach allows for the fact that higher pollution estimates are likely to have higher levels of absolute error. For example, given two modeled pollution values of 2 μg/m³ and 200 μg/m³, it is unlikely that that both would be over- or underestimated by the same absolute amount (e.g., 100 μg/m³). Instead, it is more likely that higher absolute error is found at higher pollution levels. The method allows for a relatively small number of data points and yet is simple enough to be used effectively by people who may not have an in-depth knowledge of statistical methods. One of the main differences between the two methods is that the NSCA regression-based procedure is not affected by the lack of background measurements for a pollutant: for it examines the relationship between the data points. However, one might argue that background pollution is an important element in measuring overall pollution levels and should be included when validating any model.

The NO_x model validation illustrates that results from the Indic-Airviro model (using the emissions database and weather data) are considerable overestimates when

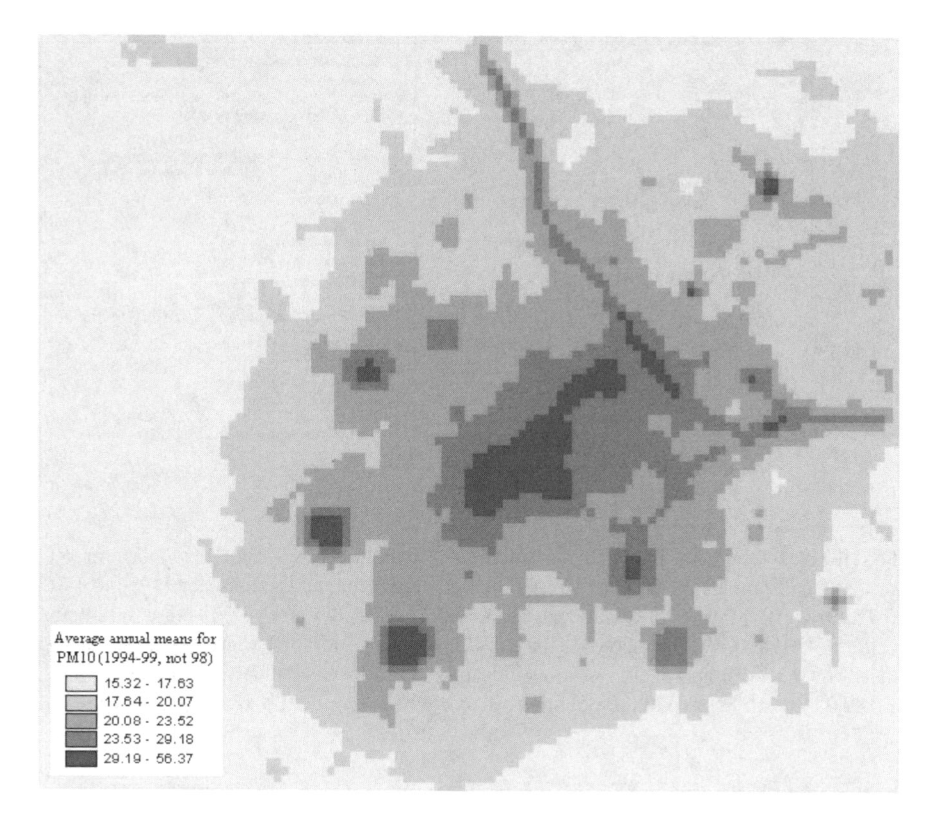

FIGURE 8.3C The average of the annual mean pollution levels, 1994 to 1999 (excluding 1998): PM_{10} ($\mu g/m^3$).

compared with monitored levels (Figure 8.4 and Table 8.1). However, pollution concentrations are all overestimated by the model at a broadly comparable level, suggesting that as relative measures of pollution concentration they are probably valid.

There is a much closer association between modeled and monitored PM_{10} values, although the Indic-Airviro model appears to underestimate pollution values slightly (Figure 8.5 and Table 8.1). There is an evident spatial pattern within the differences between modeled and monitored CO values (Figure 8.6 and Table 8.1). The Indic-Airviro model underpredicts pollution values for the city center (Data Point 1 to Data Point 3) to a greater extent than the values obtained for the Tinsley site (Data Point 4 to Data Point 8). This may reflect missing or incorrect components within the emissions database, problems with monitoring equipment, or differences in site location.

These validation results should be taken with an element of caution because the comparison is between area-based modeled air pollution (pollution for a grid cell) and point source monitoring concentration. This raises statistical issues that share common ground with the change of support problem in geostatistics (see, e.g., Haining, 2003). Some of the differences between the two sets of results will be due

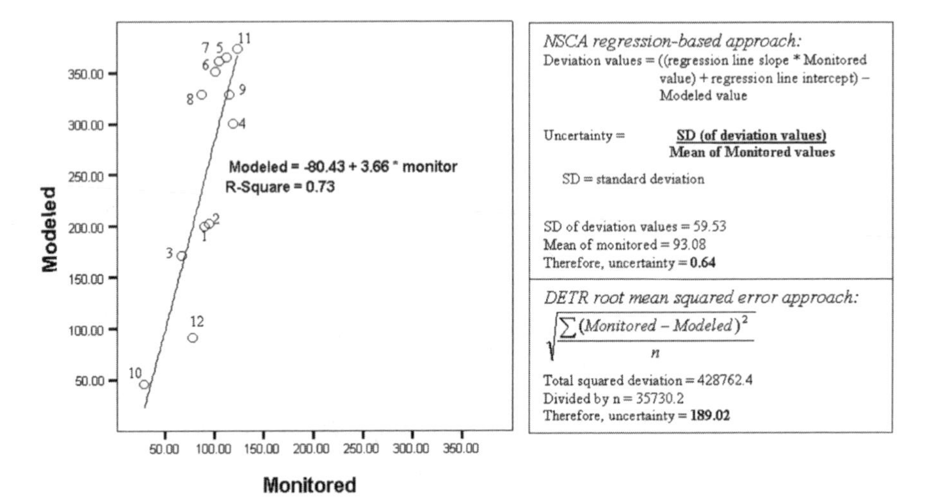

FIGURE 8.4 Graph of modeled and monitored data, workings, and examples for NO_x validation. Examples for NSCA regression-based approach: (1) Annual mean (1994 to 1999) = 42.79, 42.79 * 0.64 = 27.39, annual mean = 42.79 ± 27.39 μg/m³; (2) maximum pollution value = 420, 420 * 0.64 = 268.61, max = 420 ± 268.61 μg/m³. Examples for DETR root mean squared error approach: (1) Annual mean (1994 to 1999) = 42.79, annual mean = 42.79 ± 189.02 μg/m³; (2) maximum pollution value = 420, max = 420 ± 189.02 μg/m³.

to the smoothing effects of grid cells. All results are based on a small sample due to limitations with the monitoring data and care should be taken not to overinterpret these results.

Overall, the results generally imply that although we cannot be entirely certain of the absolute pollution values obtained, we are confident in them as relative pollution values. Order differences in the modeled pollution values are probably valid so that the model data are at least valid at the ordinal level of measurement.

However, we must add a further word of caution. When comparing model estimates to monitored levels of pollutants one should always remember that the monitors are themselves not accurate. The governmental Automated Urban Network (AUN) has an accuracy of approximately ±10 percent (SO_2, CO, NO, NO_2, and O_3) (Leicester City Council, 2000).

Wong et al. (1999) and Leicester City Council (2000) suggest that TEOM (tapering element oscillating microbalance) methods for measuring PM_{10}, as used by Sheffield City Council, underestimate particle mass compared to other techniques (such as BAM — beta attenuation monitoring). It has been estimated that TEOM estimates should be multiplied by a factor of 1.3 (Airborne Particle Expert Group, 1999), although care needs to be exercised because of the nonlinear nature of the underlying relationship.

Although monitoring sites should ideally be placed within a mixture of land uses — residential, industrial, and rural — for optimal model validation, under DETR (2000) guidelines "sites must be located where there is likely to be human

TABLE 8.1
Site Information and Validation Data

Site		NO_x		PM_{10}		CO	
		Monitored	Modeled	Monitored	Modeled	Monitored	Modeled
1	DEFRA City Center 1996	89.91	200.03	36.09	30.13	628	395
2	DEFRA City Center 1997	94.04	202.27	33.01	30.19	651	406
3	DEFRA City Center 1999	66.47	170.49	25.57	26.53	497	345
4	DEFRA Tinsley 1994	119.35	300.31			452	440
5	DEFRA Tinsley 1995	111.82	365.40			789	542
6	DEFRA Tinsley 1996	100.48	351.16			638	525
7	DEFRA Tinsley 1997	105.50	361.41			615	535
8	DEFRA Tinsley 1999	86.90	329.61			476	481
9	Groundhog 1a 1999	114.37	329.61	27.51	32.59		
10	Groundhog 1b 1999	28.50	46.27	19.06	24.72		
11	Groundhog 2a 1999	122.75	373.67	29.46	33.40		
12	Groundhog 3a 1999	76.93	91.30	22.59	23.41		

exposure over the relevant time period for each pollutant." Hence, monitoring stations are frequently unrepresentative of the study area and positioned in built-up locations (without a suitable rural station) and in areas of high pollution; in addition, there are usually far fewer monitoring sites than necessary due to the high financial costs of recording pollution levels.

8.3 LINKAGE TO CENSUS UNITS: AREAL INTERPOLATION

To compare different datasets, the spatial frameworks on which the data are collected should be the same. If data are collected using spatial frameworks that are incompatible (i.e., they do not match), then it will be necessary to achieve compatibility. The process of transferring data from one spatial framework to another is termed areal interpolation. In our example, we have air pollution levels recorded on a grid, but health, socioeconomic, and demographic data recorded by the smallest reporting unit used in the British population census, the enumeration district (ED). It seems sensible to transfer the air pollution data reported to an arbitrary grid to the ED framework.

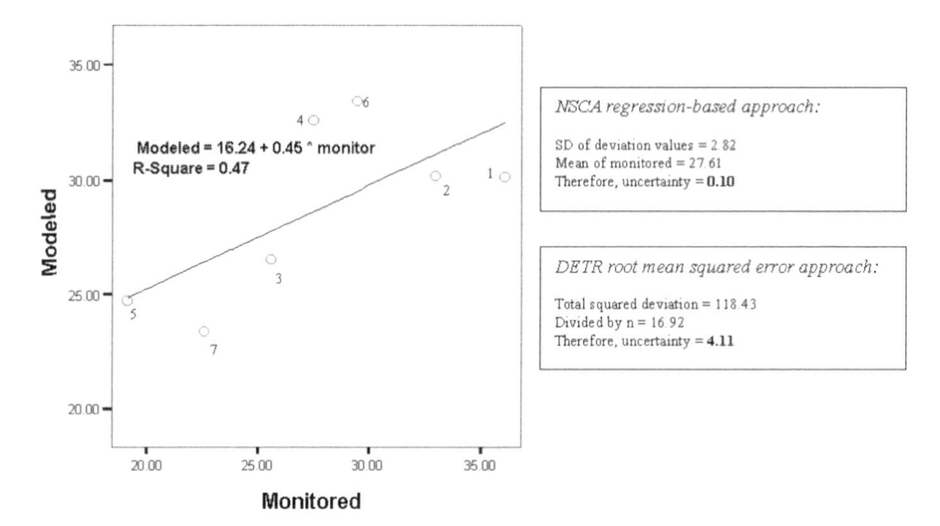

FIGURE 8.5 Graph of modeled and monitored data, workings, and examples for PM_{10} validation. Examples for NSCA regression-based approach: (1) Annual mean (1994 to 1999) = 18.97, 18.97 * 0.10 = 1.80, annual mean = 18.97 ± 1.80 μg/m^3; (2) maximum pollution value = 65.1, 65.1 * 0.10 = 6.51, max = 65.1 ± 6.51 μg/m^3. Examples for DETR root mean squared error approach: (1) Annual mean (1994 to 1999) = 18.97, annual mean = 18.97 ± 4.11 μg/m^3; (2) maximum pollution value = 65.1, max = 65.1 ± 4.11 μg/m^3.

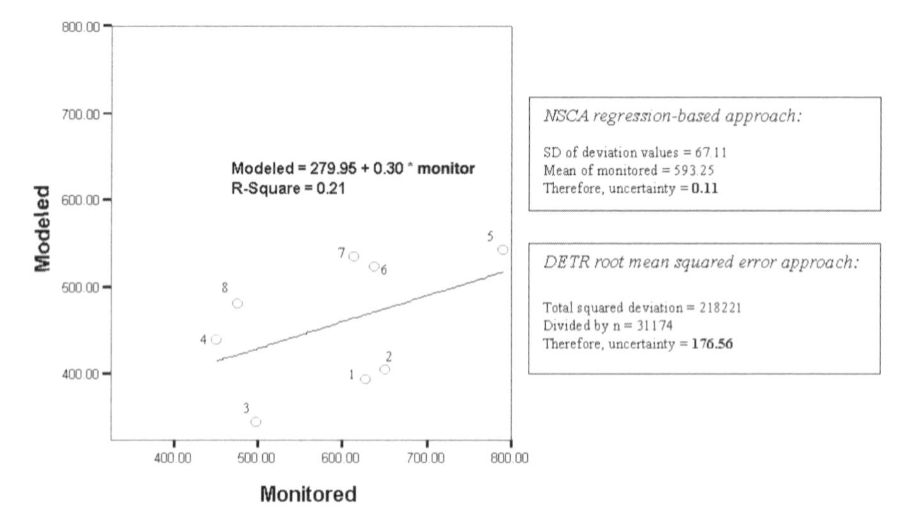

FIGURE 8.6 Graph of modeled and monitored data, workings, and examples for CO validation. Examples for NSCA regression-based approach: (1) Annual mean (1994 to 1999) = 121.36, 121.36 * 0.11 = 13.73, annual mean = 121.36 ± 13.73 μg/m^3; (2) maximum pollution value = 708, 708 * 0.11 = 80.09, max = 708 ± 80.09 μg/m^3. Examples for DETR root mean squared error approach: (1) Annual mean (1994 to 1999) = 121.36, annual mean = 121.36 ± 176.56 μg/m^3; (2) maximum pollution value = 708, max = 708 ± 176.56 μg/m^3.

The decision was made to calculate the mean pollution level for each ED. Each ED contains approximately 150 households (Rhind, 1991). Pollution estimates for the EDs should reflect the underlying population distribution within each ED, thereby giving an approximate measure of the true average exposure for people residing in each ED (Brindley et al., in press). This is likely to be particularly important where the population in an ED is concentrated in one part of the ED and there is considerable variation in pollution levels within the geographic area of the ED.

There are numerous methods of areal interpolation including area weighting, point-in-polygon, dasymetric mapping, linear regression-based analysis, the expectation maximization (EM) algorithm, and numerous surface measures. Each method encompasses advantages and disadvantages and has its own assumptions that affect the likely accuracy of the method (see Fisher and Langford, 1995; Flowerdew and Green, 1989, 1990; Flowerdew et al., 1991). For a short review, see Haining (2003).

Ideally, we want to measure people's exposure to the air pollutants. It is possible to use commercial databases for the location of postal addresses to obtain relatively fine-grained information about the location of population. In the British postcode system, the finest level of detail is the unit postcode (e.g., S10 2TN), which is used for a single large user (such as a business) or a group of approximately 12 houses (Raper et al., 1992). The British Ordnance Survey produces the Code-Point® product, which provides a precise geographical location for each unit postcode (at one meter precision) and the number of domestic and nondomestic delivery points. PostPoint® Professional, produced by MapInfo and based on Code-Point, also includes additional error checks.

Area weighting (or polygon overlay) estimates the value for the target unit as the area weighted average of the values for source units that overlap it (see example in Figure 8.7). This method assumes that the variable of interest is distributed homogeneously within the source units.

Point-in-polygon methods assign the data to representative points, for example, polygon centroids or population weighted centroids that summarize the area data (Bracken and Martin, 1989). Thus, it is assumed that all of the spatial objects are exactly located at the representative points (Sadahiro, 1999). This method is illustrated in Figure 8.8, whereby ED1 is represented by Point A and Point B summarizes the data relating to ED2.

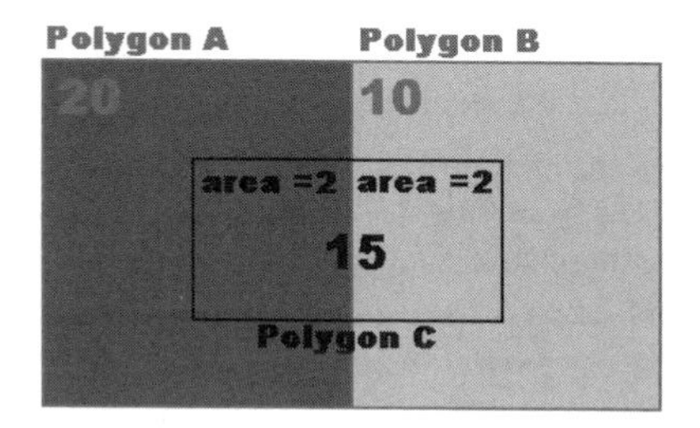

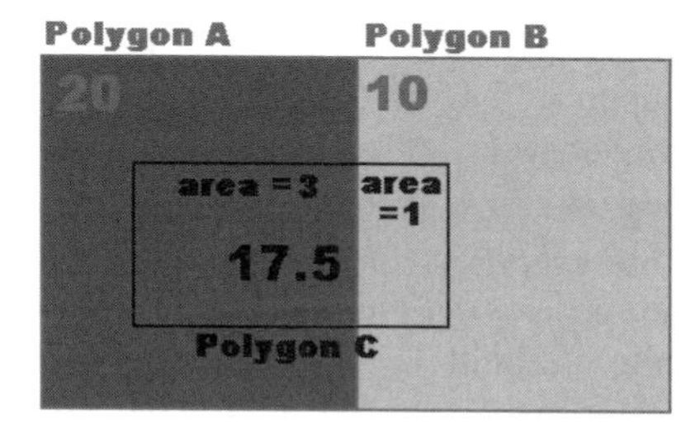

FIGURE 8.7 Area weighted interpolation.

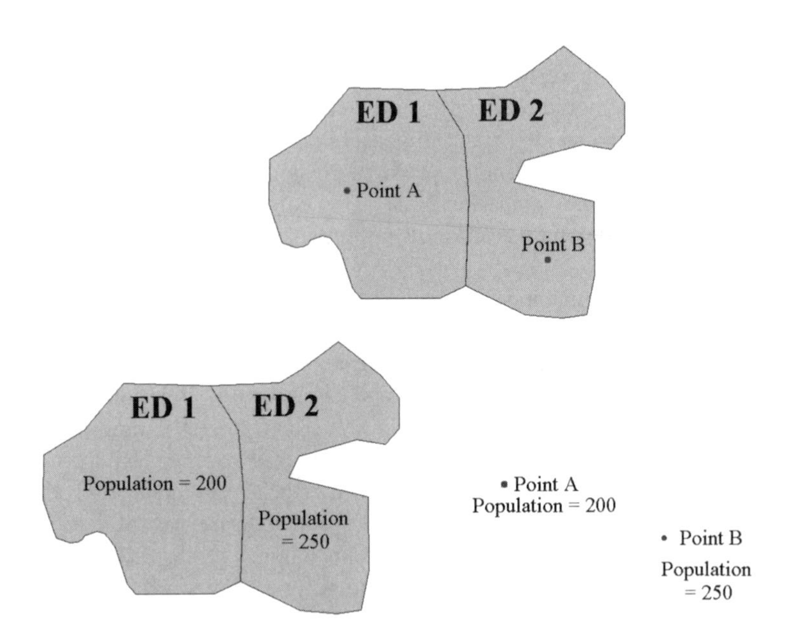

FIGURE 8.8 Point-in-polygon areal interpolation.

If health data were available at the individual level, the patient's postcode could be used to determine their geographic location. Point-in-polygon areal interpolation could be used to determine the pollution grid in which the patient's location is contained. However, if only aggregate health data is available or it is desired to use data relating to other boundaries (e.g., census data for population age and sex baselines), then the following procedure could be used to provide an estimation of people's exposure within each ED.

Using the PostPoint data, it is possible for a number of representative points to be used for a single ED. Thus, the average pollution values at every PostPoint point within each ED, weighted by the number of domestic properties, were used to estimate the average pollution exposure for each ED. Only the 1030 EDs that were completely within the study area were included. An example of the procedure is given in Figure 8.9, while Figure 8.10 illustrates the results obtained for NO_x.

A problem with this methodology is that people move around and rarely spend the majority of their time at their home location (except for the elderly age group, which is generally less mobile than other age groupings and the most likely age group to suffer from the effects of cardiovascular and respiratory disease) (National Travel Survey, 1999). Therefore, some measure is needed to capture the daily activity spaces of residents to try and measure the extent of people's mobility and the effect of this mobility upon an ED's average pollution exposure. One solution (see Brindley et al., in press) would be to construct buffers around each postcode unit, using a radius threshold. The average journey length by mode of transport as supplied within the National Travel Surveys could provide an approximate indicator for activity space (Table 8.2).

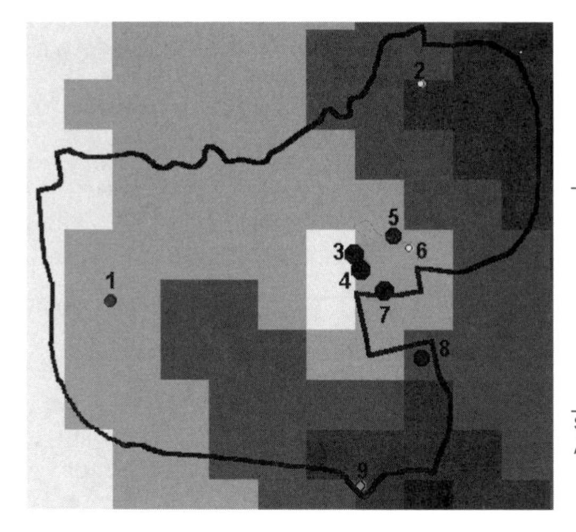

ID	Domestic properties	Pollution for grid	Dom*Poll
1	13	16.95	220.38
2	3	18.29	54.88
3	33	16.72	551.63
4	31	16.97	526.19
5	19	16.97	322.51
6	3	17.40	52.20
7	33	17.02	561.80
8	20	17.72	354.44
9	7	18.72	131.04
Sum	162		2775.06
Average		17.42	

Weighted average = 17.13

FIGURE 8.9 Example of point-in-polygon areal interpolation using PostPoint, weighted by the number of domestic properties.

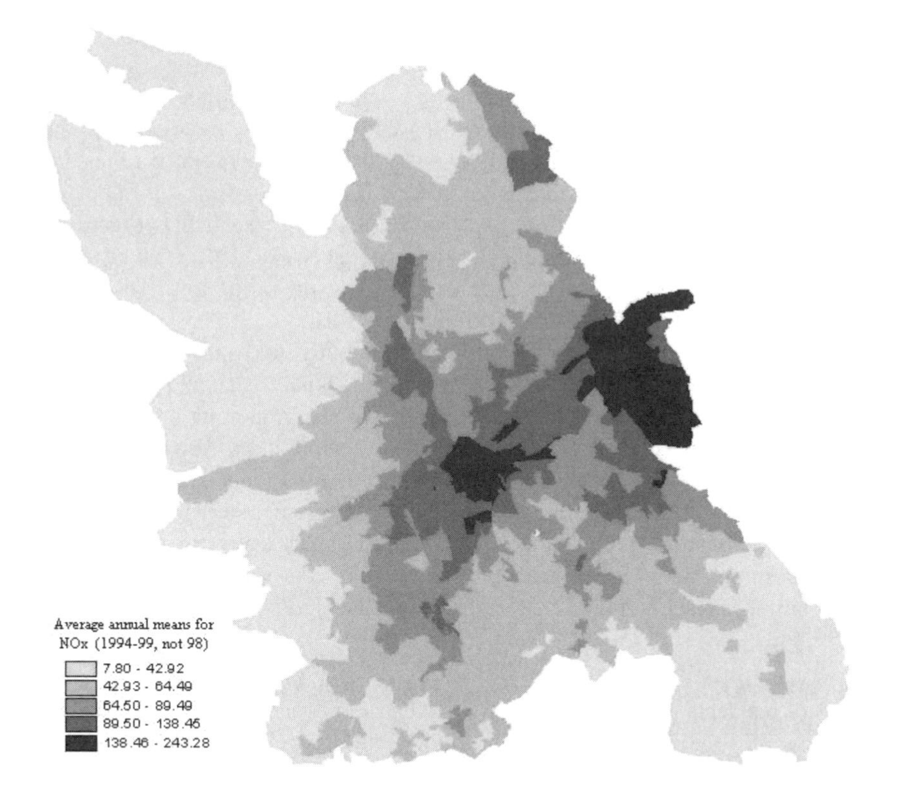

FIGURE 8.10 The NO_x average of the annual mean pollution levels, 1994 to 1999 (excluding 1998) for Sheffield enumeration districts (μg/m^3).

TABLE 8.2
Average Journey Length by Mode of Transport

	1992/1994		1997/1999	
	Miles	Kilometers	Miles	Kilometers
Walk	0.6	1.0	0.6	1.0
Bicycle	2	3.2	2.4	3.9
Car	8.5	13.8	8.6	13.8
Motorcycle	7.0	11.3	9.6	15.4
Other private	14.5	23.3	17.0	27.4
Bus (London)	3.3	5.3	3.5	5.6
Bus (other)	4.1	6.6	4.4	7.1
Nonlocal bus	60.0	96.6	61.5	99.0
Surface rail	31.2	50.2	33.7	54.2
Taxi/minicab	3.8	6.1	4.4	7.1
Other public transport	31.0	49.9	43.1	69.4
All modes	6.1	9.8	6.5	10.5

Source: National Travel Survey 1997/1999 update.

Buffers of 1 kilometer (reflecting average walking distance journey), 2 kilometers, and 4 kilometers were constructed. It was felt that any variation in pollution concentrations would be diminished seriously if spatial averages were calculated using a buffer radius greater than 4 kilometers. The buffers for each ED can then be aggregated together to form a single buffer-region for each ED (Figure 8.11). The pollution value at each postcode location within each ED buffer can be averaged and weighted according to the number of domestic properties. The spatially smoothed results for CO are illustrated in Figure 8.12.

The damaging effects of air pollution are frequently due to the combined effects of several air pollutants (Hall, 1996). Consequently, analysis should incorporate all relevant air pollutants (Brown et al., 1995). This is also important when attempting to model the complex interactions that occur between pollutants (Brown et al., 1995; Clarke, 1986; Mukherjee et al., 2000). Derwent et al. (1995) and Künzli et al. (2000) found that NO_x, CO, and PM_{10} all had a high degree of interdependence and, as such, any pollutant-by-pollutant technique could possibly overestimate effects. This makes it difficult (if not impossible) to separate the effects of any one given pollutant. This point is further demonstrated in the graphs in Figure 8.13.

8.4 AIR POLLUTION VALUES BY ED IN RELATION TO POPULATION EXPOSURE

What is the relationship between these aggregate (ED level) pollution data and the real exposure experiences of people, given that their exposure is purely identified by the location of their home address? These aggregate pollution data make no allowance for the fact that people may not continually remain in a given locality

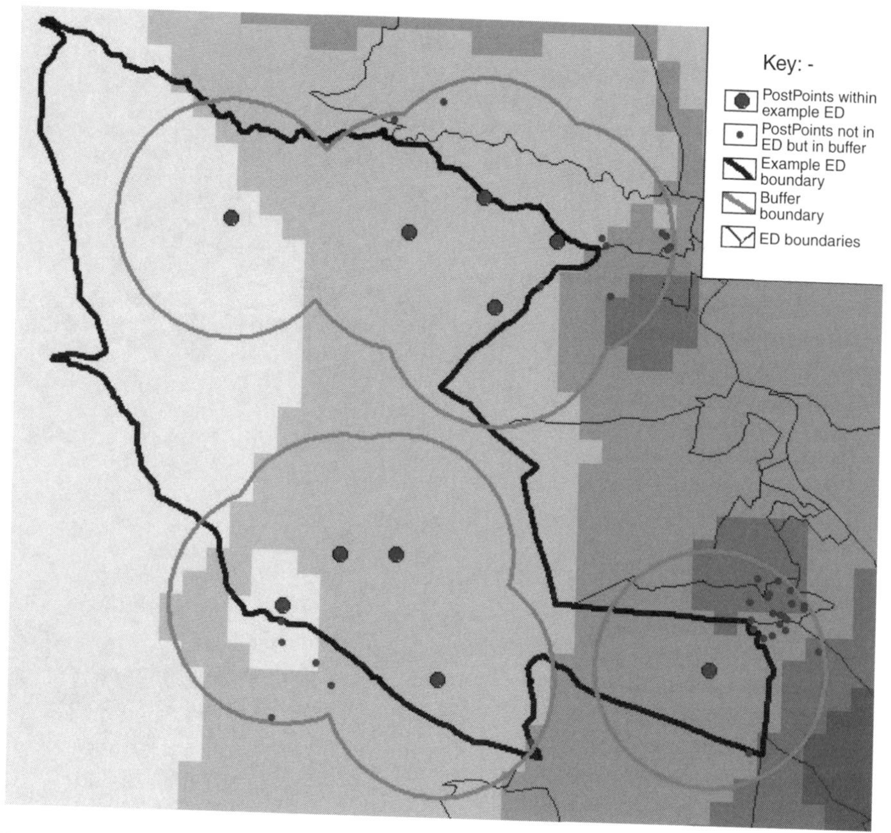

FIGURE 8.11 Methodology for constructing spatially smoothed pollution estimates.

and undertake long-term migration (as opposed to the more short-term daily migration discussed within Section 8.3). In addition, people have a tendency to spend a large proportion of their time indoors; yet modeling is usually performed to generate outdoor pollution concentrations. These issues are discussed below.

8.4.1 Long-Term Population Movements

In assigning air pollution exposures to individuals, one of the issues to consider is that over the duration of a long-term study, people will tend to move address. To gain some insight as to the size of these population movements, we used data from the Sheffield Health and Illness Prevalence Survey carried out in 1994, to then link to subsequent information to create a cohort study. A sample of 12,239 randomly selected individuals aged 18 to 94 years were followed over an eight-year period between 1994 and 2002. The sample was representative of all socioeconomic groups and the proportion of males and females was 44 and 56 percent, respectively.

This study used a record of date stamped address postcodes to identify the residential movements made by the cohort individuals over the eight-year study period. Sheffield Health Authority maintained the postcode changes and updates. To

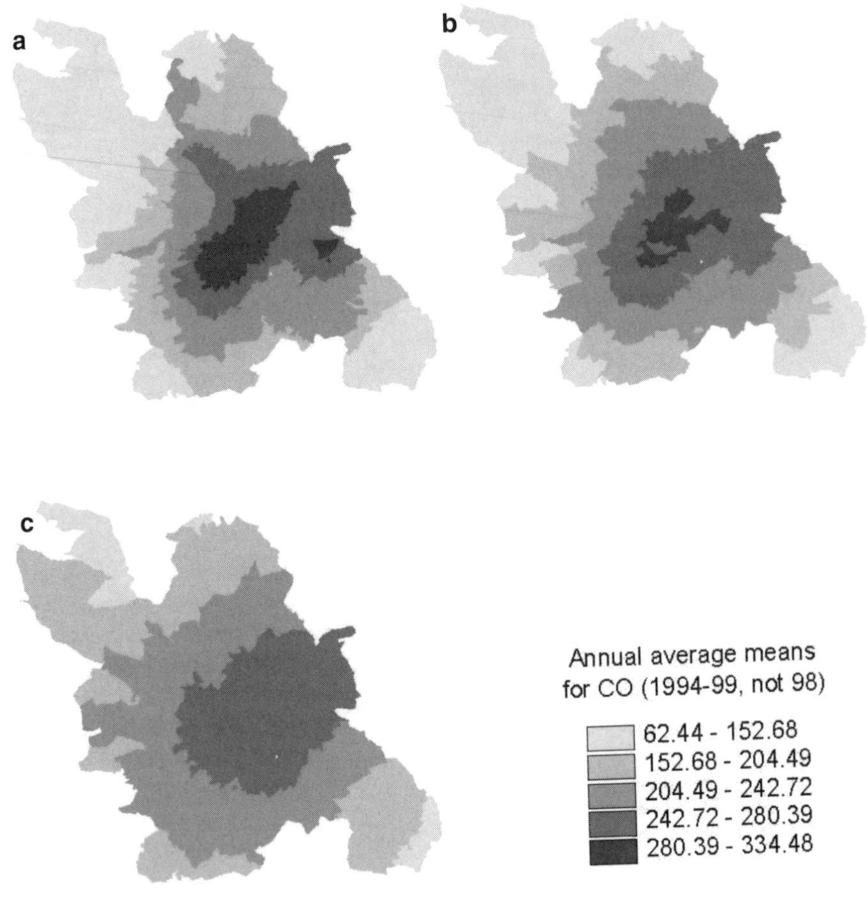

FIGURE 8.12 Spatially smoothed CO average of the annual mean pollution levels (1994 to 1999, excluding 1998) for Sheffield enumeration districts (μg/m^3). (a) 1-km spatial average; (b) 2-km spatial average; (c) 4-km spatial average.

avoid problems arising from postcode changes made for administrative reasons (i.e., the postcode of an address had been changed, but the geographical location of the address remained unchanged), a comparison of postcode coordinates rather than postcodes themselves was used to identify changes of location. Postcode coordinates were accurate to within 50 meters of the center of the postcode, which was acceptable relative to the 200-meter grid squares on which air pollutant levels were modeled.

Over the study period, 1491 people died while living in Sheffield, 1572 moved out of Sheffield, and 9176 remained alive and lived in Sheffield for the full duration of the study. Those individuals who either moved away from Sheffield or died were considered as cohort losses from the date of their move or their date of death. Of the 9176 individuals who remained residents of Sheffield over the entire study period, the number of internal address changes was tracked from the record of date-stamped residential postcodes. This data showed that of these 9176 cohort members,

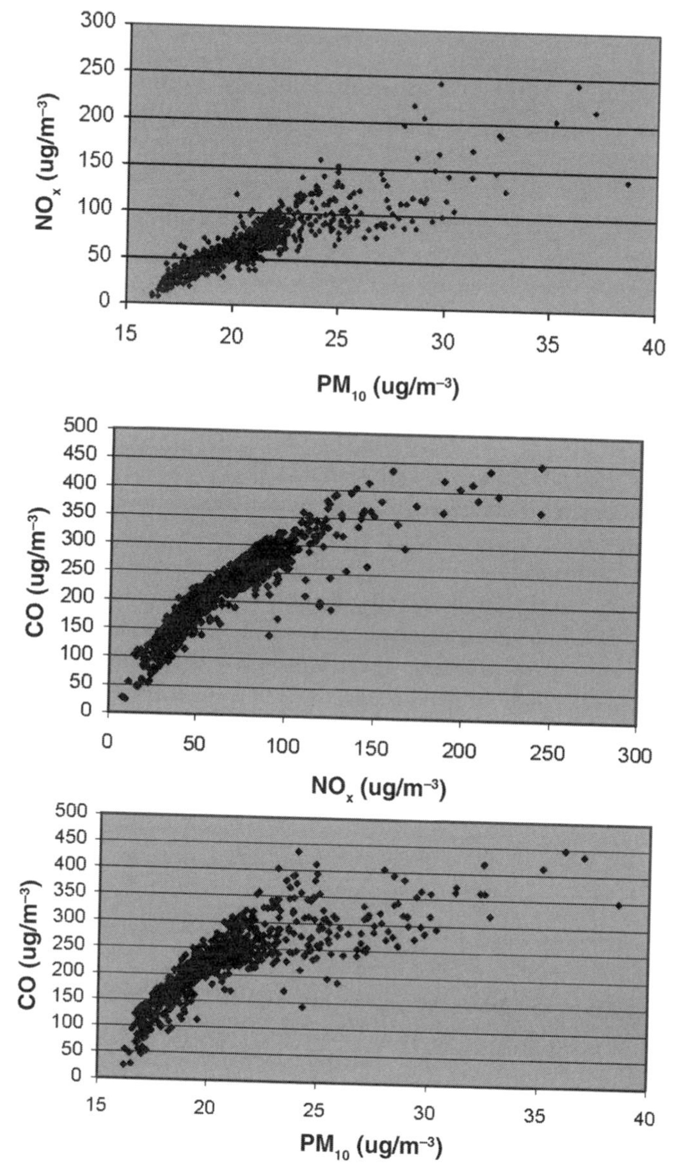

FIGURE 8.13 Scatterplots of untransformed enumeration district pollution values: pollution interdependence graphs.

approximately 70 percent did not move, 23 percent made one move, 5 percent made two moves, just over 1 percent made three moves, and less than 1 percent made four or more moves (Table 8.3). Stratification by age showed that the youngest age group (18 to 44 years) was twice more likely to make one or more moves than those aged 45 years and older. However, the proportion of individuals making more than three

TABLE 8.3
Number of Address Moves Made within Sheffield by Individuals Who Remained as Residents of Sheffield over the Full Duration of the Study

Number of Internal Moves	Male		Female		Total	
	n	Percent	n	Percent	n	Percent
0	2817	69.9	3581	69.6	6398	69.7
1	948	23.5	1167	22.7	2115	23.0
2	208	5.2	285	5.5	493	5.4
3	40	1.0	74	1.4	114	1.2
4	11	0.3	32	0.6	43	0.5
>4	4	0.1	9	0.2	13	0.1
Total	4028		5148		9176	

moves was less than 1 percent in all three age groups (Table 8.4). These figures showed a similar pattern when looked at by gender.

These data suggest that ideally, population movement should be taken into account when estimating long-term exposure to outdoor air pollution. However, this is not usually possible in ecological studies using routine data because of data constraints. The issue of potential misclassification of exposure for a significant proportion of the population therefore needs to be considered in such studies.

8.4.2 Outdoor and Indoor Pollution Levels

One of the problems of exploring the relationship of modeled air pollution and ill health is that it assumes that people are exposed only to outdoor air pollution

TABLE 8.4
Number of Address Moves Made within Sheffield by Individuals Who Remained as Residents of Sheffield over the Full Duration of the Study by Age Group

Number of Internal Moves	Age 18–44 years		Age 45–64 years		Age 65+ years	
	n	Percent	n	Percent	n	Percent
0	2559	57.9	2535	81.6	1303	79.0
1	1351	30.6	475	15.3	289	17.5
2	371	8.4	72	2.3	50	3.0
3	90	2.0	17	0.5	7	0.4
4	38	0.9	5	0.2	0	0.0
>45	11	0.2	2	0.1	0	0.0
Total	4421		3106		1649	

levels. Modeling indoor pollution levels is even more difficult and problematic than outdoor pollution, especially at a large scale. However, people generally spend between 75 and 90 percent of their time indoors (Dockery et al., 1981; Lee et al., 1997).

Indoor pollution concentrations depend not only on outdoor emissions but also on the type of cooking and heating systems, as well as ventilation. The association between outdoor and indoor pollution levels also varies with particle size (Ando et al., 1996). There has been considerable research comparing outdoor and indoor pollution concentrations and although outdoor to indoor ratios appear encouraging from a number of studies (Table 8.5), the evidence is not conclusive. There are strong associations between outdoor and indoor air pollution concentrations, although other factors also influence levels of indoor pollution.

In addition, exposures other than outdoor air pollution have important respiratory and cardiovascular effects, especially smoking and occupational exposure. Hence, it may be difficult to apportion which factors lead to higher mortality or admissions in certain circumstances. There is no easy method through which to determine how well any such aggregate measure may reflect individuals' pollution exposures, short of continually monitoring a large number of individuals.

TABLE 8.5
Comparisons between Indoor and Outdoor Pollution Concentrations

Pollutant	Source	Indoor Mean (μg/m³)	Outdoor Mean (μg/m³)	Indoor/Outdoor Ratio
CO	Valerio et al. (1997)	7.8[a]	9.55[a]	0.82
NO	Drakou et al. (1998)	56.53	70.66	0.80
NO_2	Drakou et al. (1998)	67.14	88.04	0.76
NO_x	Drakou et al. (1998)	126.98	87.74	0.68
O_3	Drakou et al. (1998)	17.54	37.14	0.47
$PM_{2.5}$	Lee et al. (1997)	25.3	26.3	0.96
$PM_{2.5}$	Fischer et al. (2000)	19	23	0.85
PM_{10}	Lee and Chang (2000)	120	134	0.90
PM_{10}	Fischer et al. (2000)	29.5	39.5	0.75
SO_2	Lee et al. (1997)	6.18	11.1	0.56

[a] Denotes units represented are median (μg/m³) values.

8.5 DISCUSSION

The continual development of complex dispersion modeling should allow for more accurate modeling of air pollution levels. Yet such models can only ever be as accurate as allowed by the specification and the quality of input data. Such modeling is most suitable for areal units (such as the grids used in this example). Validation procedures are essential in determining how reliable these estimated pollution concentrations are.

The recent rapid increase in the availability of digital data suitable for GIS has facilitated the widespread development of GIS. This has also highlighted the growing number of boundaries for which data are available. However, the problem arises as to how to compare datasets where the boundaries are incompatible (i.e., they do not match). The problem of incompatible zonal systems, where several variables needed for analysis have not all been collected on the same spatial framework, is encountered frequently within GIS. Such problems can only intensify with the creation of new boundaries, for example, output areas (instead of EDs) for the 2001 population census or new ward boundaries planned for 2004. New boundaries are not a problem themselves, but they make comparisons between datasets problematic.

There are many methods of areal interpolation and, arguably, a better estimate of people's exposure levels within an ED can be obtained if information pertaining to the populations' location within the ED is utilized rather than disregarded. For continuous data (in this example, air pollution) more information is lost because of aggregation than in the case of discrete data (Haining, 2003). No detail on the variability in pollution values within an ED can be derived from just the mean pollution value of the ED.

Within environmental epidemiology, exposure-disease relationships derived using aggregate data are conceived frequently as weaker forms of analysis due to the problems associated with ecological inference. Some of the issues associated with ecological studies are discussed in Chapter 2, but space precludes detailed treatment of the problems associated with ecological inference (including the ecological fallacy) and the modifiable areal unit problem (MAUP). For a fuller review of these problems, see Haining (2003). However, aggregate analyses may be useful in helping to identify valid hypotheses that may be followed up with other forms of epidemiological research.

Frequently, we are interested in pollution exposure levels of individuals. As individuals, we exhibit extremely complex patterns of behavior as we move within both space and time. Dispersion modeling of air pollution levels can never capture the full complexity of exposure levels: incorporating such dynamic components as when and where exercise occurs, modes of transport, and lung capacity to name just a selection of the variables that will affect the level to which people are affected by pollution levels.

Currently, we cannot continually monitor exposure levels of large numbers of people. One possibility may come with the advancement of mobile phones with access to the Internet and the ability to measure real-time positioning through global positioning systems (GPS). It may be possible for mobile phones to also monitor individual pollution exposures (Löytönen, 2001), also discussed in Chapter 17. For now, aggregate pollution values from complex dispersion modeling, such as that used in Sheffield, can provide some insight into people's pollution exposures.

ACKNOWLEDGMENTS

This research was funded by the NHS Executive Trent Research Scheme. The views expressed are those of the authors and do not necessarily reflect those of the funding organization. The authors wish to thank the Environmental Protection Service, Sheffield City Council for the provision of air pollution data. This work is based on data (digital ED boundaries) provided with the support of the Economic and Social Research Council and Joint Information Systems Committee and uses boundary material that is copyright of the Crown, the Post Office, and the ED-LINE Consortium.

References

Airborne Particle Expert Group, 1999, Department of the Environment, Transport and the Regions, the Welsh Office, the Scottish Office, and the Department of the Environment (Northern Ireland).

Ando, M. et al., 1996, Indoor and outdoor air pollution in Tokyo and Beijing supercities, *Atmospheric Environment,* 30, 5, 695–702.

Beattie, C. and Longhurst, J., 1999, Local air quality management: A best practice guide, Air Quality Management Resource Centre, University of the West of England.

Benarie, M.M., 1987, The limits of air pollution modelling, *Atmospheric Environment,* 21, 1, 1–5.

Bower, J.S. and Vallance-Plews, J., 1995, The UK National Air Monitoring Networks, paper presented at a WHO seminar, 21–23 November 1995.

Bracken, I. and Martin, D., 1989, The generation of spatial population distributions from census centroid data, *Environment and Planning A,* 21, 4, 537–543.

Briggs, D.J. et al., 1997, Mapping urban air pollution using GIS: A regression-based approach, *International Journal of Geographical Information Science,* 11, 7, 699–718.

Brindley, P. et al., 2004 (in press), Estimating Area Based Population Exposure to Pollution from Grid Based Model Results, *Computers, Environment and Urban Systems.*

Brown, J., Wasniewki, J., and Zlatev, Z., 1995, Running air pollution models on massively parallel machines, *Parallel Computing,* 21, 971–991.

Clarke, A.G., 1986, Chapter two: The air, in Hester, R.E., Ed., *Understanding Our Environment,* London: The Royal Society of Chemistry.

Collins, S., 1996, Modelling urban air pollution using GIS, in Craglia, M. and Couclelis, H., Eds., *Geographic Information Research: Bridging the Atlantic*, London: Taylor and Francis.

Collins, S., 1998, Modelling spatial variations in air quality using GIS, in Gatrell, A. and Löytönen, M., Eds., *GIS and Health*, London: Taylor and Francis.

Collins, S., Smallbone, K., and Briggs, D., 1995, A regression model for estimating small scale variations in air pollution, *Epidemiology,* 6, 4, S60.

Dabberdt, W.F. and Miller, E., 2000, Uncertainty, ensembles and air quality dispersion modelling: Applications and challenges, *Atmospheric Environment,* 34, 4667–4673.

Derwent, R.G. et al., 1995, Analysis and interpretation of air quality data from an urban roadside location in central London over the period from July 1991 to July 1992, *Atmospheric Environment,* 29, 8, 923–946.

DETR (Department of the Environment, Transport, and the Regions), 1998, *Review and Assessment: Selection and Use of Dispersion Models*, London: Stationery Office.

DETR (Department of the Environment, Transport, and the Regions), 2000, *Guidance for Review and Assessment: Monitoring Air Quality*, London: Stationery Office.

Dockery, D.W. et al., 1981, Relationships amongst personal, indoor and outdoor NO_2 measurements, *Environmental Interpretation,* 5, 101.

Dockery, D.W. et al., 1993, An association between air pollution and mortality in six U.S. cities, *The New England Journal of Medicine,* 329, 1753–1759.

Drakou, G. et al., 1998, Measurements and numerical simulations of indoor O_3 and NO_x in two different cases, *Atmospheric Environment,* 32, 4, 595–610.

Fischer, P.H. et al., 2000, Traffic-related differences in outdoor and indoor concentrations of particles and volatile organic compounds in Amsterdam, *Atmospheric Environment,* 34, 3713–3722.

Fisher, P.F. and Langford, M., 1995, Modelling the errors in areal interpolation between zonal systems by Monte Carlo simulation, *Environment and Planning A,* 27, 2, 211–224.

Flowerdew, R. and Green, M., 1989, Statistical methods for inference between incompatible zonal systems, in Goodchild, M. and Gopal, S., Eds., *Accuracy of Spatial Databases*, London: Taylor and Francis.

Flowerdew, R. and Green, M., 1990, Inference between incompatible zonal systems using the EM algorithm, North West Regional Research Laboratory: Research Report No. 6, University of Lancaster.

Flowerdew, R., Green, M., and Kehris, E., 1991, Using Areal Interpolation Methods in Geographic Information Systems, *Papers in Regional Science: The Journal of the RSAI,* 70, 3, 303–315.

Haining, R.P., 2003, *Spatial Data Analysis: Theory and Practice*, Cambridge: Cambridge University Press.

Hall, J.N., 1996, Assessing health effects of air pollution, *Atmospheric Environment,* 30, 5, 743–746.

Hedley, M. et al., 1997, Evaluation of an air quality simulation of the lower Fraser Valley — II: Photochemistry, *Atmospheric Environment,* 31, 11, 1617–1630.

Hewitt, C.N., 1991, Spatial variation in nitrogen dioxide concentration in an urban area, *Atmospheric Environment,* 25B, 429–434.

Hewitt, C.N. and Harrison, R.M., 1986, Chapter One: Monitoring, in Hester, R.E., Ed., *Understanding Our Environment*, London: The Royal Society of Chemistry.

Hoek, G. et al., 2002, Association between mortality and indicators of traffic-related air pollution in The Netherlands: A cohort study, *Lancet*, 360, 1203–1209.

Johnson, G.T. and Hunter, L.J., 1999, Some insights into typical urban canyon airflows, *Atmospheric Environment,* 33, 3991–3999.

Kühlwein, J. and Friedrich, R., 2000, Uncertainties of modelling emissions from road transport, *Atmospheric Environment,* 34, 4603–4610.

Künzli, N. et al., 2000, Public-health impact of outdoor and traffic related air pollution: A European assessment, *Lancet,* 356, 795–801.

Lee, H.S. et al., 1997, Relationship between indoor and outdoor air quality during the summer season in Korea, *Atmospheric Environment,* 31, 11, 1689–1693.

Lee, S.C. and Chang, M., 2000, Indoor and outdoor air quality investigation at schools in Hong Kong, *Chemosphere,* 41, 109–113.

Leicester City Council, 2000, Leicester air quality review and assessment, http://www.leicester.gov.uk/sys_upl/documents/departments/dpt_18.pdf, accessed 3 March 2004.

Lena, F. and Desiato, F., 1999, Inter-comparison of nocturnal mixing height estimate methods for urban air pollution modelling, *Atmospheric Environment,* 33, 2385–2394.

Löytönen, M., 2001, Mobile devices and GIS in health: New opportunities and threats, keynote address at Geographic Information Sciences in Public Health, 19–20 September 2001, Sheffield, England, http://www.shef.ac.uk/gis-unit/newpages/conferencehomepage.htm, accessed 3 March 2004.

Mukherjee, P., Viswanathan, S., and Choon, L.C., 2000, Modeling mobile source emissions in presence of Stationery sources, *Journal of Hazardous Materials,* A76, 23–37.

National Atmospheric Emissions Inventory, 1998, Regional pollutants, http://www.aeat.co.uk/netcen/airqual/emissions/den-naei.html, accessed 1 May 2003.

National Travel Survey, 1999, *National Travel Survey 1997/99 Update*, London: The Stationery Office.

Peace, H.V., Parkin, J., and Nwagboso, C., 1998, Development of a model, based on observations to predict roadside emissions from traffic flow data, *Traffic Engineering and Control UK,* 39, 11, 620–624.

Pope, C.A., 2000, Epidemiology of fine particulate air pollution and human health: Biologic mechanisms and who's at risk? *Environmental Health Perspectives,* 108, 4, 713–723.

Pope, C.A. et al., 1995, Particulate air pollution as a predictor of mortality in a prospective study of U.S. adults, *American Journal of Respiratory and Critical Care Medicine,* 151, 669–674.

Raper, J.F., Rhind, D.W., and Shepherd, J.W., 1992, *Postcodes: The New Geography,* Harlow, U.K.: Longman.

Rhind, D.W., 1991, Counting the people: The role of GIS, in Maguire, D.J., Goodchild, M.F., and Rhind, D.W., Eds., *Geographical Information Systems, Volume 2: Principles and Applications*, New York: Longman.

Sadahiro, Y., 1999, Accuracy of areal interpolation: A comparison of alternative methods, *Journal of Geographical Systems,* 1, 4, 323–346.

Schmidt, M. and Schäfer, R., 1998, An integrated simulation system for traffic induced air pollution, *Environmental Modeling and Software,* 13, 295–303.

SMHI, 2000, Indic-Airviro: Air quality management, technical profile of version 2.21.

Theurer, W., 1999, Typical building arrangements for urban air pollution modelling, *Atmospheric Environment,* 33, 4057–4066.

Tirabassi, T., 1999, New directions: Listening out for urban air pollution, *Atmospheric Environment,* 33, 4219–4220.

Valerio, F. et al., 1997, Preliminary evaluation, using passive tubes, of carbon monoxide concentrations in outdoor and indoor air at street level shops in Genoa (Italy), *Atmospheric Environment,* 31, 17, 2871–2876.

Veal, A.T. and Appleby, R.S., 1997, Comparison of ADMS urban and Indic-Airviro regional scale dispersion models, Working Group for DOE, http://www.bham.ac.uk/geography/met/task1.htm, accessed 1 May 2003.

Watkins, L.H., 1991, *Air Pollution from Road Vehicles*, London: HMSO.

Wong, T.W. et al., 1999, Air pollution and hospital admissions for respiratory and cardiovascular diseases in Hong Kong, *Occupational and Environmental Medicine,* 56, 10, 679–683.

Zannetti, P., 1990, *Air Pollution Modelling*, Boston: Computational Mechanics Publications.

9 Health and Environment Information Systems

Paul Aylin and Samantha Cockings

CONTENTS

9.1 INTRODUCTION

The effect of the environment on human health is an increasingly important issue in the political, public, and scientific arenas. Reports of disease clusters associated with environmental sources can cause great public anxiety and need to be handled sensitively and effectively. The investigation of such concerns in a timely manner requires the integration of systems, data, and expertise within short timescales.

The Small Area Health Statistics Unit (SAHSU) at Imperial College, London, has developed a tool that helps in the initial stages of such investigations. The Rapid Inquiry Facility has been developed to establish rapidly if the observed numbers for an apparent cluster are greater than would be expected for a given population.

0-415-30655-8/04/$0.00+$1.50

Environment-health relationships may operate at a range of scales, from the local to the international. As such, it is important that systems, data, and expertise be shared between and within these scales. The aim of the European Health and Environment Information System (EUROHEIS) project is to improve understanding of the links between environmental exposures, health outcomes, and risk through the development of integrated information systems for rapid assessment of relationships between the environment and health at a geographical level in various European countries.

This chapter focuses on integrated systems for the rapid initial assessment of apparent disease clusters. Illustrated by the U.K. Rapid Inquiry Facility, it describes some of the issues surrounding the establishment of similar systems in other European countries, drawing on experiences from the EUROHEIS project.

9.2 THE U.K. RAPID INQUIRY FACILITY

SAHSU holds national cause-specific data on deaths, births, cancer registrations, hospital admissions, and congenital anomalies, using the postcode of residence to locate cases to within 10 to 100 meters. Each record represents an event occurring to an individual and includes date of birth, sex, cause, or procedure, and, most crucially, a georeference in the form of a postcode. In 2000, there were around 1.6 million residential postcodes in use in the U.K. containing, on average, around 14 unique addresses each.

Denominator data is currently obtained from the 1991 Census at enumeration district (ED) level for age and sex in five-year age bands. Using annual births and deaths and a migration factor based on the estimate for the whole health authority, mid-year ED population estimates have been derived up to 2000 (Arnold et al., 1999).

SAHSU also holds a range of geographical, socioeconomic, and environmental data, all of which are geographically referenced. Using in-house database, statistics, and GIS technology and expertise, these datasets can be integrated, analyzed, and displayed. The resultant store of data is large (as shown in Table 9.1) and requires substantial hardware to cope with the analysis.

The Rapid Inquiry Facility was originally developed in the mid-1990s (Aylin et al., 1999), with the aim of facilitating the calculation of disease risk around a point source of pollution. A customized system was developed, based around the SAHSU database. The system was able to calculate, relatively rapidly, the indirectly standardized mortality ratio (SMR) (Breslow and Day, 1987) and the standardized incidence ratio (SIR), by dividing the observed number of health events by the expected number (calculated based on a set of reference rates). Reference rates were precalculated for speed, using rates from the U.K. Standard Region within which the study area was located as the reference. Using the Carstairs index (Carstairs and Morris, 1991), disease risks were also adjusted to allow for the potential confounding effect of deprivation. The Carstairs index is a small area deprivation measure derived from U.K. Census variables — overcrowding, access to a car, unemployment, and social class of head of household — that has been shown to be strongly predictive of mortality and cancer incidence (Jolley et al., 1982).

TABLE 9.1
Data Held at the Small Area Health Statistics Unit in 2002

Dataset	Years	Years	No. Records	Total (Mb)
Cancer	1974–1998	25	6,783,072	1,218
Births	1981–2000	18	14,400,364	1,426
Deaths	1981–2000	18	12,657,648	1,664
	Hospital Admissions			
England (HES)	1992–1999/2000	7	76,421,934	20,500
Scotland	1992–1999/2000	7	5,740,948	772
Wales (PEDW)	1991–2000	9	7,241,139	1,420
Northern Ireland (HIS)	1991/2–1994/5	4	1,566,000	357
Populations	1981, 1991 census		1,672,000	472
Socioeconomic variables	1981, 1991 census		1,971,000	103
Postcode data			2,041,000	688
Geographical data	[GIS datasets]			5,000
Other data				18,000

Note: HES = Hospital Episode Statistics; PEDW = Patient Episode Database for Wales; HIS = Hospital Information System.

For estimating the risk surrounding a point source, concentric bands (usually of radius two kilometers and seven and a half kilometers) were drawn around the source (specified either as a national grid reference or as a postcode that was then converted to a grid reference). The EDs that had their population-weighted centroid falling within the bands were then selected to form the study area and the risk was calculated for each of the bands. To acknowledge sampling variability, 95 percent confidence intervals for these risks were also calculated. The system could also generate contextual maps of the study area, together with basic disease maps. A description of the SAHSU approach to the analysis of data around point sources and more general geographical epidemiology can be found elsewhere (Elliott and Wakefield, 2000; Elliott et al., 1995) and in Chapter 7.

The version of the Rapid Inquiry Facility described above and in Aylin et al. (1999) was fairly restrictive for users as it was developed within a UNIX environment and required that they acquire a number of software packages and development tools, including Tcl/Tk, Oracle® PL/SQL™, ArcInfo™ AML, C, and HTML. A key part of the EUROHEIS project (described in more detail below) was to make the Rapid Inquiry Facility more generic so that users from other countries would be able to adapt and implement the system. The latest version (Cockings and Jarup, 2002), therefore, employs two relatively common and affordable software packages — ArcView® 3.2 and Oracle9i™ (a copy of Oracle Personal is sufficient) and the code has been written more generically to enable it to operate on datasets that are in the appropriate, prespecified format. The Rapid Inquiry Facility is now platform independent and more exportable for other users. Additional functionality has also been developed, including the ability to calculate directly standardized rates

(MacMahon and Trichopoulos, 1996) and extended output options such as the generation of contextual and disease maps in .jpg and .wmf format and tabular or text-based output in .html or comma-separated format. A further additional feature is the production of smoothed maps of disease risk. For small area disease mapping, large differences in health risk between small areas may arise simply due to chance, even when several years of data are used. This is particularly true when the numbers of cases are small (e.g., typically, an electoral ward will have fewer than 10 deaths from heart disease in the under-75 age group per year). The system applies empirical Bayesian smoothing (Clayton and Kaldor, 1987) to the risk estimates giving a more robust estimate of the true ward relative risks than the raw SMRs. Further details of the functionality, methodology, and system architecture of the latest version of the U.K. Rapid Inquiry Facility can be found in Cockings and Jarup (2002).

9.3 EUROPEAN HEALTH AND ENVIRONMENT INFORMATION SYSTEMS

The EUROHEIS project was conceived in 1999 as a natural extension to the Rapid Inquiry Facility project. Its aim was to improve understanding of the links between environmental exposures, health outcomes, and risk through the development of an integrated information system for the rapid assessment of spatial relationships between the environment and health. Its objectives were to develop further the U.K. Rapid Inquiry Facility system and to make its underlying concepts, methods, and techniques available to other countries. A further aim was to share expertise in the field. Partners from seven countries collaborated on the project (Table 9.2). (The National Institute of Public Health and the Environment (RIVM) in the Netherlands also joined in 2002 as a nonfunded partner.)

The European Commission, Directorate-General Health and Consumer Protection, Luxembourg funded the project under the program Action on Pollution-Related Diseases. It was constructed as a three-year program, comprising a feasibility study in year one (2000), an implementation phase in year two (2001 to 2002), and an evaluation phase in year three (2002 to 2003). This section presents results from the feasibility phase and discusses early reflections on the implementation phase.

TABLE 9.2
EUROHEIS Partners

Partner	Country
SAHSU, Dept. Epidemiology and Public Health, Imperial College	United Kingdom
National Board of Health	Denmark
National Public Health Institute	Finland
Trinity College, University of Dublin	Ireland
WHO European Center for Environment and Health, Rome	Italy
Dept. Statistics and Operation Research, University of Valencia	Spain
Dept. Epidemiology, Stockholm Center of Public Health	Sweden

9.4 REQUIREMENTS FOR HEALTH AND ENVIRONMENT INFORMATION SYSTEMS

The feasibility stage of the EUROHEIS project involved the definition of a set of data requirements for the development of integrated systems in different countries and the consideration of a range of issues associated with their implementation, including political and organizational feasibility, data access and confidentiality issues, and technical requirements.

9.4.1 Data Requirements

Informative analysis using a Rapid Inquiry Facility system requires the availability of data of a suitable quality. These requirements have already been discussed in detail elsewhere (Cockings and Jarup, 2002), thus only a brief overview is given here. Five main types of data may be identified:

1. Health
2. Denominator
3. Socioeconomic
4. Environmental
5. Geographical

A variety of health datasets may be available within different countries; typical examples include mortality registrations, cancer registrations, hospital admissions, and congenital malformations. These datasets are all routinely collected within the United Kingdom. Nonroutinely collected datasets could also feasibly be used. The key requirements are a diagnostic code, date of event, age, and sex of the person (or mother in the case of birth-related events), and some form of georeferencing.

To calculate rates of diseases or health events within geographical areas it is necessary to be able to calculate the denominator population. Denominator data are usually obtained from population data, but for some health events, an alternative denominator is more appropriate. For hospital admissions it is sometimes more meaningful to use total admissions as a denominator rather than total population. It is important to remember that any inaccuracies in estimating the denominator will affect the disease rate estimates. Denominator datasets must contain a date (to indicate when they were collected or modeled), they must be broken down by age and sex (to enable age-sex specific rates to be applied), and they must be geographically referenced. In some instances, individual level denominator data may be available; in others, only aggregated data will be available.

Variations in socioeconomic characteristics at the individual and group level frequently show strong correlations with both health and environmental factors, but the relevance of different factors varies between countries. For example, in the United Kingdom, in the context of point-source investigations and disease and exposure mapping, deprivation is the most commonly used measure of socioeconomic status of individuals or groups. Usually this is assessed by using some form of score such as the Carstairs index (Carstairs and Morris, 1991) or the Townsend index (Townsend et al., 1988), which combines different factors thought to be indicators of deprivation, such as social class and overcrowding. In Finland, people's occupations have been shown to be a useful measure of socioeconomic status relative to health (Pukkala, 1995). Whereas in Denmark, education is one of the most important variables for such studies (Lissau et al., 2001).

The environmental exposures of concern vary in different countries and through time. For example, in the United Kingdom, current concerns include traffic-related air pollution, point-source emissions (e.g., from industrial activities or incineration), electromagnetic fields, landfill and waste sites, and drinking water quality (e.g., disinfection by-products). In the wake of the bovine spongiform encephalitis (BSE) crisis, food-borne exposures are also a major focus of concern. In Spain, environmental concerns are focused on drinking water quality and air pollution. Intensive agricultural activities tend to disseminate chemical contaminants, but industrial and tourist activities are producing an excess of water consumption that tends to impoverish water resources. In main Spanish cities, air pollutants such as black smoke, total suspended particles, NO_2, SO_2, and CO are of concern for their effects on health.

The assessment of a causal relationship between a health outcome and an environmental factor is extremely problematic. Measuring individual-level exposure is rarely feasible due to its costly and time-consuming nature and because of the ethical and confidentiality issues involved. Even if individual-level exposure data are available, it is still difficult to prove a causal relationship. In countries such as the United Kingdom and the United States, confidentiality issues also restrict the availability of individual-level health outcome data. Instead, many investigations are forced to employ group level data and to undertake ecological studies. Ecological studies cannot prove causal relationships, but they may suggest associations between environmental factors and health outcomes. In such ecological studies, environmental data should be of the highest possible spatial resolution and should ideally be validated using measured data from a sample of individuals. When estimating or modeling exposure, the long latency periods associated with many of the diseases of importance in today's Western societies should be taken into account and, where possible, information on migration should be obtained to inform the exposure assessment and to aid the interpretation of results.

Many environment-health investigations use data aggregated by geographical area. This may be through choice (because it is believed that there are explicit area-level effects in operation or because decisions are needed at an area level to aid policy implementation) or through necessity when individual level data are not available (usually due to confidentiality constraints). Often, these units reflect administrative boundaries or data collection units, rather than the spatial distribution of the underlying phenomena. Interpretation should always be undertaken with this in mind. A further problem is that different datasets are often only available for non-matching sets of geographical units. Interpolation is therefore necessary to integrate the datasets onto a common set of geographical units. Again, the assumptions made in such interpolations must be borne in mind at the interpretation stage. The data requirements depend on the units selected and on the degree of interpolation required, but usually involve at least the following:

- Digital boundaries of the different geographical units
- Centroids of the geographical units (ideally population-weighted)
- Look-up tables linking the various geographical units

GIS techniques are invaluable for transferring data between sets of nonmatching geographical units. For example, grid-referenced address-based health data can be aggregated into grid squares using point-in-polygon techniques or exposure data for water supply zones can be interpolated onto another set of geographical units according to the proportion of each water supply zone's area falling within each unit (area-weighted interpolation).

9.4.2 Political and Organizational Feasibility

The organizational framework required to implement and use a Rapid Inquiry Facility as part of the decision-making process depends on the proposed usage of the system. A Rapid Inquiry Facility may be used in a number of ways, from responding to infrequent inquiries on an ad hoc basis to using the system for some sort of regular surveillance. Whatever the scale of implementation and precise purpose, the successful use of such systems for decision making requires the development of a network of key agencies and individuals involved in the investigation of relationships between the environment and health. According to Cockings and Jarup (2002), organizations likely to be involved include:

- The national bodies responsible for health and the environment
- Regional and local health authorities
- Local authorities
- Census agencies
- National statistics offices
- National, regional, and local health registries
- National mapping agencies
- Private data suppliers
- Academic, research, and quasi-public institutions

Ideally, these organizations need to be involved not only in the setting up of such systems, but also in their development and support so that data quality, methodological issues, and interpretation of results can be discussed as part of a continuous dialogue. Ideally, a team of skilled and experienced specialists in epidemiology, public health, spatial statistics, geography, GIS, environmental science, and IT is needed to support and develop these systems.

9.4.3 Data Access and Confidentiality Issues

In many countries, concerns over disclosure control mean that individual-level health and health-related data are frequently not available. Instead, the data are spatially aggregated to an area sufficient to guarantee confidentiality. The problem is that if this area is too large it will limit the usefulness of any analysis, especially for informing policy.

The purpose behind a Rapid Inquiry Facility system is to provide rapid initial assessment of potential links between the environment and health. This requires either that the various datasets are obtained from the data providers and integrated into one georeferenced system in one organization (as in the United Kingdom at SAHSU) or that the datasets can be rapidly and efficiently queried across some form of network or Internet connection. Confidentiality concerns, security considerations, dataset sizes, and ownership issues will all influence whether the datasets are held centrally or by individual organizations. A further consideration is that the integration of the datasets into one central database in one location enables the cross-referencing and crosschecking of the different datasets. Experience in the United Kingdom has shown the usefulness of this through the identification of various systematic errors in the georeferencing and coding of various datasets (as provided by the data providers). This sort of added value is a distinct advantage of having a Rapid Inquiry Facility based in one location.

9.4.4 Technical Requirements

The U.K. Rapid Inquiry Facility employs two types of software: a database management system (DBMS) and a GIS. The DBMS provides database functions, including querying and indexing, which enable the efficient searching for and retrieval of records, together with the calculation of statistics. GIS provides the ability to overlay the various georeferenced datasets and to undertake spatial analysis. In particular, it provides the means of defining areas of exposure and of identifying populations at risk. It also provides the facility for producing maps and for carrying out visual exploratory spatial data analysis. Although it is true that most GIS incorporate significant database management functions, if the datasets involved are large and if the system is to be used in a multiuser environment, then the database functions of the GIS alone may be insufficient and a dedicated DBMS may be preferable (in conjunction with GIS).

9.5 EUROHEIS PARTNER EXPERIENCES

Most of the EUROHEIS partners have gone on either to implement the U.K. Rapid Inquiry Facility or to build different systems based on the U.K. experience. This section reports briefly on some of their experiences.

9.5.1 Sweden and Spain

Sweden and Spain have implemented the U.K. version of the Rapid Inquiry Facility with some modifications. In particular, the Spanish version of the Rapid Inquiry Facility has been installed in two settings:

1. *Stand-alone PC*: Requiring the inclusion of Oracle and ArcView packages jointly with the Rapid Inquiry Facility on a stand-alone PC running Windows® 2000 operating system.

2. *Rapid Inquiry Facility satellites of a central database*: Where many PCs are connected to the central Oracle database held on a UNIX server. Data are generated and updated in this central database while individual Rapid Inquiry Facility packages are installed on different PCs.

Gathering, cleaning, and reformatting datasets to the required Rapid Inquiry Facility formats have proven to be time-consuming jobs, but a library of Oracle scripts has been developed for undertaking similar tasks in the future. Additional work has been required on the Avenue (scripting language for ArcView) scripts provided by the U.K. partner to adapt them for use with local data formats. Intensive exchange between technical staff from all partner countries has resulted in practical improvements for the future and has been a positive learning experience for all involved.

Many of the current environment-health concerns in Spain are related to exposure to different contaminants that, although spatially distributed, are not necessarily associated with a simple, definable point source of pollution. The Spanish partner has therefore extended the methodological functionality of the standard Rapid Inquiry Facility program by adding a new option that accepts levels of exposure as a covariate in the analysis, rather than defining exposure by distance to a source.

9.5.2 Finland

Prior to its participation in the EUROHEIS project, Finland had already developed a Rapid Inquiry Facility style system of its own, called the SMASH (Small Area Statistics on Health) system (Kokki et al., 2001). This system has been modified in collaboration with the EUROHEIS group. The Rapid Inquiry Facility system is also being implemented alongside the SMASH system and a comparison between the two systems will be made during the final phase of the EUROHEIS project.

9.5.3 Denmark

The integrated Rapid Inquiry Facility model developed in the United Kingdom has been the inspiration for the development of a system for investigating environment-health relationships in Denmark. Less restrictive confidentiality constraints mean that it is possible to develop a more comprehensive model in Denmark. The underlying health registers contain individual-level data that can be linked with geocoded addresses and datasets holding information on population, the environment, and the socioeconomic characteristics of individuals. The information system is being developed using ArcView 8i and database DB2 8i. The aim is to create a Web-based information system with different levels of users and different levels of authorization. The interface will be linked to the database, which will be updated periodically to ensure that the system does not lose its immediacy.

It is intended that the initial development of the system will be based on standard reports and disease mapping. The next step will be Web-based standard reports and the usage of disease mapping facilities. Finally, if a proper level of security can be obtained, the system will be accessible for different user groups with a possibility of user-defined reporting facilities. The user group will be limited to persons with the professional background and capability to handle and analyze the data.

Development of the system is based on close cooperation with a number of specialists within the fields of medicine and environment. It is seen of vital importance that the system is based on data of high quality and that methods and models are correctly incorporated in the system.

9.5.4 Italy

The Italian partner has been exploring the possibility of using the Rapid Inquiry Facility for health impact assessment. The results indicate that it is feasible to apply methods that allow the estimation of attributable risk with appropriate treatment of several sources of systematic and random error. The methods have been explored and tested, using real data from a participating country. Results suggest that it is possible to develop a tool that can be used in conjunction with data on environment and health to assist health professionals involved with health impact assessment. The tool could facilitate the evaluation of the public health implications, allow effective communication with the general public and decision makers alike, and, ultimately, assist in the development of appropriate policies.

9.5.5 United Kingdom

Further experience within the United Kingdom has revealed several limitations. The system was originally devised to facilitate rapid assessment of disease risk, automating much of the work that previously had to be carried out manually. To provide this rapid turnover of reports, few checks are made on the validity of the data and the reports are provided with this in mind. For instance, checks are made neither on the accuracy of postcodes within the study area nor on the accuracy of disease coding. In larger studies, where large areas are aggregated, a small percentage of inaccurate postcodes are unlikely to be a significant problem. The problem is that such errors are usually systematic and location-specific (e.g., due to the repostcoding of an area) and hence may give rise to significant errors in exposure classification or missed disease events in a specific locality.

There are further concerns regarding the interpretation of data. Currently, a summary document highlighting significant findings and a page of warnings on data quality are provided alongside the results from a Rapid Inquiry Facility inquiry. Generally, the local knowledge required to interpret such reports lies with the person who commissioned the study and SAHSU can add little to that local knowledge. There have been calls for greater interpretation, but this would inevitably result in an increase in the cost of the inquiries and may not be desirable scientifically. Alternatively, there have been suggestions that the tables should be provided alone with only the normal cautions provided.

9.6 THE FUTURE

The future role of the Rapid Inquiry Facility in the United Kingdom merits serious discussion. Although there are issues surrounding data quality at a local level and the interpretation of findings, the Rapid Inquiry Facility would appear to be a useful tool for public health practitioners. The Rapid Inquiry Facility is still in development and it is hoped to enhance it to respond more flexibly to increasingly complex requests relating to point and area sources and to small area disease mapping.

The lowest level of resolution of a study is currently the ED level. However, developments allowing for postcode-level analysis would give a much better resolution for point-source studies. This is not without significant challenges, including the need to apportion or disaggregate all denominator data down to postcode level. Because postcodes are phased in and out and their geographical location may change through time, there is an important temporal element to consider when using postcode level analysis. This has not really been explored in current environment-health analyses in the United Kingdom. Moreover, postcode level analysis will require an improvement in the performance of the Oracle database because it will involve a 300-fold increase in the denominator data to be referenced. Database design and tuning will therefore be an important issue.

A major advance in the interpretation of the Rapid Inquiry Facility output would be the identification of areas where data quality is known to be poor, through inaccurate denominators, poor numerator coding, or poor georeferencing. This could be aided with a more formal metadata structure to include some form of data quality indicators.

Finally, the possibility of making the current code (but not the underlying data) freely available to public health practitioners is being investigated. This would allow professionals with the necessary software and hardware to run rapid inquiries on their own data. It is likely that this would also require the establishment of a help desk to support installation and running of the system in other locations, together with a training program and support courses.

9.7 CONCLUSIONS

This chapter has explained the concepts and methods underlying the U.K. Rapid Inquiry Facility and has outlined the aims and objectives of the EUROHEIS project. It has described the requirements for developing Rapid Inquiry Facility systems and has discussed some of the issues surrounding the establishment of such systems in other countries. Finally, it has reported on early results from the feasibility and implementation phases of the EUROHEIS project.

ACKNOWLEDGMENTS

We would like to thank the EUROHEIS lead partners: Juha Pekkanen, National Public Health Institute, Finland; Christina Reuterwall, Stockholm Center of Public Health, Sweden; Marco Martuzzi, WHO Environment and Health (Rome), Italy; Alan Kelly, Trinity College Dublin, Ireland; Anthony Staines, University College, Dublin, Ireland; Arne Poulstrup, National Board of Health, Denmark; Juan Ferrandiz, University of Valencia, Spain; Sylvia Richardson, INSERM, France (now at SAHSU).

The EUROHEIS project was funded by the European Commission Public Health Directorate DG SANCO/G under a program of community action on pollution-related diseases in the context of the framework for action in the field of public health (Grant Agreement Number SI2.291820 (2000CVG2–605)).

The Small Area Health Statistics Unit is funded by a grant from the Department of Health; Department of the Environment; Food and Rural Affairs; Environment Agency; Health and Safety Executive; Scottish Executive; Welsh Assembly Government; and Northern Ireland Department of Health, Social Service, and Public Safety. The views expressed in this publication are those of the authors and not necessarily those of the funding departments.

We are grateful to the Office for National Statistics for the provision of and permission to use their data. This work is based on data provided with the support of the ESRC and JISC and uses census and boundary material, which are copyright of the Crown, the Post Office, and the ED-LINE Consortium.

References

Arnold, R. et al., 1999, *Population Counts in Small Areas: Implications for Studies of Environment and Health,* London: The Stationery Office.

Aylin, P. et al., 1999, A national facility for small area disease mapping and rapid initial assessment of apparent disease clusters around a point source: The U.K. Small Area Health Statistics Unit, *Journal of Public Health Medicine*, 21, 3, 289–298.

Breslow, N. and Day, N.E., 1987, *Statistical Methods in Cancer Research Volume II: The Design and Analysis of Cohort Studies,* Scientific Publication No. 82, Lyon, France: International Agency for Research on Cancer.

Carstairs, V. and Morris, R., 1991, *Deprivation and Health in Scotland,* Aberdeen: Aberdeen University Press.

Clayton, D. and Kaldor, J., 1987, Empirical Bayes estimates of age-standardised relative risks for use in disease mapping, *Biometrics,* 43, 671–681.

Cockings, S. and Jarup, L., 2002, A European Health and Environment Information System for exposure and disease mapping and risk assessment (EUROHEIS), in Briggs, D.J. et al., Eds., *GIS for Emergency Preparedness and Health Risk Reduction,* Dordrecht: Kluwer Academic Publishers.

Elliott, P. and Wakefield, J.C., 2000, Bias and confounding in spatial epidemiology, in Elliott, P. et al., Eds., *Spatial Epidemiology: Methods and Applications,* Oxford: Oxford University Press.

Elliott, P., Martuzzi, M., and Shaddick, G., 1995, Spatial statistical methods in environmental epidemiology: A critique, *Statistical Methods in Medical Research,* 4, 149–161.

Jolley, D., Jarman, B., and Elliott, P., 1982, Socio-economic confounding, in Elliott, P et al., Eds., *Geographical and Environmental Epidemiology: Methods for Small-Area Studies,* Oxford University Press.

Kokki, E. et al., 2001, Small area estimation of incidence of cancer around a known source of exposure with fine resolution data, *Occupational Environmental Medicine*, 58, 315–320.

Lissau, I. et al., 2001, Social differences in illness and health-related exclusion from the labour market in Denmark from 1987 to 1994, *Scandinavian Journal of Public Health,* Suppl. 55, 19–30.

MacMahon, B. and Trichopoulos, D., 1996, *Epidemiology, Principles and Methods,* 2nd ed., New York: Little, Brown and Company.

Pukkala, E., 1995, *Cancer Risk by Social Class and Occupation: A Survey of 109,000 Cancer Cases among Finns of Working Age,* Basel: Karger.

Townsend, P., Phillimore, P., and Beattie, A., 1998, *Health and Deprivation: Inequality and the North,* London: Croom Helm.

Section 3

GIS Applications in Healthcare Planning and Policy

10 Health GIS in the English National Health Service: A Regional Solution

Ralph Smith

CONTENTS

10.1 INTRODUCTION

Much has been written on the application of GIS in public health practice in recent years, but rarely do commentators suggest an appropriate place in a health service for it to operate. This chapter argues for a regional setting where public health practitioners can fully utilize GIS.

A pollution incidence of regional proportions in 1995 led to the creation of the West Midlands Health GIS service. A release of powerful solvents into a tributary of the river Severn in Shropshire, England, led to the detection of minute proportions by the public in Worcester, many miles downstream. This led to a high-profile public health situation, with subsequent research not revealing any association between

0-415-30655-8/04/$0.00+$1.50

chemicals in the water supply and any symptoms experienced by Worcestershire residents (Fowle et al., 1996). During the early 1990s, digital geographic information and its associated technology had made little headway into the British health service (Cumins and Rathwell, 1991; Gould, 1992) at local or regional levels. With GIS being recognized by the regional director of public health as an appropriate technology to support such pollution incidents and the public health function in the West Midlands in general, a project was set up based in the regional cancer registry (where it still resides). The siting of the facility in the latter organization has proved to be strong evidence that a regional solution to GIS in the National Health Service (NHS) is a sensible one.

The strength of a regional health GIS service has to be assessed in the health service structure in which it operates. The British NHS is notorious for change, including the way it carves up countries geographically to administer a health service. Higgs and Gould (2001) document this succinctly when putting GIS in a health information context. At a national level in the 1990s, the next hierarchy down from the Department of Health in Government was a regional setup based on 13 regions, which over the years got whittled down to 9. As a parallel to this, within a region, for instance the West Midlands, healthcare commissioning was undertaken by health authorities, which numbered 22, 18, 15, and finally 13 over a period of 7 years. These authorities were the traditional home for health GIS, so with all the disruption of change and mergers, the application of geographic information (GI) to healthcare issues progressed slowly. However, regional institutions — Regional Health Authorities (RHA) and latterly NHS Executive Regional Offices — were more stable entities geographically. Mimicking this regional stability were cancer registries, which were coterminous with the original set of RHAs and indeed retained their geographic jurisdiction despite reorganization elsewhere. The picture painted above reveals several problems that a regional GIS service can overcome.

Expertise in GIS and the manipulation of geographic data are scarce, especially when applied to health and health-related data. Any such expertise will get diverted to more pressing duties as authorities get reorganized. A dedicated regional service based in a stable environment is more likely to survive and retain expertise.

Economies of scale can be exercised in terms of software, hardware, and data. Only recently has GIS software and hardware become affordable to small organizations. Often, health authorities could only prioritize purchasing geographic information that pertained to the population for which they were responsible. Many issues that face public health professionals mean that intelligence is needed way beyond the border of an authority. A regional service, adequately funded, can address these cross-border issues on behalf of, or in conjunction with, smaller health organizations. A regional service can purchase and maintain a set of basic geographic information because national datasets are now just as affordable as regional ones. All this has to be seen in the context of an absence (at the time of writing) of an agreement between the health service and Britain's national mapping agency (Ordnance Survey) concerning access to affordable geographic information.

Similar barriers exist to the full utilization of health event and health-related attribute datasets. Most of the vital health databases that are patient based are geographically referenced by full postcode (e.g., mortality, hospital admission, and cancer registrations) and are best accessed at a regional level. Furthermore, specialist health regional databases can often be higher in quality and more varied, such as those pertaining to the perinatal audit, breast screening quality assurance, and communicable disease. Access at a regional level encourages local collaboration and takes advantage of valuable local knowledge of the data.

A recent change in the structure of the NHS (Department of Health, 2001) has done away with the regional tier of the health service. The main public health function now resides in the primary care trust (PCT), and with over 300 of these in existence (in England), any public health GIS expertise will be diluted. A regionally based health GIS service is essential to maintain the use and interest in this technology, with the advent of the Public Health Observatory[1] movement promising to maintain a high profile for health GIS. English Public Health Observatories are now eligible to join the Pan Government Agreement for improved access to Ordnance Survey data, but they operate on small budgets. Their capacity to provide a thorough regional health GIS service will be limited. The place for a regional health GIS service is accentuated by the desire of all government organizations to work in a collaborative nature. Local government associations, government offices for the regions, regional development agencies, regional observatories, and even charities all utilize a regional framework in which to operate. If data sharing and multiagency working in pursuit of the public's well-being is going to be successful, a health GIS service has to operate at a regional scale.

10.2 REGIONAL APPLICATIONS OF HEALTH-BASED GIS

Higgs and Gould (2001) set out three broad examples of applications of health-based GIS:

1. Health outcomes and epidemiology
2. Overlap and intersection between health outcomes and healthcare delivery
3. Healthcare delivery

The three examples outlined below follow this broad classification and illustrate where the West Midlands Health GIS service has been able to use its regional remit to overcome some of the issues listed above and capitalize on the advantages of a regionally based service also described above.

10.2.1 HEALTH OUTCOMES AND EPIDEMIOLOGY: HEALTH AROUND A FOUNDRY

Acting as a complimentary service to local public health expertise, the West Midlands Health GIS service was able to augment an ecological study of respiratory disease experience of children around a source of air pollution (Olowokure et al., 2002a). This is a much-researched area offering many sophisticated solutions. However, a simple approach is often the most pragmatic for a public health department to assess

[1] Association for Public Health Observatories, http://www.pho.org.uk/, 30 January 2004.

a situation and satisfy the concerns of local residents. In Sandwell Health Authority, there had been historic concern surrounding an established foundry, with heightened concern over child respiratory health. The foundry in question had undergone a recent intervention to reduce emissions so a before-and-after study was conducted to establish the baseline respiratory health of the area and to assess if there had been a change following the intervention. By constructing concentric circles around the point source of emissions and then summarizing the prevailing wind as coming from the west, the easternmost bands of the circles could be used to capture population denominator information and the health events (Figure 10.1). The West Midlands Health GIS service was able to coordinate the people and the data vital to this study, with the respiratory health data coming from a hospital episode statistics safe haven project based in the West Midlands. Several health and local authorities were involved in the study so cross-border issues were addressed. The study found that after the intervention the respiratory health of 5 to 9 year olds had improved downwind of the foundry. Subsequent studies based on data from local schools were also supported, as the spatially referenced school questionnaire information easily integrated into the GIS framework (Olowokure et al., 2002b).

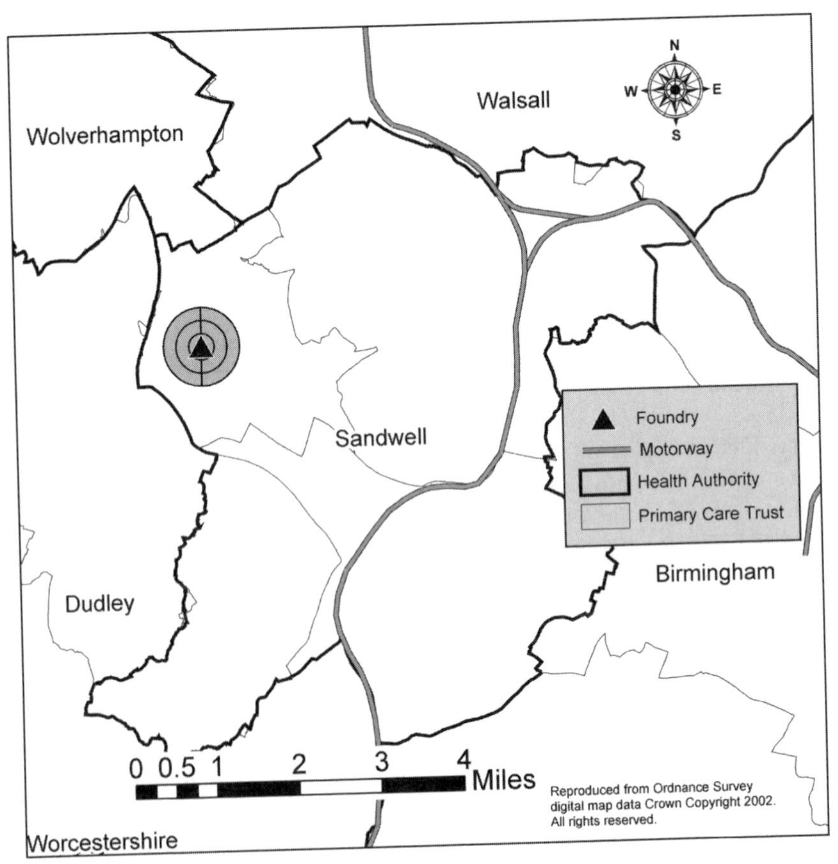

FIGURE 10.1 Position of foundry and concentric circles used in the analysis.

10.2.2 Overlap and Intersection between Health Outcomes and Healthcare Delivery: Health Needs Assessment

The NHS Plan proposed diagnostic and treatment centers (DTCs) (Department of Health, 2000a). They intend to act as new centers of excellence for elective treatment leaving hospitals capacity to cope with emergency procedures and thus reduce waiting times. The basis on which NHS local health economies bid for DTC funding was grounded in operational criteria. However, to make an informed choice on the best location for a scarce resource, managers were keen to assess the relationship between DTC and wider determinants of health including socio-economic factors.

Shifting the Balance of Power (Department of Health, 2001) for England created four directorates of health and social care (DHSC) (which have subsequently been abolished). The West Midlands was one of three health regions that made up the Midland DHSC and was in a position to capitalize on its geographic information databases and analytical expertise to provide intelligence on DTC bids across the directorate. The West Midlands Health GIS service was key in integrating hospital episode statistics derived day case rates (at a unit postcode level) and standard measures of deprivation to examine the hinterlands of the proposed DTC by thematically mapping small area information. There is a known inverse relationship between deprivation and the utilization of emergency hospital procedures so the pattern of deprivation around a DCT was essential knowledge.

More-sophisticated spatial analysis was available as the distance people traveled to proposed-DTCs was investigated by locating electoral wards within 5, 10, and 15 kilometers of a DTC and determining how many of the bidding hospital's patients were presently coming from those wards. The latter was an effort to identify a crude catchment area to assess if there was a genuine local pressure on existing sources: a situation that could be ameliorated by a successful bid for a DTC. The output of this geographic analysis was used in the process of deciding which bids to become DTC were successful.

Figure 10.2 illustrates the geography of directorates and the pattern of proposed DTC on a backdrop of small area deprivation.

10.2.3 Healthcare Delivery: Cancer Networks

As discussed in the introduction, health geographies vary and are subject to change over time. Keeping abreast of these ever-changing geographies can be made easier by using GIS mapping. Most health boundaries are made up of recognized administrative areas so it can be a relatively easy task to identify these and construct the unique health boundaries. In Great Britain, the Office for National Statistics is responsible for maintaining and disseminating the constitutions of health service areas. However, there are some health boundaries that apply to niche sections of the NHS that are poorly documented and thus their geographic relationship with complimentary health organizations is not fully understood.

The West Midlands Regional Health GIS service played a full part in constructing and visualizing the administrative boundaries of cancer networks. The latter were

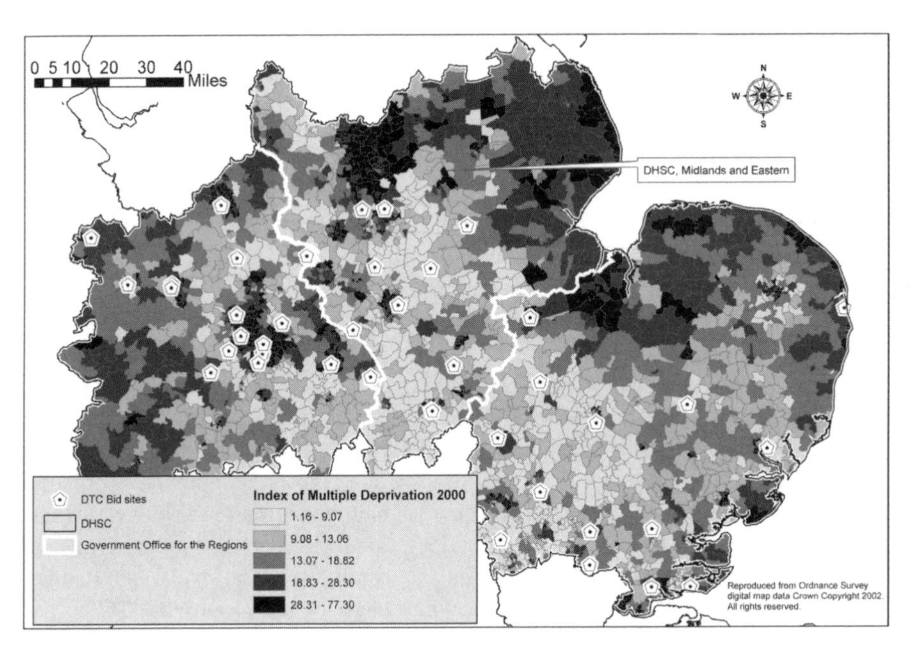

FIGURE 10.2 DTC bids in the DHSC, Midlands, and Eastern and the relationship with small area deprivation.

proposed in the NHS Cancer Plan (Department of Health, 2000b) as an organizational model for cancer services, based on the notion of managed networks of health services with the patient as the focus. This starting point inevitably means that any boundaries that can be drawn from such managed networks will have complex interactions with other geographies. As mentioned earlier, the PCT is currently the dominant health geography. In the West Midlands, the geographic information representing them has been constructed and maintained since the inception of primary care organizations. They proved to be valuable building blocks when it came to constructing a set of cancer network boundaries to provide valuable visualization to see how health agencies related to one another and as a means of constructing reference tables for population denominators. Cross-regional patient movement (and subsequent flows of information between regional organizations) was better understood through this work. Both local and regional agencies need to collaborate for the good of the cancer patient where cancer networks straddle regional boundaries. Figure 10.3 illustrates how cancer networks are managed outside the West Midlands health region but involve both PCTs and hospital trusts within the region. Other providers of cancer-related health services, such as breast screening unit areas (used to invite residents for screening) and hospices, can be added to a cancer network-based GIS project to explore the complex relationship needed to deliver the NHS Cancer Plan.

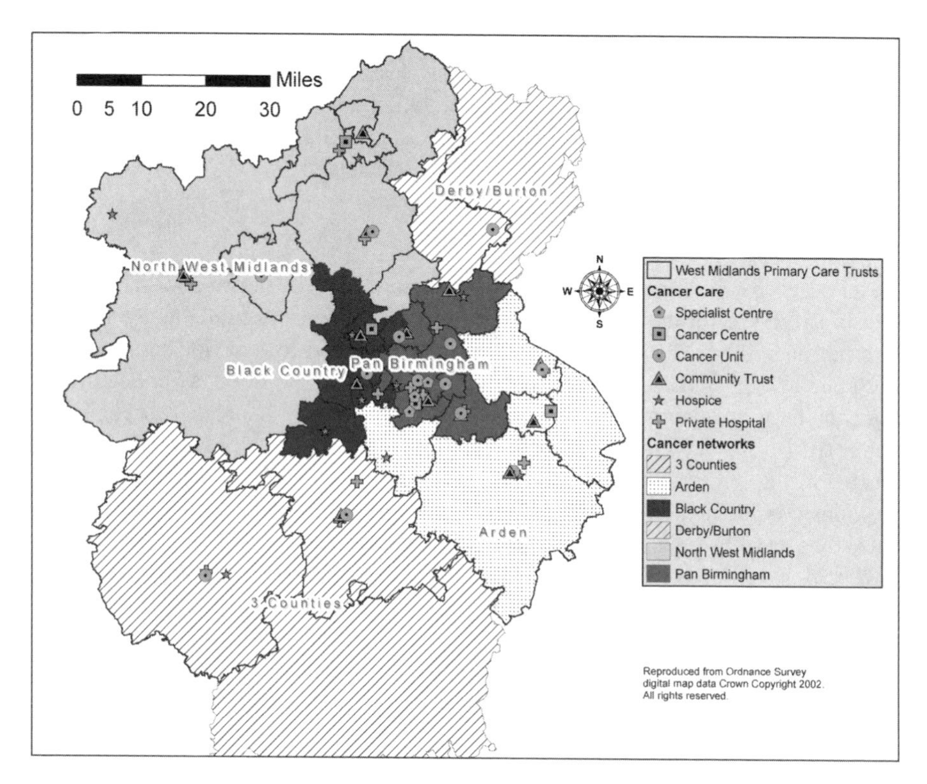

FIGURE 10.3 Cancer networks and cancer service in the West Midlands.

10.3 PUBLIC HEALTH INTERNET MAPPING

The first part of this chapter argued for a regional solution to the provision of a public health GIS service. The rapid advancements in Internet mapping and GIS have the ability to leapfrog the region as a natural setting and provide a national or more global picture. However, although the technology, digital boundaries, and methodology to query large national databases are more or less in place, consistent and timely databases will more often exist at a regional level. The development of regional data and intelligence Web portals with GIS functionality will help to prolong a regional approach to GIS in public health practice.

One of the main functions of public health GIS, that of descriptive health thematic mapping, is increasingly being provided over the Internet. Internet mapping and GIS are offered as solutions by almost all of the desktop GIS vendors, and customized solutions are available through Web-based programming languages.

Increasingly sophisticated Internet technology is being applied to the management and visualization of health and health-related data via the World Wide Web. Current sites addressing the location of health services and the management and dissemination of health statistics in the United Kingdom can be divided into three categories:

1. Those that identify location-based health services
2. Those that use geographic features to locate and access aggregate health event data in the user's locale (often, small area based)
3. Those that enable the integration and visualization of health services and statistics through the medium of thematic mapping

10.3.1 Identifying Location-Based Health Services

Despite geographic information not featuring in any NHS information policy, the flagship Web site for the NHS informs citizens on the services available by utilizing Internet mapping.[1] All NHS facilities can be referenced to their locations using a postcode, with the NHS Information Authority's Organisation Codes Service investing heavily in maintaining the positional accuracy of such resources. Its geographic potential is exploited when combined with topographic large-scale national mapping to inform the public on where NHS services are located. A third party presently provides this facility, as the NHS is unable to access affordable geographic digital data. The establishment of a framework to enable the provision of geographic information to NHS organizations, in the same way that central and local government enjoy, will take the utilization of health GIS a significant step forward.

10.3.2 Accessing Health Data through Geographic Selection

10.3.2.1 Primary Care

Health-related Internet mapping services in England that facilitate access to health data by geography include the National Database for Primary Care Groups and Trusts based at Manchester University.[2] With primary care being the focus of NHS service provision, information based on the relevant geography is vital. This site not only integrates disparate sources of data pertaining to primary care boundaries, it enables users to identify, quickly and intuitively, which datasets are related to their geographical area of interest. The service is backed up by a database project that is able to create unique nationwide primary care databases that have a spatial dimension. The Internet mapping technology can then be used to disseminate these data.

10.3.2.2 Neighborhood Statistics

The Neighbourhood Statistics Service (NeSS) from the U.K. Office for National Statistics provides a similar geographically based tool for users to pinpoint vital data by location (ONS, 2003). Following a review of information sources needed to address social exclusion issues, vital information was sourced and supplied based on standard geography via the Internet. Web-based GIS is used as a tool whereby basic geographic querying functionality is used to locate, integrate, and disseminate

[1] http://www.nhs.uk/, accessed 30 January 2004.

[2] National Primary Care Research and Development Centre, http://www.primary-care-db.org.uk/, accessed 30 January 2004.

national datasets. Although the health content is presently limited to hospital episode statistics and mortality, the site's strength is its integration of health-related variables that have strong links to the determinants of health. With NeSS now being the prime tool for the dissemination of the 2001 population census for England and Wales, the accompanying small area health-data holdings are also being expanded in areas such as life expectancy, smoking cessation, healthy lifestyles, and avoidable mortality (ONS, 2002).

The above two examples show how Internet mapping is acting as an enabling technology to disseminate standard national health databases and to improve accessibility to not only health professionals, but also the public and the wider research community. The ability to facilitate such open access will foster an understanding of health geographies, improve data sharing practices and metadata standards, and enhance the usability of geographic query tools.

10.3.3 Visualizing and Disseminating Health Data

Core GIS functionality such as thematic mapping, spatial integration of databases, and route or network analysis is now being enabled via Internet GIS. This provides useful tools for areas such as health needs assessment and target monitoring. Several services are establishing themselves to provide these functions.

10.3.3.1 Regional Internet Mapping

The MAIGIS (Multi-Agency Internet Geographic Information Service) project set out to integrate and supply health and health-related data to public health professionals and those concerned with public health issues in the West Midlands (Theseira, 2002). Using thematic mapping it has been able to bring together previously hard-to-obtain datasets and nationally collated information (such as that available at NeSS, see Section 10.3.2.2) in a common geographical framework. On top of this, administrative boundaries important to professionals in the West Midlands are available to put the data in context. Initially funded via the Department of Health Public Health Development Fund, this project will go on to establish an integrated service, complementing the West Midlands Public Health Observatory's information provision strategy.

10.3.3.2 Local Internet Mapping

In a similar vein to MAIGIS, the Community Health Information Profile[1] in north-west England focuses on the local scale to provide public health intelligence for the cities of Manchester, Salford, and Trafford (Community Health Information Profile, 2003). Relevance to and ownership by the community is at the heart of this project, with community and voluntary services representatives having a large part to play in deciding which health data are important (Moran and Butler, 2001). A subregional approach is taken here in addressing community profiles for three adjacent health economies. As well as core public health datasets, this site provides health and

[1] Community Health Information Profile, http://www.healthprofile.org.uk/, accessed 30 January 2004.

health-related geographies particular to the local area based initiatives (Health Action Zone and Single Regeneration Budget areas) and the location of basic health and related services available to communities such a pharmacies, doctors, leisure facilities, and unique community-derived databases. The Internet mapping technology allows customized report writing as well as thematic mapping.

10.4 SUMMARY AND CONCLUSIONS

The projects described in Section 10.2 carried out by the West Midlands Health GIS service provide evidence that a NHS-based healthcare GIS service is effective at the regional level. As well as complementing other regionally based partner organizations and data sources, a regional health GIS service can maintain and disseminate constantly changing health geographies, provide centralized GIS expertise, and complement local public health GIS capacity. Basic spatial epidemiology can be facilitated, as well as the integration of local, regional, and extraregional health event and geographic data. The power of spatial visualization can be used to understand complex regional and cross-regional interrelationships between NHS and private and community services that need to work together to deliver NHS policy.

The ability to visualize and disseminate health data using Internet mapping has led to greater care and preparation of the information. Standards concerning data manipulation and statistical reporting have been addressed and improved. Metadata concerning these data has also been prioritized as nonhealth professionals need to know where data are coming from and how they should be interpreted. It has highlighted the need for users to become more spatially aware and for Internet mapping providers to appreciate how users use and interpret their tools and data.

The proliferation of Internet mapping services providing health and health-related data will meet the basic information needs of professionals involved in public health practice. However, there remains a need for a regionally based health GIS service that can support or provide more-specialized facilities, advice, guidance, and customized geographic information to the region it serves.

References

Cumins, P. and Rathwell, T., 1991, *Geographical Information Systems and the National Health Service,* Association for Geographic Information (AGI): An Education, Training & Research Committee Publication.

Department of Health, 2000a, *NHS Plan,* London: Stationery Office.

Department of Health, 2000b, *NHS Cancer Plan,* London: Stationery Office.

Department of Health, 2001, *Shifting the Balance of Power,* London: Stationery Office.

Fowle, S.E. et al., 1996, An epidemiological study after a water contamination incident near Worcester, England, in April 1994, *Journal of Epidemiology and Community Health,* 50, 18–23.

Gould, M.I., 1992, The use of GIS and CAC by health authorities: Results from a postal questionnaire, *Area,* 24, 4, 391–401.

Higgs, G. and Gould, M.I., 2001, Is there a role for GIS in the "new NHS"? *Health and Place*, 7, 247–259.

Moran, R. and Butler, D.S., 2001, Whose health profile? *Proceedings of the First International Conference: Geographic Information Sciences in Public Health,* Sheffield, U.K.

Olowokure, B. et al., 2002a, Impact of an intervention to reduce outdoor air pollution on hospital admissions for asthma in children, *Journal of Epidemiology and Community Health,* 56, Suppl. II, A14.

Olowokure, B. et al., 2002b, Respiratory health in children downwind of an iron foundry, *Proceedings of the European Respiratory Society, Stockholm,* p. 206s.

ONS, 2002, *Neighbourhood Statistics: Focusing on Local Statistics,* Census Advisory Group Paper AG(02)16, http://www.statistics.gov.uk/census2001/advgroups.asp, accessed 3 March 2003.

ONS, 2003, Neighbourhood Statistics Service, http://www.neighbourhood.statistics.gov.uk/, accessed 3 March 2003.

Theseira, M., 2002, Using Internet GIS technology for sharing health and health related data for the West Midlands region, *Health and Place*, 8, 37–46; also http://maigis.wmpho.org.uk/, accessed 3 March 2003.

11 GIS in District Public Health Work

Edmund Jessop

CONTENTS

11.1 INTRODUCTION

This chapter gives examples of how GIS is currently used in district public health work. All but the last of these applications are within the reach of an ordinary public health department. They need no special resources beyond a standard personal computer, a basic mapping package, and people who are willing to learn. Staff members who have basic computer skills, especially with spreadsheets, can learn to use mapping packages fluently in two or three months. The cost of setting up a system is around £15,000: £2,000 for the hardware (including a good color printer) and about £4,000 to £5,000 each for the mapping package, the map data files, and some statistical analysis software.

Here, district is taken to mean public health work with populations of about 250,000 to 1,000,000. The functions of district public health departments change as health services are reorganized, but the basics remain the same: protecting the health of the local population and ensuring that local services are responding to health needs. The examples are drawn from West Surrey, an affluent district in southeast England.

GIS can display data or analyze data and it is convenient to separate these two uses. In the first three examples, GIS simply displays data.

0-415-30655-8/04/$0.00+$1.50

11.2 BOUNDARY MAPS

By far the most common request of anyone running GIS is "Can I have a map of...?" Such maps are necessary to sort out jurisdiction and responsibility, particularly when working with other agencies. Which social services department? Which housing authority?

Ironically, boundary maps are of less use, at least in the U.K. National Health Service, in identifying who has responsibility for health services. Hospital catchments have never been allocated geographically and, nowadays, primary healthcare responsibilities are assigned by choice of family doctor (GP), not by place of residence. Nonetheless, a broad indication of the coverage of primary care trusts and the location of hospitals remains the starting point for anyone wanting to understand local health services. The precise coverage of a GP practice or primary care trust could be displayed by mapping each patient's home postcode as a dot on a map, but in practice, there is little call for such maps.

Facilities such as hospitals and health centers can readily be shown on these maps, together with main roads. In general, GIS does not show street names. This limits their use in helping people to find the route to any particular facility – an old-fashioned street map works better. Interactive systems allow people to type in an address to find the nearest doctor, dentist, or walk-in clinic, but such systems are difficult to design and build.

Display maps have been used for 150 years to picture the spread of communicable disease. The geography of most outbreaks is obvious, but occasionally a map display is necessary, particularly if contamination of drinking water is suspected. A display that overlays the local water supply catchments on the cases of disease can quickly provide evidence to confirm or refute suspicions of waterborne disease. Snow's famous cholera maps are at http://www.ph.ucla.edu/epi/snow.html.

Bhopal et al. (1992) showed that sophisticated analyses could reveal unsuspected clusters of Legionnaires' disease. Cluster analysis is discussed further in Section 11.8.

11.3 AREA MAPS

Area maps show how health differs from place to place. Mortality maps are a popular feature of annual reports from directors of public health. These maps are typically based on electoral ward populations of about 10,000 people, which make them slightly problematical statistically. The area rates displayed purport to show the death rate of residents in each area, so the numerators are based on small numbers of events. In addition, the denominator populations are not known accurately — for example, reports published in 2001 will be reliant on 1991 census data. In practice, these maps serve their purpose: to display for public health action, not to analyze with statistical precision.

The Health for All database of the World Health Organization's European Region allows easy comparison of a range of international health data. All of this data can be downloaded freely from http://www.euro.who.int/eprise/main/WHO/InformationSources/Data/20011012-1. Looking at international comparisons may not seem like district public health work, but it is. The information is important for public health advocacy. For example, a display map of breast cancer mortality in countries in Europe shows why breast cancer is a particular priority for the United Kingdom.

This database also allows easy comparison of time trends in different countries. A striking comparison is the change in life expectancy for England versus Denmark over the past 30 years. The stagnation of health improvement in Denmark during the 1980s and early 1990s is all too plain. Healthy areas may need to be reminded that there is nothing inevitable about improvement in health.

11.4 SPIDER MAPS

District public health departments have a duty to check how well local organizations are serving the public. One aspect of this is the interplay between local hospitals, particularly in urban areas where more than one hospital may serve the same catchment population.

The approximate catchment area of a hospital can be displayed by drawing a line from the patient's home postcode to the hospital of treatment. The mapped data can be selected by specialty, calendar period, or any other data item. Where catchment zones overlap greatly, such displays help to start discussions about clinical collaboration between hospitals. An example of this type of map is shown in Figure 11.1.

These striking displays would look even better in color. One drawback is that the eye is drawn to the very long lines representing a handful of patients who have been admitted to hospital far away from their home address. These lines may simply

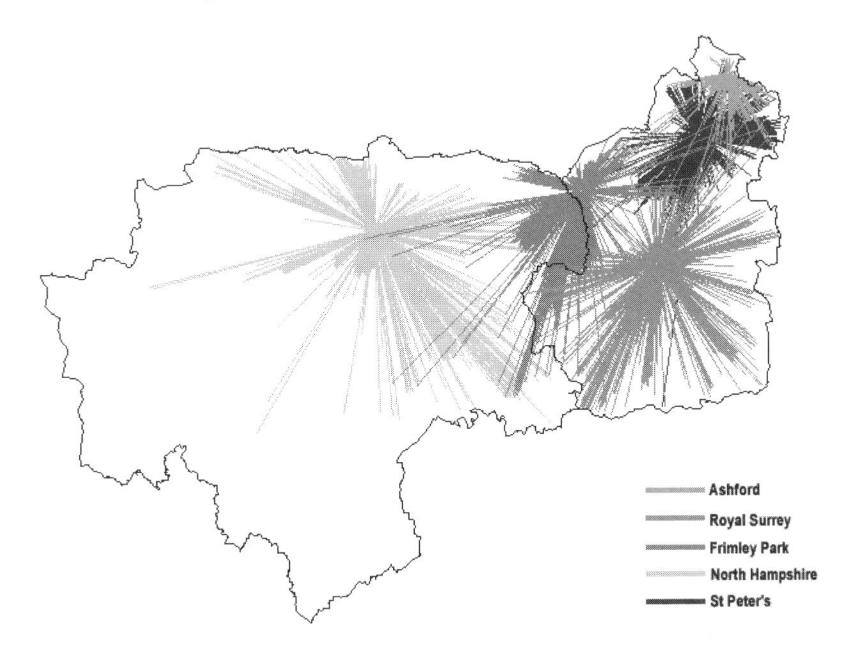

FIGURE 11.1 Admissions of West Surrey residents to local hospitals for general surgery, October 1998 to December 1998.

represent people who have fallen ill while staying away from home or on a shopping trip. Such rare events may reveal nothing about clinical practice or patient preference.

Hospital admission data uses a strong personal identifier — exact postcodes of residence for individual patients. One needs to assemble data from several hospitals to establish complete patterns of hospital use throughout an area. This raises problems of confidentiality.

In the next three examples (Section 11.5 to Section 11.7), GIS is used for analysis of spatial data. In each case, the task is to assess or improve the functioning of local health services.

11.5 TRAVEL TIME ZONES

Small hospitals face increasing difficulty in maintaining 24-hour cover for surgical emergency admissions. This translates quickly into public debate about A&E closure and concerns that patients may die before they can reach a hospital.

GIS provides a quick way to look at the effect of different A&E options. The first step is to decide on a standard for travel time. There is a belief (actually rather difficult to substantiate from the research literature) that surgical emergency patients must have their operation within a "golden hour" from the onset of symptoms. Time needs to be allowed for the ambulance to reach the patient; there is more delay in the hospital in getting that patient from the front door to the operating theater. In West Surrey, we thought that 30 minutes was a reasonable standard for the ambulance travel time. This ambulance drive time determines the location of surgical facilities.

Travel times are available in commercial packages such as MapInfo DriveTime™ software. The average speed can be specified. Historic data from Surrey Ambulance Service show that ambulances on emergency runs with sirens and flashing blue lights average 30 miles per hour under all conditions, even motorway gridlock (they use the hard shoulder).

By combining census data with GIS information on road travel times, one can readily count the number of people who live within 30 minutes by ambulance of various hospitals in the district. This permits a first assessment of the effect of different options for A&E closure. In principle, the calculations can be done manually, but the great ease of GIS encourages one to look at a much greater number of possible scenarios and options. In addition, the maps are generated electronically, which makes them easy to incorporate into documents and presentations (see Figure 11.2 for an example).

11.6 REGRESSION ANALYSES

Equity is an important goal in public health. We try to ensure that everyone has equal access to hospitals. Geographical equity implies that there is no variation in hospital admission rates from different parts of the district, except where justified by greater or lesser burdens of disease. Most illness is strongly associated with age and deprivation, so age and deprivation can be used as proxies for many diseases.

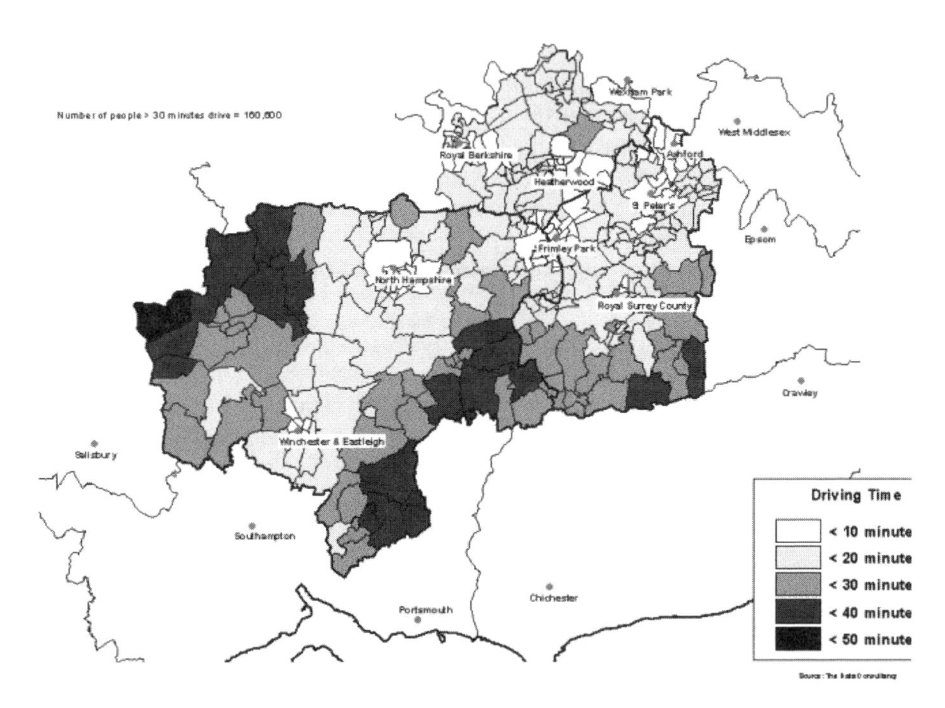

FIGURE 11.2 Mean drive times to the nearest hospital, all hospitals included. With permission of the West Surrey Health Authority.

Hence, the equity question can be written as follows: Are age-standardized admission rates from different parts of the district as predicted from their deprivation scores?

The multiple regression analysis needed to answer this question is complicated by the problem of spatial autocorrelation: adjacent areas tend to be similar to each other and so their data are correlated (Griffith, 1987). This contravenes the requirement for statistical independence in ordinary least squares regression. Standard techniques and statistical packages cannot make allowance for autocorrelation, but GIS can. We used ArcInfo™ and S-Plus® software with the geographical analysis module.

The GIS can be used to map the results of the regression analysis. Mapping is often more thought provoking than simply setting the same data out in a table.

11.7 OPERATIONAL REAL-TIME GIS

Patients with life-threatening illness need prompt treatment. From this obvious fact, we usually conclude that they should be taken as quickly as possible to the nearest hospital. This is a fallacy; the nearest hospital may be so busy that on arrival at the hospital the patient has to wait an hour or more to receive medical attention. Therefore, the patient may actually get treated more promptly if taken to a hospital that is farther away, but less busy. This has led to the concept of emergency capacity management. The Emergency Capacity Management System in Surrey uses real-time information to direct ambulances to the hospital best able to receive the patient, not necessarily the nearest one. All hospitals send regular updates to the ambulance control room with information on how busy they are. GIS displays travel times to each hospital from any location in the district. Isochrone zones indicate the best choice of hospital for any patient at any time. This GIS was written specifically for the task.

Although the GIS underpins the system, it was in many ways the easiest part of the system to set up. Much more difficult and time consuming was the business of agreeing rules between all the participating hospitals and monitoring compliance.

11.8 CLUSTER DETECTION

A district public health department may investigate a putative cluster of disease. Usually concerns are raised about environmental causes — pollution of air or water. Schulte et al. (1987) provides a good review of the issues.

The key question in responding to a possible cluster is how many resources to commit to the investigation. The full investigation of a cluster is hugely time consuming and far beyond the capacity of a district department. It makes sense to have a stepped or graded response.

The first step is to manage the emotional issues: meet the people who are expressing concern and hear from them firsthand.

The next step is to check plausibility of the concerns. A local councilor asked about a cluster (three cases) of multiple sclerosis on a housing estate. Residents were worried about contamination of their drinking water. We know enough about multiple sclerosis to give immediate reassurance; no further resource need be committed to the investigation. Two caveats must be noted at this point. First, reassurance is only effective if its source is palpably trustworthy and trust is built by a good relationship. Second, plausibility is judged by current knowledge, so reassurance is only as good as the strength of current knowledge. It is always essential to search the literature before giving reassurance.

This second step also involves examining available information more closely. In particular, are all cases in the cluster actually the same disease? Lay people may regard cancer as a single disease, so a cluster may include a wide range of different neoplasms. A cluster of brain cancer may turn out to include a single case of primary malignant disease of the brain together with an assortment of metastatic cancers of the brain derived from primary disease in lung, breast, or bowel. Of course, sometimes a single toxin can produce a variety of ill effects (e.g., radiation-induced cancers or the effects of tobacco smoke). Further information is also needed about the locality, both present and past. The local authority's environmental health department is the best source of this information.

The third step is a simple analysis of available data, probably in the form of comparing area rates of death, hospital admission, and cancer registration. Even if the first two steps are negative, analyzing routine data may be a necessary part of reassuring local people that their concerns have been taken seriously. It is always wise to agree with local people about the choice of disease, area, and time period for analysis.

Once the cloud of rumor and emotion has cleared away, the precise disease or syndrome identified and all cases verified, mathematical analysis is needed. Such analyses are best left to specialized units or academic departments: it is important to know the limits of one's own competence and the mathematics of cluster analysis can be extremely difficult. In England, the Department of Health funds a Small Area Health Statistics Unit to do this work (Aylin et al., 1999). An alternative is for district departments to collaborate in funding a collective resource for expert GIS, as had been done in the Trent region of England.

The final step in cluster investigation is a case-control study, perhaps followed in extreme examples by continuous monitoring of a cohort.

Most cluster investigations are reactive: concerns are raised by local people or perhaps by a local clinician. Should district departments use their GIS to search routinely for clusters? There is some precedent for this. In England and Wales, the Office for National Statistics monitors area counts of congenital disease. Local public health departments are notified when the expected count for specific malformations is exceeded on a simple cumulative sum analysis. To my knowledge, this system has not revealed any hitherto unsuspected threats to health. The surveillance system has great sensitivity, but far too little specificity to be useful. Surveillance for disease clusters would face the same problem with an almost infinite variety of disease and area combinations to screen.

11.9 CONCLUSION

GIS skills should be available in every department of public health. The most common use is display of data to inform, educate, or persuade. District departments need GIS for analysis infrequently, but basic geographical analyses are fundamental to monitoring access to health services. Concerns about clusters are common and the key question for local departments is how many resources to commit to the investigation. A graded or stepped response is best. Detailed statistical analysis of clusters should be left to GIS experts.

References

Aylin, P. et al., 1999, A National Facility for Small Area Disease Mapping and Rapid Initial Assessment of Apparent Disease Clusters around a Point Source: The U.K. Small Area Health Statistics Unit, *Journal of Public Health Medicine,* 21, 289–298.

Bhopal, R.S., Diggle, P., and Rowlingson, B., 1992, Pinpointing clusters of apparently sporadic cases of Legionnaires' disease, *British Medical Journal,* 18, 1022–1027.

Griffith, D.A., 1987, *Spatial Autocorrelation,* Washington, D.C.: Association of American Geographers.

Schulte, P.A., Ehrenberg, R.L., and Singal, M., 1987, Investigation of occupational cancer clusters: Theory and practice, *American Journal of Public Health*, 77, 52–56.

12 Using GIS to Assess Accessibility to Primary Healthcare Services

Andrew Lovett, Gilla Sünnenberg, and Robin Haynes

CONTENTS

12.1 INTRODUCTION

The principle of equal access to health services for those in equal need is one of the guiding tenets of the National Health Service (NHS) in the United Kingdom. Nevertheless, health services are inevitably located in particular places and are therefore more accessible to nearby residents than those living farther away. Variations in proximity are, obviously, only one element of accessibility to health services (Ricketts and Savitz, 1994), but the physical difficulties of overcoming distance tend to be particularly important in rural regions. Poor physical accessibility reduces the use of services and may lead to poorer health outcomes (Carr-Hill et al., 1997; Deaville, 2001; Jones and Bentham, 1997; Joseph and Phillips, 1984). Low utilization of primary healthcare services is of particular concern because of the gatekeeper role of general practitioners (GPs) in terms of referral to hospitals. Since the late 1990s, these issues of access have received renewed attention in the United Kingdom as part of broader debates regarding social exclusion and the future of rural areas (e.g., DETR, 2000a; Social Exclusion Unit, 2002). As a consequence, there have been substantial initiatives to improve aspects of public transport provision (Countryside Agency, 2002; DETR, 2000b), efforts to include an accessibility dimension in measures of multiple deprivation (DETR, 2001) and more thorough monitoring of changes in patterns of service availability (Countryside Agency, 2001a).

0-415-30655-8/04/$0.00+$1.50

Alongside this evolving policy context, developments in GIS and digital map databases have made it possible to calculate measures of physical accessibility such as travel time in a more automated and sophisticated manner than was previously practical (e.g., Higgs and White, 1997; Naude et al., 1999). Another innovation has been the use of GIS to assess accessibility by public transport, taking into account the spatial distribution of bus routes and frequency of services (Higgs and White, 2000; Martin et al., 2002; O'Sullivan et al., 2000). This chapter discusses the issues involved in undertaking such accessibility assessments with GIS, using examples from studies of primary healthcare services in eastern England (Lovett, Sünnenberg, and Haynes, 2003; Lovett et al., 2002, 2003). The next section reviews the data typically required, followed by a consideration of modeling techniques and some examples of how results can be presented. A final section summarizes the current state-of-the-art use of GIS to measure accessibility and identifies some directions for further research.

12.2 DATA SOURCES

Conducting an accessibility assessment typically requires four main types of information:

1. Locations of relevant service delivery points (e.g., GP surgeries)
2. Distribution of the resident population in the surrounding area
3. Details of the road network
4. Patterns of public transport provision

Data on the locations of facilities such as GP surgeries, pharmacies, or dentists are usually straightforward to obtain from organizations such as Primary Care Trusts (PCTs) or other NHS sources. To use these positional details reliably in a GIS it is important to georeference them as accurately as possible using sources such as postcode directories or ADDRESS-POINT® software from the Ordnance Survey (Martin and Higgs, 1996). Another consideration is to ensure that facilities are sufficiently comparable in terms of the services they provide. For instance, dental practices can vary considerably in the categories of patients they will treat under the NHS and GP surgeries may range in size from large health centers to outlying consultation facilities (OCFs) that are typically open for only a few hours each week. Finally, it is often necessary to take into account facilities situated outside the particular district or region under focus, but which local residents use. If such facilities are ignored, then there can be significant boundary effects in any subsequent accessibility calculations. Figure 12.1 illustrates this point by showing a map of pharmacies in the counties of Norfolk, Suffolk, and Cambridgeshire (hereafter referred to as East Anglia) as of autumn 1997. Many such facilities were located in towns or large villages situated close to county borders and served populations living either side of these boundaries.

A second key requirement is information on the distribution of the population. In many cases, the most obvious data source is the decennial census such as that in 2001 (Rees et al., 2002). Population totals can be assigned to point locations (e.g.,

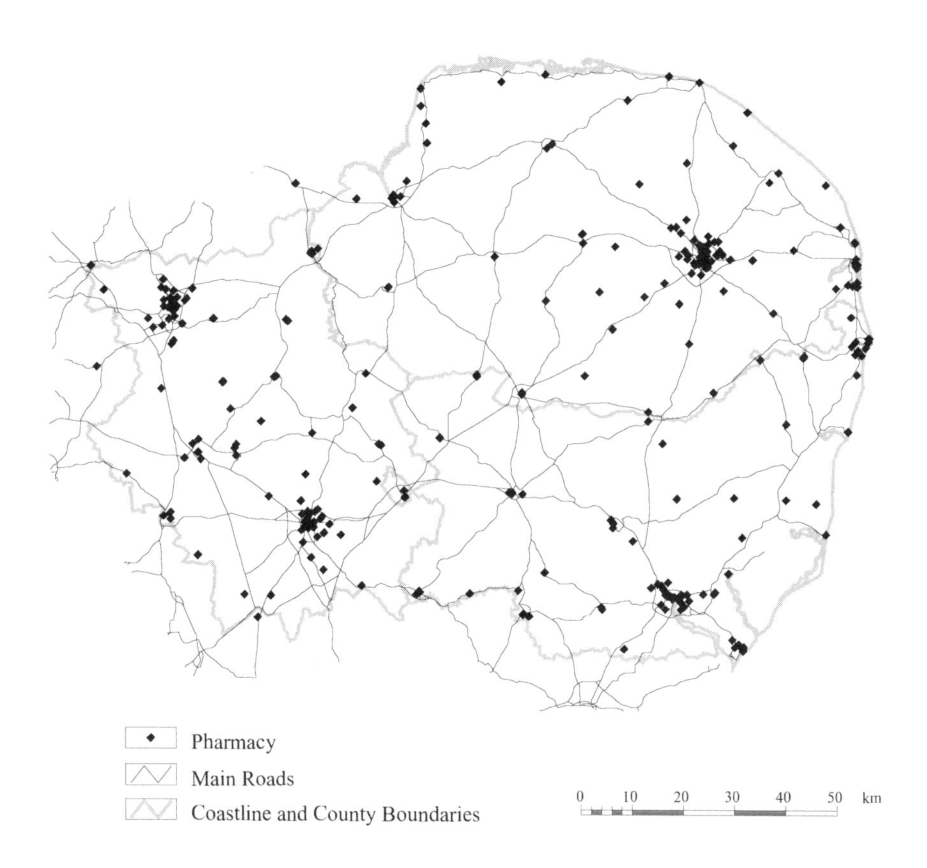

FIGURE 12.1 The locations of pharmacies in East Anglia, Autumn 1997.

the centroids of output areas) and may be interpolated to produce surfaces in the form of raster grids (Bracken and Martin, 1995; Martin et al., 2002). These approaches will be satisfactory for many purposes, but there are several other means of making local population estimates (Simpson, 1998) and in a NHS context one alternative that merits particular attention is the use of GP patient registers. There are important confidentiality and data quality issues regarding the use of such registers (Lovett et al., 1998), but if they can be made available then there may also be substantial advantages. These include the continuously updated nature of the information (especially valuable in the years between censuses), an ability to relate any accessibility measures to the practices that patients are actually registered with, and usually a higher level of geographical detail than is possible with census products. The geographical resolution of population data is a key consideration in accessibility research, because analyses based on centroids of zones such as census output areas or parishes inevitably tend to overconcentrate residents in locations where services are more likely to be present. Figure 12.2 illustrates this point by comparing population distributions for the district of South Norfolk derived from 1991 Census population surface models and postcoded patient register data. The more dispersed distribution of the population outside urban centers and villages is readily apparent in the patient register map (Lovett et al., 2002).

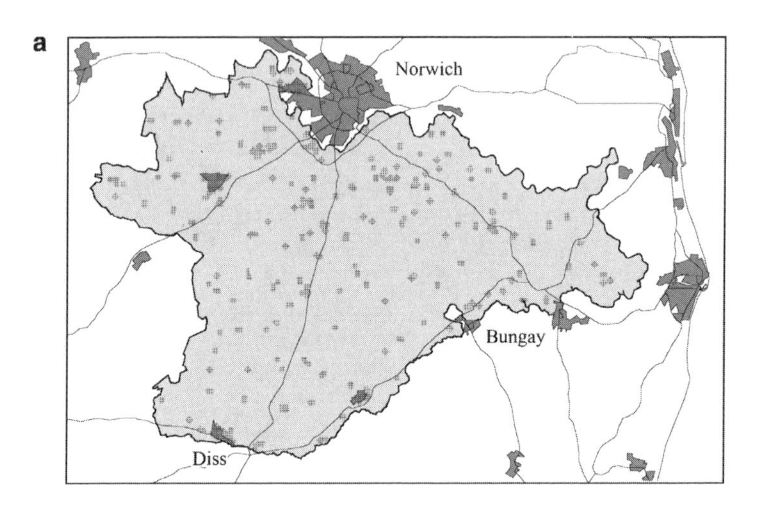

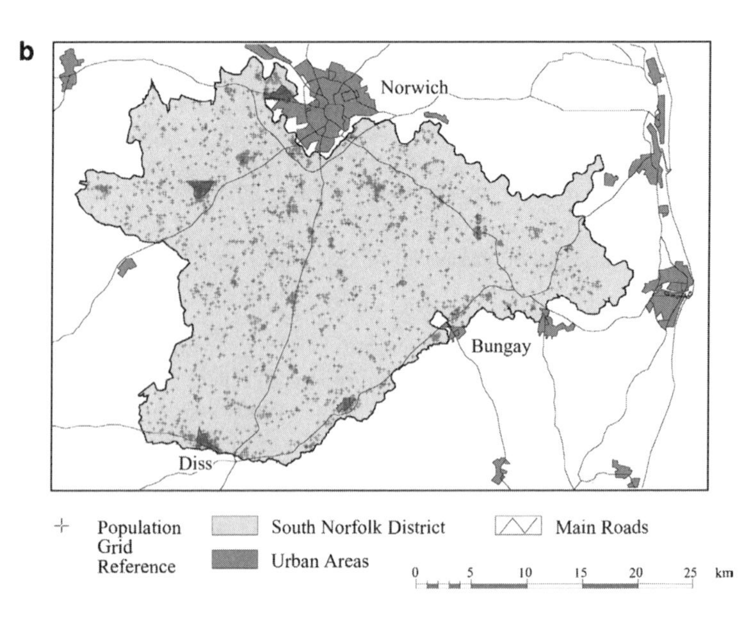

FIGURE 12.2 A comparison of population distributions in South Norfolk: (a) Population distribution from 1991 Census Surface Model; (b) population distribution from 1997 FHSA Patient Register. Reprinted from Lovett, A.A. et al., 2002, Car travel time and accessibility by bus to general practitioner services: A study using patient registers and GIS, *Social Science & Medicine*, 55, 97–111. With permission.

Digital road network data for the United Kingdom can be obtained from the Ordnance Survey and a number of commercial data providers. From the perspective of accessibility modeling, it is important that such details identify different classes of road (e.g., dual carriageway A-road, single carriageway B-road, etc.) and ideally distinguish between sections in urban or rural areas. These characteristics matter because of their influence on the typical speed of travel along individual stretches of road. Unfortunately, there is no standard way of calculating appropriate speeds for different types of road. A pragmatic approach is to use the national speed limits, but methods that are more refined are possible using monitoring information on typical road speeds published by the Department for Transport (http://www.dft.gov.uk) or collected by local authority highways departments. Table 12.1 shows a set of speeds derived from sources that were used in a number of East Anglian studies (e.g., Bateman et al., 1999; Lovett et al., 2002); it appears to provide reasonably robust results when compared to local experience.

Integrating details of bus services or community transport schemes into GIS-based accessibility assessments is often a time-consuming exercise. It is relatively straightforward to obtain details of service frequencies and routes from published timetables or Internet sources (e.g., http://www.ukbus.co.uk), but considerable work may be required to convert this information into a digital format that can be used within GIS. The simplest approach is to classify areas such as parishes in terms of the level of service available to the majority of the population (e.g., Higgs and White, 2000; Countryside Agency, 2001a), but for more detailed assessments (including consideration of journey times) it is necessary to define individual routes (e.g., O'Sullivan et al., 2000). This process usually involves digitizing or editing routes onto the digital road network and then adding attribute details such as journey times or service frequencies (e.g., Lovett, Sünnenberg, and Haynes, 2003; Martin et al., 2002). Figure 12.3 shows an example of the output from this type of exercise with bus routes in South Norfolk symbolized according to service frequencies. In this particular case, no attempt was made to record the locations of bus stops, but these details would become important for analyses on an intraurban scale. It is also worth recognizing that bus timetables are revised quite regularly, so the task of keeping such a database current can be substantial.

TABLE 12.1
Road Speed Estimates Used in East Anglian Travel Time Calculations

	Average Road Speed (miles per hour)	
Road Type	**Rural**	**Urban**
A-Road Dual Carriageway	54	28
A-Road Primary Single Carriageway	45	25
A-Road Single Carriageway	32	18
B-Road Dual Carriageway	36	18
B-Road Single Carriageway	24	12
Minor Road	14	11

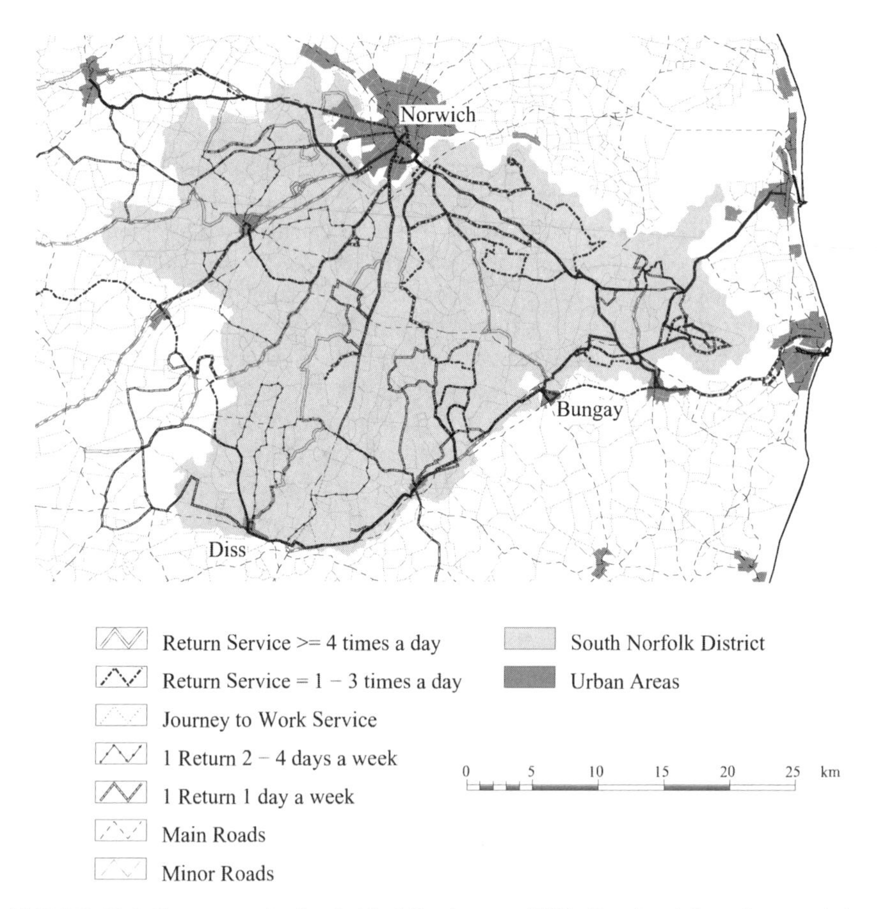

FIGURE 12.3 Bus routes in South Norfolk, Autumn 2000. Reprinted from Lovett, A.A., Sünnenberg, G., and Haynes, R.M., 2003, Accessibility to GP surgeries in South Norfolk: A GIS-based assessment of the changing situation 1997–2000, in Kidner, D. et al., Eds., *Innovations in GIS 9: Socio-Economic Applications of Geographic Information Science*, London: Taylor and Francis, 181–198.

Community transport schemes are a component of public transport provision whose importance has grown appreciably in recent years. According to the Countryside Agency (2002), the percentage of rural parishes with a community transport service increased from 21 percent in 1997 to 48 percent in 2000. Such provision can take a variety of forms, with community car schemes typically involving volunteer drivers using their own cars to provide door-to-door journeys for people without transport and dial-a-ride services being based on minibuses or taxi-style vehicles (Countryside Agency, 2001b). Most community transport schemes have defined catchment areas and so representing levels of coverage within a GIS using ward or parish boundaries is not especially difficult. However, it does need to be recognized that many such schemes depend heavily on volunteer staff and consequently service availability (as well as cost) may vary according to the locations and other commitments of potential drivers (Lovett, Sünnenberg, and Haynes, 2003).

12.3 METHODS

Once the necessary data have been compiled and assembled within GIS, a number of accessibility measures can be calculated (Cromley and McLafferty, 2002; Handy and Niemeier, 1997; Ricketts and Savitz, 1994). The simplest approach is to calculate straight-line distances from points representing the distribution of the population to the locations of the nearest primary healthcare facilities. This method can provide a useful indicator of access in some circumstances (Phibbs and Luft, 1995), including an assessment of the extent to which facilities are within a feasible walking range, but for many purposes it does not take sufficient account of constraints in the availability and nature of transport infrastructure. It has also been found that associations between straight-line distance measures and health outcomes can be rather different to those observed when more sophisticated measures of access are used (e.g., Martin et al., 2002), so the extent to which one can act as a surrogate for the other may be questionable.

The development of GIS, particularly tools for network analysis (Lupien et al., 1987; Waters, 1999) has made it much easier to calculate access measures based on road travel times. These take account of variations in transport infrastructure (e.g., road quality or the presence of bridges) in a much more satisfactory way than straight-line distances. The key concept underpinning the calculation of journey travel times is that of minimizing impedance. Within GIS, a road network is usually stored as a set of digitized lines (arcs) that connect to each other at nodes (see Figure 12.4). The nodes typically represent junctions or points where a road changes from one type to another (e.g., from single to dual carriageway). Each arc or node can have a series of attributes (e.g., a road type and speed as listed in Table 12.1) and these can be used to calculate new variables such as the length of time required to travel along the section of road:

$$\text{car travel time (in minutes)} = \frac{\text{length of road section (in miles)}}{\text{speed (miles per hour)}} \times 60$$

The travel time represents an impedance measure that can be stored as an attribute for each network element and many desktop GIS programs now include shortest path algorithms (Dunn and Newton, 1992), which can identify a route between a specified origin and destination (e.g., patient location and GP surgery) that minimizes the total travel time incurred. Extensions to this approach include

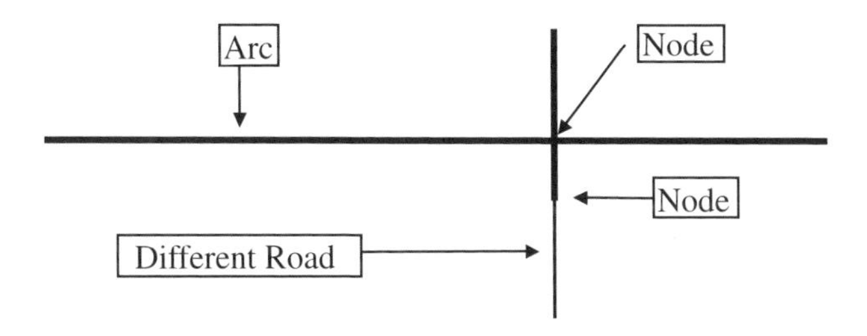

FIGURE 12.4 Schematic diagram of road network elements.

batch-processing capabilities to calculate times from multiple origin locations and, if there are many possible destinations, it is possible to define shortest travel time catchment areas around each facility.

When travel times have been calculated for point locations representing the distribution of the population it is straightforward to use overlay operations within GIS to match the results to areas and derive population-weighted average travel times for administrative units such as wards or parishes. Another useful approach is to create a map of contour lines showing equal travel time (known technically as isochrones, see Brainard et al., 1997). This is best done by generating a triangulated irregular network (TIN) from the point values and then extracting contours from TIN. It is also important to ensure that the points from which TIN is generated are relatively evenly spaced across the region of interest. If they are just concentrated in urban centers (where healthcare facilities are more likely to be situated), then the absence of intermediate data points may mean that areas of poorer accessibility between settlements are not identified. One solution to such a potential problem is to include travel times for nodes on the road network in the TIN generation process.

Travel time calculations can also be used to measure accessibility by bus. There are often, however, considerable variations in the times that different buses take to cover the same route (e.g., this may depend on the number of intermediate stops). This means that calculating average bus travel times for sections of road may be rather misleading and instead it is more appropriate to add specific timetable information for individual services onto the vector representations of bus routes. Such an approach is quite feasible (e.g., O'Sullivan et al., 2000; Martin et al., 2002), but it is clearly demanding in terms of the effort required for data entry and updating if the number of services involved is large.

Another approach to bus accessibility is to focus on the frequency of service rather than the actual travel time involved. This method has been used in several East Anglian studies; it involves first categorizing routes according to the frequency of service (see Figure 12.3). A GIS can then be used to determine whether residents could realistically walk to a bus route that would take them close to any particular type of primary healthcare facility. Figure 12.5 illustrates the steps involved through an example concerning access to a GP surgery in the center of the town of Bungay (on the Norfolk-Suffolk border).

The procedure automated within the GIS involves taking the surgery location and defining an 800 m radius buffer zone around it. A radius of 800 m (approximately half a mile) is used to represent a distance that the great majority of the population would find acceptable to walk. The GIS then selects all bus routes with a particular service frequency (e.g., at least four return journeys per day) that pass through the buffer zone. Next, a second buffer zone extending 800 m each side of the relevant routes is determined and the GP patient register postcodes within this corridor are identified. Residents with these particular postcodes are subsequently classified as populations with the relevant level of bus access to the surgery being examined. The procedure is repeated for all other surgeries, and again for routes with lower service frequencies, so that ultimately all residents are categorized according to the best level of bus access to a GP surgery available to them. Refinements to the method

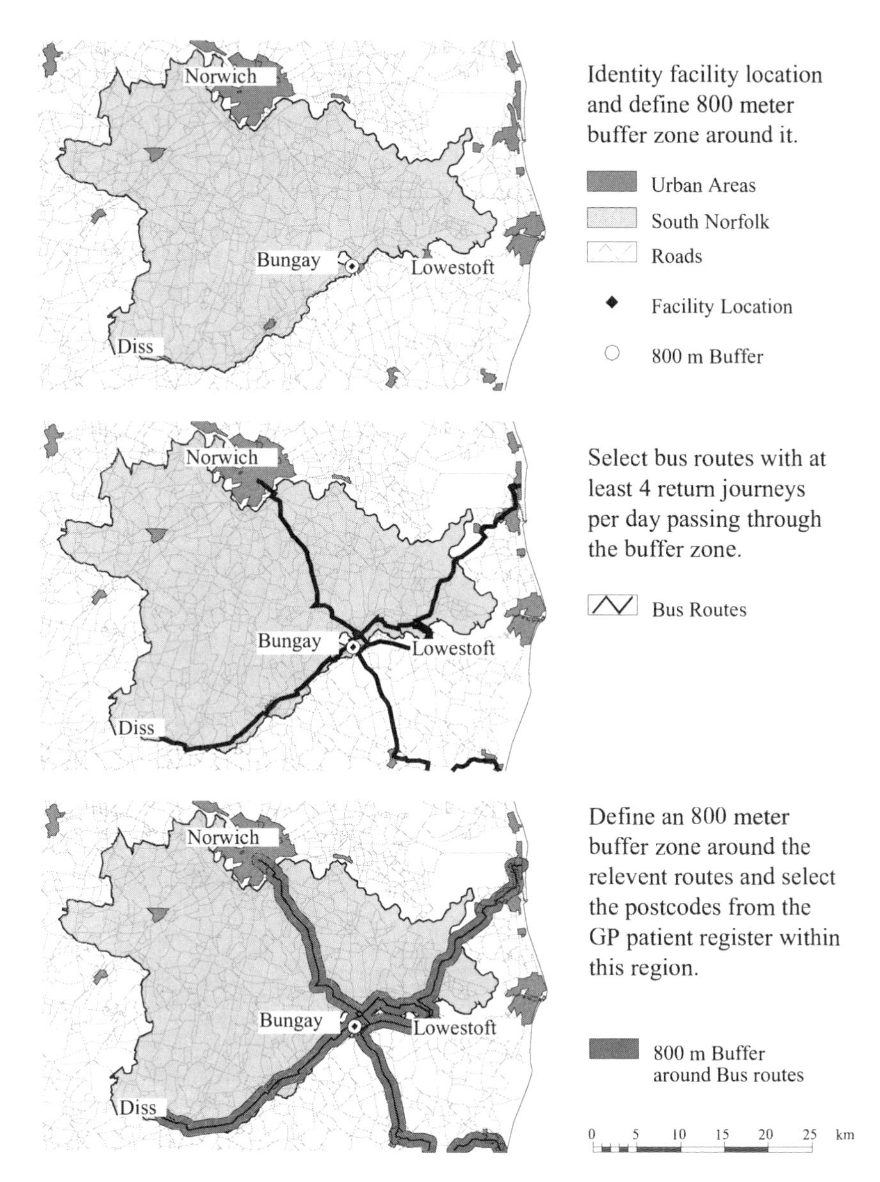

FIGURE 12.5 A method to evaluate accessibility by bus. Reprinted from Lovett, A.A. et al., 2002, Car travel time and accessibility by bus to general practitioner services: A study using patient registers and GIS, *Social Science & Medicine*, 55, 97–111. With permission.

include the use of different walking distances and consideration of the scope for reaching destinations by means of several connecting buses. Another extension involves determining whether the nearest facility (e.g., in terms of straight-line distance) of a particular type can be accessed by bus, rather than one that might be many miles away (Lovett et al., 2003).

12.4 PRESENTATION OF RESULTS

Figure 12.6 shows a typical outcome of GIS-based travel time calculations, namely a shaded isochrone map. The example in this case concerns car travel times to NHS dentists in East Anglia as of Autumn 1997. There are prominent star-like patterns around many cities and towns, reflecting the manner in which travel times are faster along major roads and reinforcing the limitations of using straight-line distances as an access measure. With GIS, it is also easy to calculate either population totals for travel time zones or average travel times (usually population-weighted) for administrative units such as wards or parishes.

Table 12.2 provides an example of the former output and compares car travel times to different types of primary healthcare facilities for GP patients in East Anglia. Around 60 percent of patients in 1997 were within 5 minutes travel of each type of facility, but at the other end of the scale 2.5 percent were more than 15 minutes away from a main/branch surgery with the proportion rising to over 7 percent for NHS dentists and pharmacies.

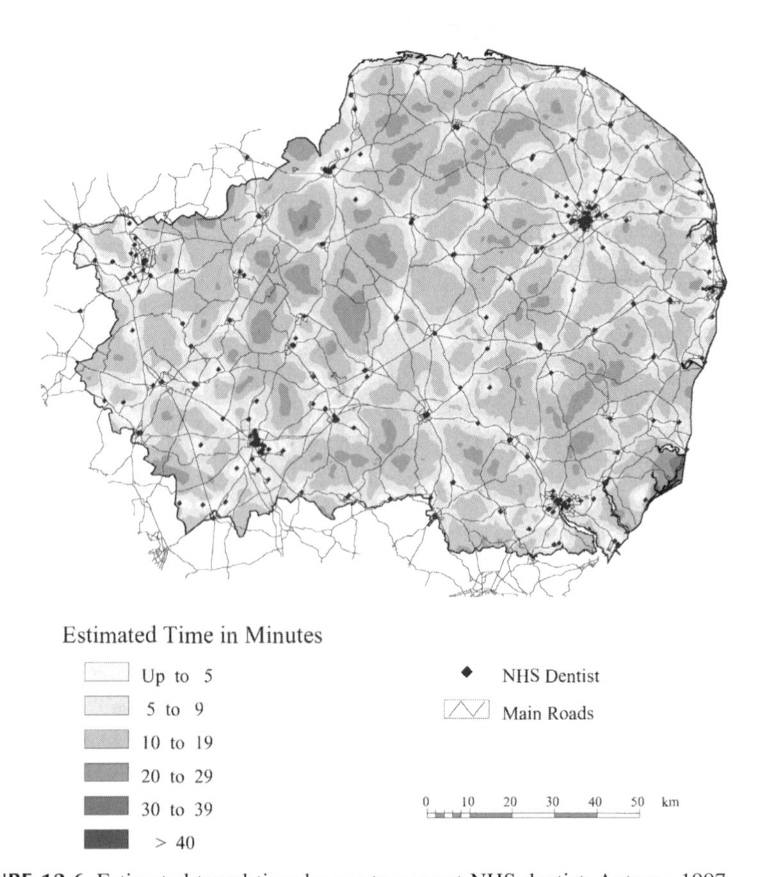

FIGURE 12.6 Estimated travel time by car to nearest NHS dentist, Autumn 1997.

TABLE 12.2
GP Patients in Car Travel Time Bands to Different Primary Healthcare Facilities

Car Travel Time (min)	Main or Branch Surgery	All Surgeries and OCFs	NHS Dentist	Pharmacy
Under 5	1,424,595	1,473,453	1,282,098	1,212,148
5 to 9.99	493,355	480,739	464,767	532,876
10 to 14.99	159,314	140,688	221,588	229,308
At least 15	53,266	35,650	162,077	156,198
Total	2,130,530	2,130,530	2,130,530	2,130,530

Note: Data refers to Autumn 1997.

Source: Reprinted from Lovett, A.A. et al., 2002, Car travel time and accessibility by bus to general practitioner services: A study using patient registers and GIS, *Social Science & Medicine*, 55, 97–111. With permission.

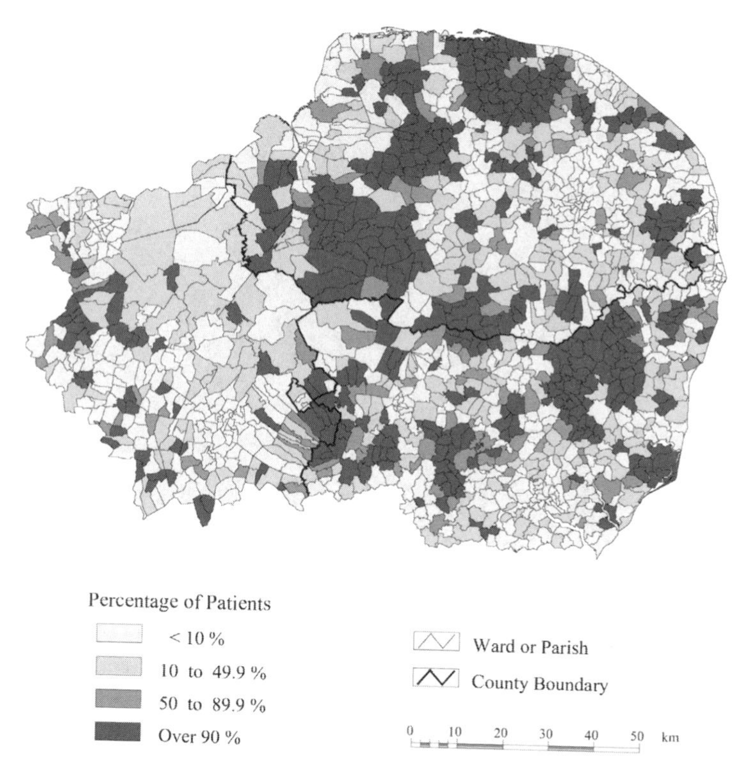

FIGURE 12.7 Percentage of patients with no weekday bus service to a GP surgery, Autumn 1997.

An example of the results from the bus accessibility method shown in Figure 12.4 is presented in Figure 12.7. This map displays the percentage of GP patients in each administrative area (ward or parish) identified as being outside walking range of a return weekday bus service that could take them to a main or branch GP surgery.

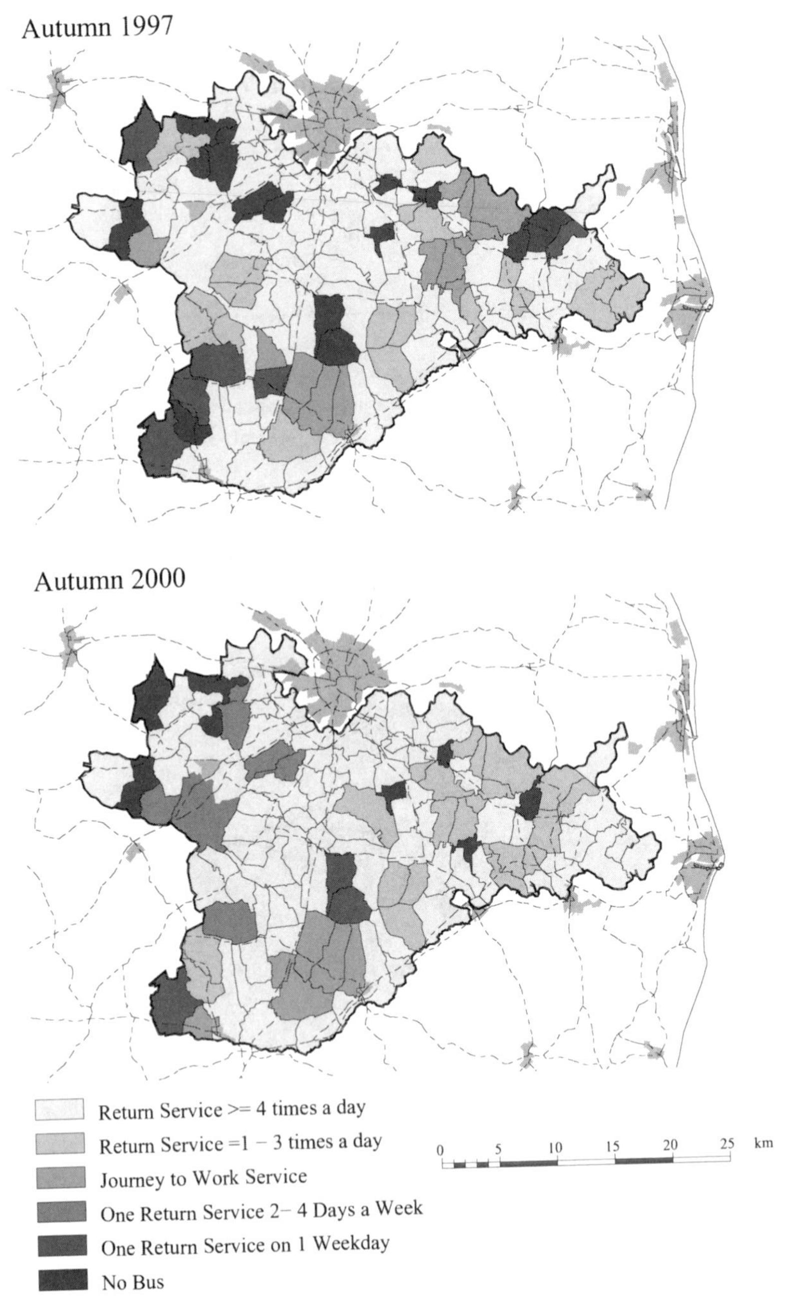

FIGURE 12.8 Classification of South Norfolk parishes by bus provision, 1997 and 2000. Reprinted from Lovett, A.A., Sünnenberg, G., and Haynes, R.M., 2003, Accessibility to GP surgeries in South Norfolk: A GIS-based assessment of the changing situation 1997–2000, in Kidner, D. et al., Eds., *Innovations in GIS 9: Socio-Economic Applications of Geographic Information Science*, London: Taylor and Francis, 181–198.

It is apparent from the map that in Autumn 1997 there were several clusters of parishes, particularly in western Norfolk and northern Suffolk, where high proportions of patients had poor bus provision. Several of these areas have since experienced improvements in services, a point illustrated by Figure 12.8, which shows a classification of bus provision for the parishes of South Norfolk in Autumn 1997 and Autumn 2000. Table 12.3 shows population totals (derived from GP register data) for the parishes at the two dates and highlights the particular reduction in numbers within the poorer bus service categories.

Several issues arise when combining measures of travel time and public transport provision to produce overall assessments of variations in accessibility. If car and bus travel times have been calculated, then they can be summed to derive an overall indicator (e.g., Martin et al., 2002). It is, nevertheless, questionable whether car and bus times are directly comparable and, more importantly, it is arguable that simply summing such measures can obscure some important differences in accessibility problems between areas. In the East Anglian studies, it was found more informative to cross-classify areas in terms of their average travel time and bus frequency to produce maps of the type shown in Figure 12.9. This type of classification can be readily extended to include information on community transport provision and may be supplemented by the calculation of socioeconomic or health variables for categories of areas. Table 12.4 provides an example of such information for East Anglian parishes identified as being more than 10 minutes car travel time from a GP surgery and further subdivided by their bus and community transport provision. One particular feature of the results is that among these rural parishes the highest levels of several health needs indicators were found in the most inaccessible locations, a trend consistent with the inverse care law (Hart, 1971).

If data from GP patient registers are available then it is also possible to compute accessibility measures for individual practice lists. Table 12.5 illustrates this option

TABLE 12.3
Classification of Parishes in South Norfolk by Bus Service for Majority of Residents

Category of Bus Service	Population		Total (%)	
	1997	2000	1997	2000
4 return daytime services per weekday	86,243	93,020	79.6	82.0
1 to 3 return daytime services per weekday	9,515	7,610	8.8	6.7
Journey to work service per weekday	6,078	6,303	5.6	5.6
1 return daytime service 2 to 4 days per week	—	3,310	—	2.9
1 return daytime service on 1 weekday	3,098	1,324	2.9	1.2
No bus service	3,380	1,813	3.1	1.6
Total	108,314	113,380	100.0	100.0

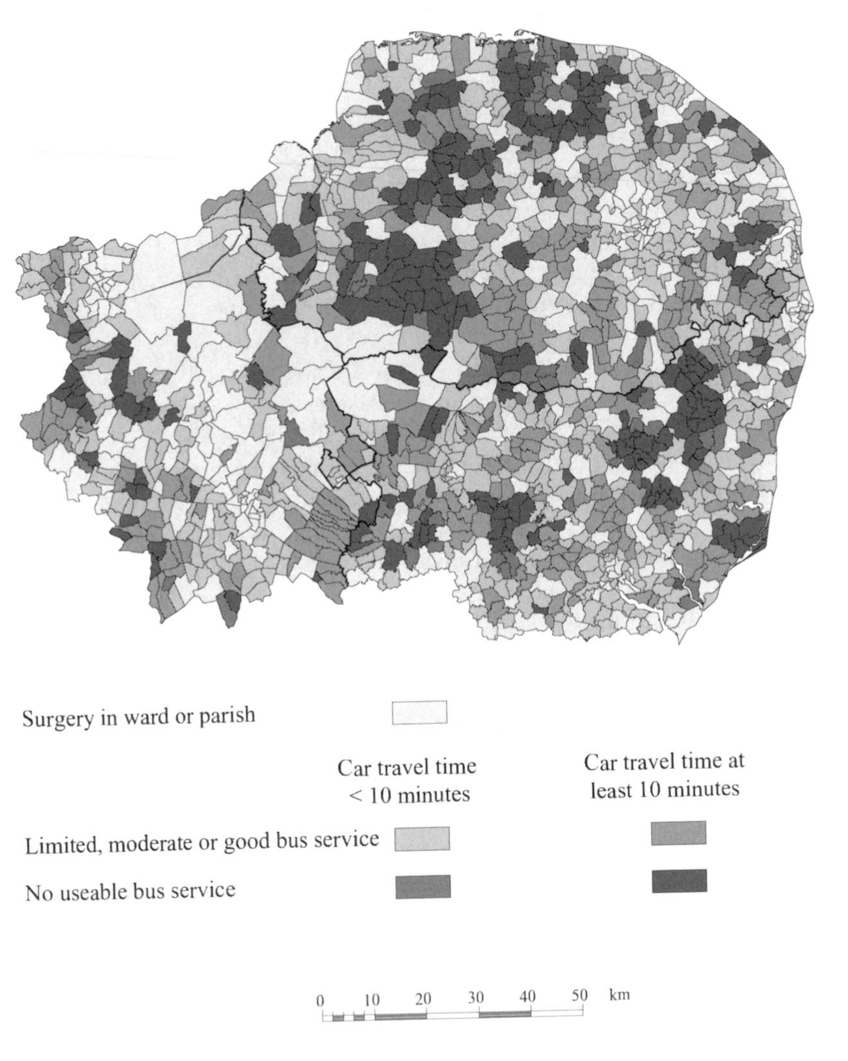

FIGURE 12.9 A classification of areas in East Anglia by accessibility to GP surgeries. Reprinted from Lovett, A.A. et al., 2002, Car travel time and accessibility by bus to general practitioner services: A study using patient registers and GIS, *Social Science & Medicine*, 55, 97–111. With permission.

using information for several Norfolk practices on the percentages of patients with poorer accessibility (i.e., longer car travel times and limited or no bus provision) in 1997 and 2000. The contrasts between practices and over time are evident, demonstrating the usefulness of such information for primary healthcare planning and management (Lovett, Sünnenberg, and Haynes, 2003).

TABLE 12.4
Characteristics of Parishes More than 10-Minutes Car Travel Time from a GP Surgery

Category of Public Transport Provision	GP Patients in 1997	1991 Population without a Car (%)	1991 Population Aged 75 (%)	Townsend Deprivation Index	Long-Term Illness Ratio
Good bus service every weekday	24,810	8.4	7.1	–2.79	69.1
Moderate bus service every weekday	70,743	7.2	6.3	–2.81	68.1
Limited bus service every weekday	35,647	7.4	6.0	–2.01	68.5
No bus service every weekday, but some community transport	34,779	7.5	6.8	–2.32	71.5
No bus service every weekday and no community transport	19,447	9.0	7.4	–1.25	76.3

Source: Reprinted from Lovett, A.A., Sünnenberg, G., and Haynes, R.M., 2003, Accessibility to GP surgeries in South Norfolk: A GIS-based assessment of the changing situation 1997–2000, in Kidner, D. et al., Eds., *Innovations in GIS 9: Socio-Economic Applications of Geographic Information Science*, London: Taylor and Francis, 181–198.

TABLE 12.5
Patients with Potential Accessibility Difficulties for Selected Norfolk GP Practices

GP Practice	Registered Patients in Poorer Accessibility Categories (%)	
	1997	2000
A	14.0	1.0
B	0.2	0.2
C	3.6	2.4
D	10.0	4.9
E	6.5	5.8
F	25.7	23.6
G	7.0	8.0

Source: Reprinted from Lovett, A.A. et al., 2002, Car travel time and accessibility by bus to general practitioner services: A study using patient registers and GIS, *Social Science & Medicine*, 55, 97–111. With permission.

12.5 CONCLUSIONS

This chapter has discussed recent developments in the use of GIS to assess variations in accessibility to primary healthcare services. It is apparent that GIS has made it much easier to calculate travel times along road networks and this approach is certainly superior to reliance on straight-line distances in the great majority of circumstances. Another feature of recent studies has been efforts to model accessibility by public transport and these have varied from classifications of areas by levels of bus provision to the detailed representation of bus routes as features in vector networks. It is fair to say that there is still work to be done in terms of identifying more-effective ways of modeling variations in accessibility by bus over large regions, and there is need for more sophisticated treatment of the services provided by community transport schemes, particularly taking account of the availability of volunteer drivers relative to travel demand. Finally, the issue of how to combine such different measures of accessibility in an overall indicator that could be directly used by NHS or local authority staff merits attention. This is not a straightforward matter, but the use of space-time prism concepts (Miller, 1991; O'Sullivan et al., 2000) is one approach that deserves further investigation.

On a practical level, the quality of results that can be obtained from an accessibility modeling exercise is dependent on the nature of the available data. As discussed above, details of facility locations, road networks, and population distributions are relatively straightforward to obtain, though in the context of primary healthcare there are particular advantages if GP patient registers can be used as a source of demographic information. Now, the major challenge is incorporating details of public transport provision within a GIS. Current approaches are too labor intensive to be used on a routine basis and it is therefore important to start integrating timetable information systems (e.g., http://www.journeyweb.org.uk) with GIS so that service details can be seamlessly transferred from one to the other. Only through such integration will it really become feasible to model accessibility by public transport in both a continuously updated and detailed manner. Such an improvement in databases will also provide the platform for developments in modeling techniques and further enhance the contribution that GIS can already make to the evaluation of accessibility to primary healthcare services.

ACKNOWLEDGMENTS

The research described in this chapter was undertaken during parts of projects funded by South Norfolk Council, Norfolk Rural Community Council, Mid Suffolk Council, and the NHS Executive Eastern Region. We would like to thank all the local authority or health service staff in East Anglia who assisted with data or guidance on various matters. For census products and digitized boundaries, we acknowledge the source, The 1991 Census, Crown Copyright, ESRC Purchase.

References

Bateman, I.J., Lovett, A.A., and Brainard, J.S., 1999, Developing a methodology for benefit transfers using geographical information systems: Modelling demand for woodland recreation, *Regional Studies*, 33, 191–205.

Bracken, I. and Martin, D., 1995, Linkage of the 1981 and 1991 Censuses using surface modelling concepts, *Environment and Planning A*, 27, 379–390.

Brainard, J.S., Lovett, A.A., and Bateman, I.J., 1997, Using isochrone surfaces in travel-cost models, *Journal of Transport Geography*, 5, 117–126.

Carr-Hill, R., Place, M., and Posnett, J., 1997, Access and the utilisation of healthcare services, in Ferguson, B. et al., Eds., *Concentration and Choice in Health Care*, London: Financial Times Healthcare.

Countryside Agency, 2001a, *Rural Services in 2000*, Cheltenham: Countryside Agency.

Countryside Agency, 2001b, *Great Ways to Go: Good Practice in Rural Transport,* Cheltenham: Countryside Agency.

Countryside Agency, 2002, *State of the Countryside 2002*, Cheltenham: Countryside Agency.

Cromley, E.K. and McLafferty, S.L., 2002, *GIS and Public Health*, New York: Guildford Press.

Deaville, J.A., 2001, *The Nature of Rural General Practice in the U.K.: Preliminary Research*, Newtown: Institute of Rural Health and the General Practitioners Committee of the BMA.

DETR (Department of Environment, Transport, and the Regions), 2000a, *Our Countryside: The Future: A Fair Deal for Rural England*, London: The Stationery Office.

DETR (Department of Environment, Transport, and the Regions), 2000b, *Transport 2010: The 10 Year Plan*, London: The Stationery Office.

DETR (Department of Environment, Transport, and the Regions), 2001, *Measuring Multiple Disadvantages at the Small Area Level: The Indices of Deprivation 2000*, London: The Stationery Office.

Dunn, C.E. and Newton, D., 1992, Optimal routes in GIS and emergency planning applications, *Area*, 24, 259–267.

Handy, S.L. and Niemeier, D.A., 1997, Measuring accessibility: An exploration of issues and alternatives, *Environment and Planning A*, 29, 1175–1194.

Hart, J.T., 1971, The inverse care law, *Lancet*, 1, 405–412.

Higgs, G. and White, S.D., 1997, Changes in service provision in rural areas. Part 1: The use of GIS in analysing accessibility to services in rural deprivation research, *Journal of Rural Studies*, 13, 441–450.

Higgs, G. and White, S.D., 2000, Alternatives to census-based indicators of social disadvantage in rural areas, *Progress in Planning*, 53, 1–81.

Jones, A.P. and Bentham, G., 1997, Health service accessibility and deaths from asthma in 401 local authority districts in England and Wales, 1988–1992, *Thorax*, 52, 218–222.

Joseph, A.E. and Phillips, D.R., 1984, *Accessibility and Utilization: Geographical Perspectives on Health Care Delivery,* New York: Harper & Row.

Lovett, A.A., Sünnenberg, G., and Haynes, R.M., 2003, Accessibility to GP surgeries in South Norfolk: A GIS-based assessment of the changing situation 1997–2000, in Kidner, D. et al., Ed., *Innovations in GIS 9: Socio-Economic Applications of Geographic Information Science*, London: Taylor and Francis.

Lovett, A.A. et al., 1998, Improving health needs assessment using patient register information in a GIS, in Gatrell, A.C. and Löytönen, M., Eds., *GIS and Health*, London: Taylor and Francis.

Lovett, A.A. et al., 2002, Car travel time and accessibility by bus to general practitioner services: A study using patient registers and GIS, *Social Science & Medicine*, 55, 97–111.

Lovett, A.A. et al., 2003, Public transport and accessibility to services in two districts of East Anglia, in Higgs, G., Ed., *Rural Service Provision*, London: Pion.

Lupien, A.E., Moreland, W.H., and Dangermond, J., 1987, Network analysis in geographic information systems, *Photogrammetric Engineering and Remote Sensing*, 53, 1417–1421.

Martin, D. and Higgs, G., 1996, Georeferencing people and places: A comparison of detailed datasets, in Parker, D., Ed., *Innovations in GIS 3*, London: Taylor and Francis.

Martin, D. et al., 2002, Increasing the sophistication of access measurement in a rural healthcare study, *Health & Place*, 8, 3–13.

Miller, H.J., 1991, Modelling accessibility using space-time prism concepts within geographical information systems, *International Journal of Geographical Information Systems*, 5, 287–301.

Naude, A., de Jong, T., and van Teeffelen, P., 1999, Measuring accessibility with GIS tools: A case study of the Wild Coast of South Africa, *Transactions in GIS*, 3, 381–395.

O'Sullivan, D., Morrison, D., and Shearer, J., 2000, Using desktop GIS for the investigation of accessibility by public transport: An isochrone approach, *International Journal of Geographical Information Science*, 14, 85–104.

Phibbs, C.S. and Luft, H.S., 1995, Correlation of travel time on roads versus straight-line distance, *Medical Care Research and Review*, 52, 532–542.

Rees, P., Martin, D., and Williamson, P., Eds., 2002, *The Census Data System*, Chichester, U.K.: Wiley.

Ricketts, T.C. and Savitz, L.A., 1994, Access to health services, in Ricketts, T.C. et al., Eds., *Geographic Methods for Health Services Research*, Langham, MD: University Press of America.

Simpson, S., Ed., 1998, *Making Local Population Statistics: A Guide for Practitioners*, Wokingham: Local Authorities Research and Intelligence Association.

Social Exclusion Unit, 2002, *Making the Connections: Transport and Social Exclusion*, London: The Cabinet Office.

Waters, N.M., 1999, Transportation GIS: GIS-T, in Longley, P.A. et al., Eds., *Geographical Information Systems: Volume 2, Management Issues and Applications*, New York: Wiley.

13 GIS in Public Healthcare Planning: The United States Perspective

Gregory A. Elmes

CONTENTS

13.1 INTRODUCTION

GIS plays a variety of roles in the planning and management of the dynamic and complex U.S. healthcare system. Although still at an early stage of integration into public healthcare planning, GIS has shown its capability to answer a diverse range of questions relating to the key goals of efficiency, effectiveness, and equity of the provision of public health services. Unquestionably, GIS will play a significant part in the reorganization of U.S. public health planning in the twenty-first century (Kamel Boulos, et al., 2001; Yasnoff and Sondik, 1999), especially in response to sweeping changes taking place in the handling of health information. Exactly what

0-415-30655-8/04/$0.00+$1.50

roles it will take on and to what degree GIS will affect structural change is subject to debate (Richards et al., 1999a,b). Consequently, the principal goal of this chapter is to consider the uses of GIS for public healthcare planning in light of the nature of the U.S. healthcare system and against the background of current endogenous and external forces.

GIS is only one component of health information technology that is transforming the U.S. healthcare system, a system that is notoriously dependent on many independent individuals working with diverse sources of data and traditional means of generating information. Linking health data with geographic, demographic, social, economic, and environmental data through a common geographic footprint (Goodchild, 1999) creates considerable benefits for different components of the health system. These benefits result from adopting digital methods in public health planning, such as in the recording of vital statistics and mapping disease (Curry, 1999). The scope of public health planning is being extended by the realization of a broader set of GIS abilities that allow for the analysis of complex situations. The presentation of these abilities to a wide public health audience provides a better understanding of geographic patterns, spatial associations, and related phenomena (Thrall, 1999). Mathematical and statistical modules embedded in GIS enable the testing of hypotheses and the estimation, explanation, and prediction of spatial and temporal trends (Kuldorff, 1999; Lawson et al., 2000). Increasingly, these modules are being tailored to the specific needs of public health practitioners.

GIS will become more significant in public heath if only because of the size of the market. Yet despite the heavily privatized nature of the U.S. healthcare system, government entities have been extremely important as early adopters and promoters of GIS (Richards et al., 1999a). While the regulatory and enforcement activities of government have not mandated the use of GIS, federal and state agencies have demonstrated GIS to be a successful means to monitor, assess, and evaluate responses to legislation (Davis, 2001; U.S. National Cancer Institute, 1999). Similarly, for many of the same reasons that other private businesses have found it beneficial, the large for-profit sector of the healthcare system is taking up GIS to reduce costs and increase profits (Hecht, 1994; Miller, 1994).

This review of GIS in public health planning begins by describing some broad characteristics of the U.S. health system. The second section investigates the range of GIS operations embedded within the core functions of public health services and the cycle of healthcare planning. The third section focuses on the public sector and provides examples from national, state, and local scales. The promotion of GIS by the Centers for Disease Control and Prevention (CDC) is examined, together with the National Cancer Institute (NCI), the National Association of City and County Health Organizations (NACCHO), and other entities. External influences will be addressed, notably those arising from the U.S. legal code. Other influences to be considered include national health policy, the national electronic data and dissemination systems, and health assessment initiatives. The chapter will conclude with a view to the future by considering the directions and trends in GIS technology, as they relate to public health priorities in the U.S.

13.2 THE U.S. HEALTHCARE SYSTEM, PUBLIC HEALTH PLANNING, AND ROLES FOR GIS

Responsibility for strategic healthcare planning lies at the federal, state, and local levels of authority and in the private sector. Policies set out in *Healthy People 2010* (HHS, 2000) are extremely influential at the national level. The 467 objectives of *Healthy People 2010* work down via state channels to day-to-day management and practice in the local health districts. The following section focuses on the U.S. health setting and core functions of public health.

In 2002, as in 1932 when the first official estimate was made by the Committee on the Cost of Medical Care, the U.S. economy was able to support the provision of satisfactory, affordable healthcare to all people (U.S. Public Health Service, 1999). The political and economic reality is that the nation chooses not to provide such coverage. The U.S. public spends absolutely and relatively more on healthcare than any other nation — $4300 per capita in 2000, 14 percent of the gross domestic product (GDP) (Thorpe and Knickman, 2002) — yet there remains an underserved population of more than 44 million people who have no health coverage (WHO, 2000). Rodwin (2002) distinguishes the U.S. system from others by its emphasis on private providers. The predominant method of payment for health services is by patients and private third-party insurers, a model characterized by Gatrell (2002) as "anti-collectivist." With the notable exception of Medicare, there is no national health insurance. Medical care payments for the elderly, military, and indigent poor are derived from federal sources. Although Medicare boasts enrollment of more than 90 percent of those over 65, it provides limited benefits to enrollees (Sultz and Young, 2001). Primarily dependent on personal responsibility for health costs, the United States suffers from enormous social and geographical inequities in delivery of and access to healthcare (see Gatrell, 2002). Providing and financing healthcare delivery is one of the most disputed and persistent political problems in the United States.

Kovner and Jonas (2002) define three broad objectives for the U.S. healthcare system:

1. Ensure access to basic healthcare for all
2. Attain universal health insurance coverage
3. Regulate private providers more effectively

Achieving these objectives requires the accurate and repeated measurement of what constitutes basic and necessary healthcare, the unequivocal assessment of system performance, and the identification and provision for those who do not have access to care. GIS has demonstrated the capacity to address the important geographical and spatial components — needs assessment, coverage, access, delivery, and evaluation — and to be capable of being integrated into comprehensive health information systems. There is growing evidence that incentives to integrate GIS within healthcare information systems will lead to an improved healthcare system (Pollard, 2002; Singer and Ryff, 2001).

One way to integrate GIS is to place it in the cycle of strategic public health planning. Since public health organizations deliver services to ever changing populations, they must build in flexibility to remain pertinent to their mission. Constantly updated demographic and epidemiological information is vital to the task. Jaeger (2001) emphasizes the need to develop effective public health strategies and structures compatible with long-term survival of the organization. Figure 13.1 modifies the strategic planning process through the inclusion of GIS operations at different stages of the cycle. The *Healthy People 2010 Toolkit* (U.S. Dept. of Health and Human Services, 2000) provides a candidate strategic planning process to be modified to include GIS functionality. Illinois has a multiorganizational approach to strategic planning, reaching across public health agencies, business, labor, health management organizations (HMOs), insurers, and other interested groups (Illinois Public Health Futures, 2002). The information required by the goals of geographic access to primary care physicians and to a data-driven health policy demands a geographical dimension. Whether GIS finds an established place in these strategic planning activities remains to be seen.

The U.S. Public Health Service (1999) Steering Committee (USPHSSC) has identified ten essential services provided by public health practitioners and agencies. GIS functions can be linked to these essential public health services as geographical and spatial factors can be recognized readily in all ten. Richards et al. (1999e) have illustrated the manner in which practitioners may apply GIS. As Table 13.1 illustrates, GIS functions in public health planning range from

System performance (Handler et al., 2001)
Market research (Lang, 2000)
Facilities management (Ibaugh et al., 1995; Isken and Rajagopalan, 2002; Poage, 2000; Rushton, 1999)
Site location (Duarte, 1998)
Patient records (Lee and Irving, 1999; Shull et al., 1998)

to

Epidemiology (Goswami et al., 2002)
Intervention (Cruz et al., 2001; Reissman et al., 2001; Rogers, 1999a)

Potential users of GIS range from health planners to business managers, financial planners, and health center administrators in the private sector engaged in profit maximizing strategies and niche market analysis. The rise to prominence of healthcare organizations (HCOs), managed care organizations (MCOs), and HMOs has increased attention to under- and overutilization of medical services and cost containment (Wennberg and Cooper, 1999).

Compared with other application areas such as natural resource management, urban planning, and transportation planning, the healthcare profession has been relatively late in adopting GIS. Richards et al. (1999b) observe, “Many state and local public health practitioners have not yet started to explore how GIS can be used to help improve performance of essential public health services.” The origins of GIS in public health in the United States lie predominantly in the academic

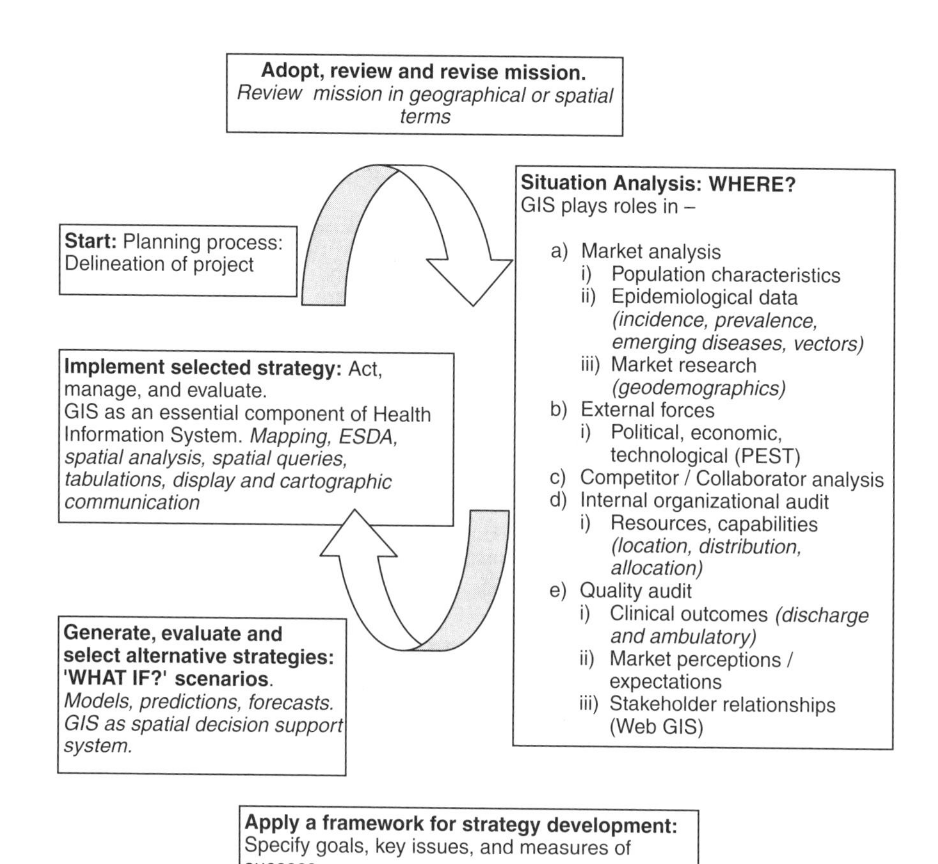

FIGURE 13.1 The strategic planning cycle in public health framed for GIS. Adapted from Jaeger, F.J., 2001, Strategic planning: An essential management tool for health care organizations and its epidemiological basis, in Oleske, D., Ed., *Epidemiology and the Delivery of Health Care Services: Methods and Application,* 2nd ed., New York: Kluwer Academic and Plenum.

study of epidemiology and disease distributions (Clarke et al., 1996; Croner et al., 1996; Gatrell and Senior, 1999; Khan, 1999). As with other rapidly expanding fields of knowledge, progress is often documented in hard-to-retrieve grey publications. Articles in sources such as the *Proceedings of the Workshop on Automated Cartography and Epidemiology, 1976* and the *Proceedings of the International Symposium on Computer Mapping in Epidemiology and Environmental Health, 1995* are oriented to the research community and not toward the practical needs of healthcare workers. As in other spheres, a few individual champions have pioneered and promoted the use of GIS within public health. Several of these advocates were instrumental in the organization of a milestone GIS and

TABLE 13.1
Illustration of Possible GIS Uses for Essential Public Health Services

Essential Public Health Services	Public Health Use of GIS
Monitor health status to identify community problems	Teenage pregnancy rate mapping by school district for community involvement and intervention targeting.
Diagnose and investigate health problems and health hazards in the community	Spatial analysis of discharge and ambulatory care records for specific ICD-10[a] or DRG[b] codes. Linkage of workplace or residential exposure to usual clusters or increased cases. Intervention and evaluation.
Inform, educate, and empower people about health issues	Spatial data exploration/data mining of lifestyle segmentation data to identify neighborhoods with at-risk populations (e.g. excess tobacco use). Development of area-specific prevention campaigns.
Mobilize community partnerships and action to identify and solve health problems	Immunization rate levels increased by identifying churches and schools for health promotion and matching geographic patterns of available workforce to minimize travel distance of children and nurses.
Develop policies and plans that support individual and community health efforts	Geocoding of Medicare residents and healthcare facilities. Optimization of facility utilization based on insurance coverage, health status, travel times, and access to public transportation.
Enforce laws and regulations that protect health and ensure safety	Match enforcement and regulatory agencies to service areas. Assign environmental complaints to correct service area. Automated geocoding and address correction.
Link people to needed personal health services and ensure the provision of healthcare when otherwise unavailable	Meeting health needs of non-English speaking people. Matching patient with same language provider. Providing travel details in patient's native tongue.
Ensure a competent public health and personal care workforce	Direct distance education to public health practitioners by identifying groups of specialists; by mapping high-risk areas, high prevalence, or emerging disease; and by locating individuals responsible. Identify practitioner deficiencies by area and mount campaigns to recruit for deficit regions.
Evaluate effectiveness, accessibility, and quality of personal and population-based health services	GIS maps of service provided and expenditures of service delivery facilities linked to demographic and community information sources to allocate resources, evaluate effects on specific preventable health outcomes.
Research for new insights and innovative solutions to health problems	Population and residential land use forecasting. Time-series, high-resolution imagery integration to generate community health reports and needs prioritization and planning. Integration of spatial statistics and modeling modules. Mobile GIS for on-site geospatial data acquisition and analysis. Enhanced reality for disaster management and training.

[a] International Classification of Diseases.

[b] Diagnosis-Related Groups.

Adapted from Richards et al., 1999e; Thrall, G.I., 1999, The future of GIS in public health management and practice, *Journal of Public Health Management Practice*, 5, 4, 75–82; and U.S. Public Health Service, 1999, Core public health functions, USPHS Steering Committee, Public health in America, Washington, D.C.: GPO, http://www.health.gov/phfunctions/public.htm.

Community Health Roundtable in 1998 (Richards et al., 1999a). In the same way, the landmark Third National Conference on Geographic Information Systems in Public Health, 1998, in San Diego owes much to a few prescient and persistent individuals (Williams et al., 1998).

In *GIS and Public Health,* the first GIS textbook specifically targeted at public health practitioners, Cromley and McLafferty (2002) detail the fundamentals and applications of GIS. Documenting the rise of GIS in public health applications during the late 1990s, Cromley and McLafferty explain the rapid expansion by the development of digital databases and specific health-related applications. They emphasize the central role of the federal government in stimulating the diffusion of GIS applications into the health sector and give prominence to GIS in environmental epidemiology, the mapping of infectious and vector-borne diseases, and the determination of access and location of health services. The value of GIS is quickly emerging in community health, an area of interest fed by the recent engagement of grassroots movements with public-participation GIS for the greater involvement of people to determine their health status and care (Buchanan et al., 2001). In a more popular vein, Lang (2000) has contributed *GIS for Health Organizations*, which publicizes ESRI's entry into the healthcare market and provides several examples of GIS use in the private sector. Conferences and Web communications, however, continue to play a significant role in the popularization and dissemination of GIS technology, methods, and advances. Most influential is the bimonthly newsletter, *Public Health GIS News and Information,* edited by Croner at the National Center for Health Statistics (NCHS). Additionally, a special issue of the Annual Review of Public Health features GIS.

13.3 EXAMPLES OF GIS FOR PUBLIC HEALTH PLANNING

Effective applications of GIS to public health planning are found in federal, state, and local institutions and authorities. The programs Epi Info™/Epi Map (Centers for Disease Control, 2002), GATHER (Geographic Analysis Tool for Health and Environmental Research) (Agency for Toxic Substances and Disease Registry, 1998), the Dartmouth Atlas of Health Care (2002), and NACCHO illustrate the advance of GIS into agencies at the national scale. Local health district applications are too numerous to be represented in this small space. Counties in Georgia and Oregon, detailed below, provide characteristic examples. Information collaboration is being promoted as a model for wider adoption (Lasker, 1997; Nyman, 1997) and consortia in San Diego, CA, and in Louisville and Jefferson County, KY, are illustrative of this trend (e.g., http://www.sandag.org and http://www.lojic.org/lojicdoc/data-doc/lojicmap/lojic.pdf).

Private sector ventures into public health information systems span scales of application from the individual local firm or facility to businesses of regional and national scope.

13.3.1 Examples at the Federal and National Scale

13.3.1.1 Epi Map 2000 (CDC, 2000)

The Centers for Disease Control and Prevention are national leaders in the introduction of GIS for public health purposes by demonstration, education, research, and software development. Epi Info 2002 developed by the CDC, is personal computer software designed for epidemiologists, public health professionals, and other medical professionals to gather primary data, merge it with existing secondary data, and produce epidemiological statistics, tables, graphs, and maps (Dean, 1999a). Epi Info is compatible with Microsoft® Access, structured query language (SQL), and open database connectivity (ODBC) databases. It can be programmed with Visual Basic® 6 and HTML and used on Web browsers. Windows®-based user interfaces can be designed for standard questionnaires or for particular data entry needs. The low end of current generation personal computers meets the hardware requirements, ensuring widespread use even in budget-strapped health departments.

Data from Epi Info 2002 is processed with Epi Map 2002 for spatial analysis and map display. Epi Map is an ArcView®-compatible GIS, which has been developed using ESRI's MapObjects® software (Ralston and Xin, 2000; see also Vinod, 2002). Users can develop GIS applications and analytical modules, which can easily be shared in the broader community. Tutorials are included with the software and the CDC frequently offers telebroadcasts and video seminars available on the Web. Given its free availability and the CDC imprimatur, the uptake of Epi Map will be extensive in the health community. Although users may initially focus on Epi Info, the ease with which spatial analysis and cartographic output can be accomplished will ensure the spread of spatial uses. The latest version of the CDC's Epi Info was released on September 16, 2002, and can be downloaded from http://www.cdc.gov.

13.3.1.2 Geographic Analysis Tool for Health and Environmental Research

Congress created the Agency for Toxic Substances and Disease Registry (ATSDR) in 1980 as the primary agency within the U.S. Public Health Service to implement the health-related sections of laws that protect the public from hazardous wastes and environmental spills of hazardous substances. ATSDR is commissioned under the Comprehensive Environmental Response, Compensation, and Liability Act of 1980 (CERCLA), commonly known as the Superfund Act

> to assess the presence and nature of health hazards at specific Superfund sites, to help prevent or reduce further exposure and the illnesses that result from such exposures, and to expand the knowledge base about health effects from exposure to hazardous substances (Heitgerd, 2001).

GATHER is a Web-based GIS designed to meet the mandate of ATSDR to monitor the performance of environmental clean up ordered under Superfund legislation.

Using Toxic Release Inventory data (Stockwell et al., 1993) and geographical and demographic data from the U.S. Bureau of Census, GATHER is able to display map layers for areas around Superfund sites and to perform simple spatial queries and analysis. GATHER suffers from the problems associated with the positional accuracy of public-domain spatial data and large variations exist in coding and positional accuracy because the data are reported from many sources. The use of census information is also problematic in this context, as the demographic data are available for area rather than point locations and the areal units generally represent place of residence rather than schools and workplaces within the population's activity space.

Until there is greater public understanding about the spatial and temporal limitations of available data, of scale, and of methods of analysis, investigating the causal relationships of exposure to toxic substances and health outcomes will continue to pose difficulties. Nevertheless, ATSDR personnel have long been at the forefront of GIS development and dissemination in public health. They can be credited with introducing the technology and educating many health professionals in its appropriate use. Recently extended to other CDC divisions, GATHER provides the Web-enabled user with basic information and the dissemination of location-specific cartographic and tabular information.

13.3.1.3 The Dartmouth Atlas of Health Care

The primary objective of the Dartmouth Atlas project is to describe the allocation and use of medical services and facilities both at the national level and for small areas representing service catchments (Goodman and Wennberg, 1999; Wennberg and Cooper, 1999). GIS is used within the multidisciplinary project to combine healthcare claims databases (e.g., Medicare) with spatial data (e.g., zip code boundaries) to create 3436 healthcare service areas (HSA) for the United States, which reflect functional regions. HSAs are grouped further into 306 hospital reference regions (HRR), representing the utilization patterns of patients of the healthcare facilities they use most frequently. Beyond regionalization, GIS is used for map comparison, overlay, spatial query, and analysis to examine the regional variations in the overuse, underuse, and misuse of medical services.

The Dartmouth Atlas project has provided evidence of significant geographical variation in the consumption of healthcare resources. According to Wennberg and Cooper (1999) "in health care, geography is destiny. The amount of health care consumed by Americans is highly dependent on where they live." The Dartmouth Atlas team has highlighted six themes based on the compilation of data, which have been studied in-depth:

1. Comprehensive centers of medical excellence demonstration project
2. Unwarranted variations in healthcare
3. Determining whether more healthcare is better
4. Reforming the Medicare program
5. Care at the end of life
6. Shared decision making

The published maps and the data used to create them are available at the Dartmouth Atlas Web site (http://www.dartmouthatlas.org/). Additionally, users can perform their own analyses using the project's data. The Dartmouth Atlas is informative, educational, and an interactive research tool. GIS applications are increasingly being grafted on to electronic atlases developed to detect patterns in disease (Gunderson, 2000), mortality rates (Pickle et al., 1996), gender, age, and ethnicity (Casper et al., 2000, 2001). These are available online with varying degrees of analytical capability.

13.3.1.4 The National Association of City and County Health Officials

National professional organizations have strong agenda-setting capabilities and influence political forces in healthcare planning. One of these, the National Association of County and City Health Officials, is a national nonprofit organization representing all local governmental public health agencies, including counties, cities, townships, and tribal reservations (Bouton and Fraser, 1999). NACCHO promotes its agenda in Congress and provides education, information, research, and technical assistance to local health departments. A major goal is support of information technology partnerships among local, state, and federal agencies. To this end, NACCHO has published protocols for the use of GIS, as well as guidelines for excellence in public health (NACCHO, 2000). One guide (NAACHO, 1996) demonstrates how a local health department can use GIS to protect the community from toxic substances in the environment. Another illustrates local public health agency GIS projects (NAACHO, 1999) using case studies on environmental justice, water supply protection, and sanitation management to demonstrate practical models for GIS implementation. The NACCHO Web site also supports an online tutorial for an introduction to GIS concepts and use (Meuser, 2001).

The National Association for Public Health Statistics and Information Systems (NAPHSIS) is an organization for public health professionals interested in the use of public health information. While not espousing GIS directly, NAPHSIS promotes standards for electronic vital statistics registries, directly affecting spatial data handling (Lorence et al., 2002). Because obtaining accurate addresses for vital statistics is crucial for their use, integrating an electronic registry with an address-matching program serves to verify address accuracy while generating the corresponding Federal Information Processing Standard (FIPS) codes. A comparison of best practices in California, Minnesota, New Hampshire, New Jersey, New York City, and New York state is available at the NAPHSIS Web site (www.naphsis.org/).

Many other professional organizations have an influence on the degree of GIS uptake in healthcare through education and advocacy. Examples include the American Public Health Association (APHA), the Association of State and Territorial Health Officials (ASTHO), the National Association of Counties (NACo), the National Academy of Public Administration (NAPA), National States Geographic Information Council (NSGIC), and the Urban and Regional Information Systems Association (URISA). Cross-membership in these organizations is frequent, resulting in the advancement of common purposes and memoranda of agreement that can promote jointly held aims, enabling faster adoption of standards, data policies, and technologies (NSGIC, 2002).

13.3.2 GIS at Regional and State Scales

13.3.2.1 NCI: Long Island Breast Cancer Study (LIBCS)

NCI has developed a prototype GIS for health (GIS-H) for breast cancer studies as part of the Long Island Breast Cancer Study Project (http://www.healthgis-li.com). The LIBCS Project was congressionally mandated in 1993, following evidence that breast cancer rates on Long Island, New York, were significantly higher than the national rate. GIS-H provides researchers with the means to study possible relationships between purported environmental exposures and the spatial distribution of breast cancer rates (see Rushton et al., 2000, Appendix A, for a list of GIS functions in GIS-H). Further development of GIS-H will be a collaborative effort between private industry, federal, state, and local government with members of the community and academia.

Despite efforts at integrating local knowledge, GIS-H relies heavily on federal, state, and local government databases. Many of these data sources do not provide sufficient spatial and temporal resolution for precise scientific inquiry into causal relationships between environmental exposures and disease rates. As a result, the use of GIS-H as a scientific instrument has become contentious. Critical reviews in the mass media have questioned the scientific credibility of the enterprise (CDC, 2002). To benefit from the LIBCS experience, the U.S. Census and other agencies have benchmarked GIS-H with an eye to generalization and wider adoption of the tools (Broome, 1999).

With regard to the use of GIS at the state level, departments of health are using GIS to monitor childhood vaccinations, infectious diseases, and legally reportable infectious diseases (including tuberculosis, HIV, and sexually transmitted diseases) and to develop strategies for preventing and controlling disease (Becker et al., 1996; Zenilman et al., 2002). For example, the recent outbreak of West Nile disease spawned applications in many states, chiefly used to disseminate incidence by county. The Behavioral Risk Factor Sample Survey (BRFSS), Health Care Financing Administration (HCFA, 1999) — now the Centers for Medicare and Medicaid Services (CMS) — data and many registries of disease are maintained and analyzed at the state level through GIS. Several states can be identified as being in the vanguard of GIS applications in healthcare planning, such as Minnesota and South Carolina. Missouri has adopted LandView® IV, a GIS initially developed by the National Oceanographic and Aeronautical Administration (NOAA), to provide public health information about and for local communities (McFaul, 2002). Until recently, state health departments focused on the use of GIS to produce maps for reporting infectious and chronic disease distributions, disease prevention activities, facility utilization, and behavioral risks. Today these same maps are ubiquitously available on the Web.

Collaborative information sharing across many agencies is common practice. In Minnesota, the planning agency, land management, environmental information, and MetroGIS (stakeholders in the Twin Cities) collaborate under the auspices of the Minnesota Governor's Council on Geographic Information (LaVenture, 2002). A pair of initiatives — the National Electronic Disease Surveillance System (NEDSS,

1999) and the Assessment Initiative — drives the participation of public health agencies in information partnerships.

Local governments are major users of GIS (Devasundaram, 1999), which is made clear by a comparison of market segments. Of a $2 billion market for GIS in North America in 1998, state and federal government accounted for $80 million (ranked eighth in expenditures), whereas local government spent $576 million for GIS (ranked first) (Warneke et al., 1998). GIS is evidently in place in local city and county agencies and departments, but is not yet as widely used by local health districts as by other local bodies. At the local and county level, local health districts deliver the majority of public health services and bear considerable responsibility for surveillance, reporting, and enforcement of public health regulations. The United States contains 3500 counties, varying in population from Los Angeles (9.7 million in 2001) to Slope, ND (754 in 2001), therefore it is impossible to generalize about the local health district use of GIS. Dekalb and Fulton counties in Georgia (Atlanta metropolitan area) and Clackamas County, OR, are among those cited for advanced GIS capabilities (Lapierre et al., 1999; Melnick et al., 1999; Roper and Mays, 1999). Barndt (1999) describes an innovative grassroots application of GIS for maximizing access to mobile facilities by underprivileged people in Milwaukee through the identification of the location of individuals in need of care, public transportation routes, and path minimizing algorithms.

Cromley and McLafferty (2002) report it is difficult to ascertain the extent and degree of GIS adoption in the United States by private (for-profit and not-for-profit) firms because of the lack of documentation. In the private sector, geodemographics firms provide high spatial resolution, lifestyle segmentation data, which permit extremely detailed assessments of the market (Weinstein, 1994; Weiss, 1999). Analyses of facility utilization, patterns of medical procedures, drug prescription frequency, and analysis of service provision are essential information for profitable activity. In efforts to contain the cost of care to insurers, MCOs and HMOs monitor and control payment for medical treatment, a task that inevitably requires spatial analysis (McDermott, 1998; Perkins, 1999). Lang (2000) gives examples of pharmaceutical sales territory identification by Health Products Research, the siting of assisted living centers by a market research firm for a nursing home provider, and locating vacant beds in Loma Linda Medical Center. Johnston and Schonhaut (2002) describe managing client access and facilities for Kaiser Permanente, a southern California HMO. As private firms become more deeply involved in providing public health services, their primary interest in minimizing costs and maximizing profits will chiefly influence their use of GIS.

13.4 IMPLICATIONS OF CERTAIN FEDERAL LAWS AND INITIATIVES

This section considers some federal laws, regulations, and executive decisions, which have the potential to affect (directly or indirectly) the use of GIS in public health planning. The most important legislation for users of public health information is the Health Insurance Portability and Accountability Act (HIPAA), which was signed into law by President Clinton in 1996. The rise of managed care coupled with the commercial use of health data by states and private companies led to demands for greater regulation of this most sensitive information. Before the creation of the HIPAA regulations, no comprehensive federal health privacy law existed in the United States. In general, medical records were less well protected than credit reports (Martinez, 2002). As medical information is among the most sensitive and personal information collected, new information sharing and communications technology raised concerns about the confidentiality and transferability of personal data. Under Title II of the Act, the privacy rule applies to personal health information in electronic, written, oral, and any other form. While not explicitly referenced in HIPPA, GIS greatly enhances the ability to identify (or misidentify) personal information through spatial integration of data. GIS data pertaining to HIPPA regulations include patient or provider name, driver's license number, phone or fax number, patient ID, social security number, address (either street or e-mail), health plan ID number, photographs, and other biometric identifiers, e.g., finger or voice prints.

More directly affecting the public health community will be the creation of a Homeland Security Department and laws promulgated in association with its broad mission (National Strategy for Homeland Security, 2002). The proposed breadth of the national strategy incorporates many functions that affect public health. Chief elements of the national homeland strategy are development of the geospatial framework, the National Spatial Data Infrastructure (NSDI), and the GeoSpatial One-Stop initiative. With the burden of developing and paying for Homeland Security most likely to fall to the state, many states are considering how best to manage GIS. The Federal Geographic Data Committee documents on its Web site necessary elements of spatial data and analysis for responding to the disaster management cycle. It can be anticipated that public health organizations will reap dividends from new data and the results of spatial analyses associated with emergency preparedness and response (see Choi, 2002, for an example related to anthrax).

13.5 PROMISES AND PITFALLS: TRENDS AND DIRECTIONS IN GIS FOR PUBLIC HEALTH PLANNING

Several influences affect current trends and directions in the development of GIS applications for public health planning. From the academic perspective, Rushton et al. (2000) presented the need for improved space-time data models, as well as enhanced communication between researchers and practitioners and an expanded focus on social and spatial diversity as the principal challenges for the increased uptake of GIS in public health. Technological opportunities embrace software, hardware, the Internet, and networking; however, technical education and staffing are troublesome issues for public health agencies. Data issues, a particular problem, include access to accurate spatial data and the emergence of national, regional, and local partnerships for data sharing. Other important external forces are associated with new government regulation, both prior to and following the terrorist attacks of September 11, 2001.

As new versions of GIS software appear every 18 to 24 months, the industry is quickly expanding into the public health market niche with customized products (Turner and Bowers, 2000). Web mapping is growing in concert with the unfolding of the broadband infrastructure necessary for the fast delivery of large volumes of geospatial data (Foresman, 1999). On the Web, commercial geocoding services are now available and meet a major need in local health districts, especially where expert staff are limited. Until the telecom industry brings much needed innovation and standardization in mobile telephone transmission reliability and coverage, hand-held hardware is unlikely to predominate over personal computer applications of GIS in the United States. The next generation of mobile technology will open many more options for real-time geospatial data acquisition and analysis, especially in the area of location-based services. Given the commercial impetus, a strong probability exists for the widespread availability of spatial statistical and analytical Web-based services in the near future.

The integration of data, information, and knowledge has become a principal theme in medical informatics (Pollard, 2002); regulation of the dissemination of spatial data and the development of data sharing partnerships will be a significant theme. As a check on these trends, the confidentiality of individual health and household information will be firmly regulated by HIPPA and through possible extensions of the Patriot Act. Federal Geographic Data Committee's (FGDC's) Geospatial One-Stop provides standards for the geospatial framework data, implements an index to geospatial data holdings at federal and nonfederal levels, and stimulates interaction in the health community about existing and planned spatial data collections, but it is difficult to anticipate the level of adoption.

Data quantity and quality will improve. The lack of current, accurate, large scale, low cost base maps essential for developing integrated health information systems is a perennial problem, not restricted to the public health field. Some types of geodata are new to healthcare planning, although long used in other domains. For example, digital orthophotographs, available through NSDI, do much to remedy the deficiencies in content and currency of spatial data. Long subject to a lack of accurate location data, health and vital statistics registries will improve because of better geocoding and initiatives like NEDSS (http://www.cdc.gov/od/hissb/act_int.htm). When completed, NEDSS will integrate and electronically link together a wide variety of health surveillance undertakings and will facilitate more accurate and well-timed reporting of disease information to CDC and state and local health departments. Major survey instruments, such as the BRFSS, have substantially increased the intensity of locational sampling to meet substate significance levels (http://www.cdc.gov/brfss). The drive for community level geodata exists in the private geodemographics sector, but public domain equivalents may need to be created (Dean, 1999b; CDC, 2000). Because minimization of data expenditures in the short term will be at the cost of interoperability in the long term, a forward-looking policy regarding maintainable and interoperable geospatial data will increase the network effect and free up its huge capabilities.

Contrasting with these positive trends are the real and perceived limitations of GIS. The sheer invisibility of "geography" both as an academic discipline and as an analytical perspective in the United States cannot be overstated (Dobson, 2002). The novelty of a geographical focus on problems and solutions may be one reason why GIS has seen such a general boom in business. The relative invisibility of geographical approaches is especially pronounced in a medical sector dominated by individual transactions and responsibilities. Nevertheless, heightened concerns for equity and spatial justice are encouraging the interweaving of issues of social diversity and community economics and stimulating the need for an increased geographic specificity (Maantay, 2002; Stoe and Oberle, 1999). As the quest for better health information continues, issues of small area statistics (Lawson, 2001; Wittie et al., 1996), ethnicity (Logan and Freeman, 2000), and gender (White and Cerny, 1999; Wood and Coggan, 2000; Vlassoff and Garcia-Moreno, 2002) rise to the forefront in geographical analysis. In the absence of an emphasis on geography's contribution to spatial problem solving, however, much of the potential benefit of GIS to public health may be squandered.

State and local public health staff are already overburdened and performing their existing duties conflicts with the additional requirements for implementing, maintaining, and using a GIS. Training and user support is a major financial burden, especially for small institutions. Clearly, an increased level of GIS education is necessary within schools of public health to ameliorate the situation (EPA, 1999). Additionally, inexpensive training is being designed especially for public health personnel. ATSDR, CDC, EPA, NAACHO, and the University of Iowa (Rushton and Armstrong, 1997) provide workshops, telecasts, Web-based tutorials, and CD-ROMs tailored to public health workers. A limited realignment of the public health workforce will certainly occur to meet information technology needs, but the extent will be restricted because more urgent workforce needs exist, for example in nursing, rural physicians, and ancillary staff.

In 1999, Richards et al. (1999c) confidently predicted that by the year 2010, "GIS applications in public health will no longer consist of the ad hoc approaches we have seen in the 1990s." Yet the fragmented and highly politicized nature of the healthcare system argues against the smooth integration of GIS into routine public health practice. From the hospital to the federal agency, a multiscale complex exists, composed of multiple authorities, and characterized by a lack of common direction and overlapping (and sometimes competing) missions. Although the trajectories of the public health sector and of the national information infrastructure will no doubt converge, the potential contribution of GIS use appears to be diminished by the sheer magnitude of the current crises in healthcare costs, medical coverage, and malpractice insurance. Nevertheless, public health measures relating to Homeland Security, coupled with the necessary digital transformation of information practices of the entire healthcare system, could dramatically increase the pace of GIS uptake, with critical consequences for public health planning.

References

Anell, A. and Willis, M., 2000, International comparison of health care systems using resource profiles, *Bulletin of the World Health Organization*, 78, 6, 770–778.

Annual Review of Public Health, 2003. Special issue on GIS in public health, Vol. 24, Palo Alto, CA, http://publhealth.AnnualReviews.org/current.shtml

Banta, J., 1997, Using ArcView in managed care, *Proceedings of the 17th Annual ESRI User Conference,* San Diego, CA.

Barndt, M., 1999, Enterprise GIS: The potential and limitations in community health GIS applications, *URISA '99 Annual Conference Proceedings*, Chicago, IL.

Becker, K.M. et al., 1998, Geographic epidemiology of gonorrhea in Baltimore, Maryland, using a geographic information system, *American Journal of Epidemiology,* 147, 7, 709–716.

Bouton, P. and Fraser, M., 1999, Local health departments and GIS: The perspective of the National Association of County and City Health Officials, *Journal of Public Health Management and Practice*, 5, 4, 33–41.

Broome, F., 1999, Benchmark testing of GIS capabilities for epidemiologic studies of breast cancer on Long Island, Geography Division, U.S. Bureau of Census, Washington, D.C., http://www.naccho.org/files/documents/GISbenchmarkNCI.pdf.

Buchanan, D. et al., 2001, The Holyoke Community Health Planning Commission: A model of academic-practice-community collaboration in Massachusetts, *Public Health Reports*, 116, 5, 499–502.

Cahill, D. and Chermak, M., 1997, Changing the face of healthcare networks, *Business Geographics*, 5, 6, 34–36.

Casper, M. et al., 2000, *Heart Disease in Women: An Atlas of Racial and Ethnic Disparity in Mortality*, Morgantown, WV: Office for Social Environment and Health Research, http://www.cdc.gov/cvh/maps/cvdatlas/index/htm.

Casper, M. et al., 2001, *Heart Disease in Men: An Atlas of Racial and Ethnic Disparity in Mortality,* Morgantown, WV: Office for Social Environment and Health Research, http://www.cdc.gov/cvh/mensatlas/.

CDC, Centers for Disease Control and Prevention, 2000, Community Indicators of Health-Related Quality of Life — United States, 1993–1997 *MMWR Weekly*, April 7, 2000, 49(13), 281–285.

CDC, Centers for Disease Control and Prevention, 2002, *Public Health GIS News and Information*, May 2002, Number 46, 22.

Choi, S., 2002, Using GIS as a teaching tool in public health, *Proceedings 22nd Annual ESRI International User Conference*, San Diego, CA, July 8–12, 2002.

Clarke, K.C., McLafferty, S.L., and Tempalski, B.J., 1996, On epidemiology and geographic information systems: A review and discussion of future directions, *Emerging Infectious Diseases*, 2, 2, 85–92.

Cromley, E.K. and McLafferty, S.L., 2002, *GIS and Public Health,* New York: The Guildford Press.

Croner, C.M., Sperling, J., and Broome, F., 1996, Geographic information systems (GIS): New perspectives in understanding human health and environmental relationships, *Statistics in Medicine*, 15, 17/18, 1961–1977.

Cruz, T., Whitney, K.A., and Runge, J.W., 2001, *Health Care: Targeting Areas for Intervention*, Caribbean GIS Conference: URISA.

Curry, R., 1999, You want 75,000 unique maps by when? *Proceedings of the 19th Annual ESRI User Conference*, July 1999, San Diego, CA.

Curtis, G., 2002, GIS use in a public health emergency, *Proceedings 22nd Annual ESRI International User Conference*, San Diego, CA, July 8–12, 2002.

Davis, S.I., 2001, Brownfields and other distressed communities: Assessing neighborhood characteristics, *Journal of Environmental Health*, 64, 1, 47–48.

Dean, A.G., 1999a, Epi Info and Epi Map: Current status and plans for Epi Info 2000, *Journal of Public Health Management Practice,* 5, 4, 54–57.

Dean, L., 1999b, Revitalizing communities with geographic information systems (GIS): HUD's Community 2020 Software, *Journal of Public Health Management Practice,* 5, 4, 47–53.

Devasundaram, J.K., 1999, An automated geographic information system for local health departments: Geographic information systems in public health, Part 1, *Journal of Public Health Management and Practice*, 5, 2, 70–72.

Dobson J., 2002, Geographer questioned at the Pearly Gates, *GeoWorld*, 15, 9, 26–27.

Duarte, P., 1998, Procedures for utilizing GIS spatial analytical tools to locate a hospital in rural South Carolina, *URISA '98 Annual Conference Proceedings*, Charlotte, NC.

English, P. et al., 1999, Examining associations between childhood asthma and traffic flow using a geographic information system, *Environmental Health Perspectives*, 107, 9, 761–767.

EPA, U.S. Environmental Protection Agency, 1999, Annotated bibliography developed for the graduate level introductory GIS classes taught at EPA, EPA/600/R-99/088, June 1999, National Center for Environmental Assessment, Office of Research and Development, Washington, D.C.: GPO.

Foresman, T.W., 1999, Spatial analysis and mapping on the Internet, *Journal of Public Health Management Practice*, 5, 4, 57–64.

Gatrell, A. and Senior, P.M., 1999, Health and health care applications, in Longley, A. et al., Eds., *Geographical Information Systems: Principles, Techniques, Applications, and Management,* 2nd ed., New York: John Wiley and Sons.

Gatrell, A.C., 2002, *Geographies of Health: An Introduction,* Oxford: Blackwell Publishers.

Goodchild, M.F., 1999, What is a geolibrary? *Distributed Geolibraries: Spatial Information Resources,* summary of a workshop panel on distributed geolibraries, Mapping Science Committee, Commission on Geosciences, Environment, and Resources, National Research Council, Washington, D.C.: National Academy Press.

Goodman, D.C. and Wennberg, J.E., 1999, Maps and health: The challenges of interpretation, *Journal of Public Health Management Practice*, 5, 4, xiii–xvii.

Goswami, E. et al., 2002, Spatial characteristics of fine particulate matter: Identifying representative monitoring locations in Seattle, WA, *Journal of Air Waste Managagement Association*, 52, 3, 324–333.

Gundersen, L., 2000, Mapping it out: Using atlases to detect patterns in health care, disease, and mortality, *Annals of Internal Medicine*, 133, 2, 161–164.

Handler, A., Issel, M., and Turnock, B., 2001, A conceptual framework to measure performance of the public health system, *American Journal of Public Health*, 91, 8, 1235–1239.

Hecht, L.G., 1994, Healthcare systems should adopt spatial applications, *GIS World*, 7, 3, 18.

Heitgerd, J.L., 2001, Using GIS and demographics to characterize communities at risk: A model from ATSDR, *Journal of Environmental Health*, 64, 5, 21–23.

HHS, U.S. Department of Health and Human Services, 2000, *Healthy People 2010: Understanding and Improving Health*, 2nd ed., Washington, D.C.: U.S. Government Printing Office, http://www.health.gov/healthypeople/.

Ibaugh, A., Rushton, G., and Ruskin, J. 1995, A spatial decision support system for improving the coordination and delivery of health care services, *Proceedings of the 1995 Annual Urban and Regional Information Systems Association,* San Antonio, TX, 1, 20–33.

Illinois Public Health Futures, 2002, http://app.idph.state.il.us/phfi/default.asp.

Isken, M.W. and Rajagopalan, B., 2002, Data mining to support simulation modeling of patient flow in hospitals, *Journal of Medical Systems*, 26, 2, 179–197.

Jaeger, F.J., 2001, Strategic planning: An essential management tool for health care organizations and its epidemiological basis, in Oleske, D., Ed., *Epidemiology and the Delivery of Health Care Services: Methods and Application,* 2nd ed., New York: Kluwer Academic and Plenum.

Johnston, J. and Schonhaut, S., 2002, Spatial analysis of hospital/patient relationships across transportation networks, *Proceedings 22nd Annual ESRI International User Conference*, San Diego, CA, July 8–12, 2002.

Kamel Boulos, M.N., Roudsari, A.V., Carson, E.R., 2001 Health geomatics: An enabling suite of technologies in health and healthcare, *Journal of Biomedical Informatics* 34, 3, June 2991, 195–219.

Khan, O. A., 1999, Geographic information systems, *American Journal of Public Health,* 89, 7, 1125.

Kohn, M., 2002, Oregon NEDSS, *Proceedings of Data Management, Integration, and Dissemination for Public Health Action Conference*, Minneapolis, MN, January 2002.

Kovner, A.R., and Jonas, S., 2002, *Jonas and Kovner's Healthcare Delivery in the United States,* 7th ed., New York: Springer Publishing.

Kulldorf, M., 1999, Geographic information systems (GIS) and community health: Some statistical issues, Geographic information systems in public health, Part 1 (special issue), *Journal of Public Health Management and Practice,* 5, 2, 100–106.

Lang, L., 2000, *GIS for Health Organizations*, Redlands, CA: Environmental Systems Research Institute.

Lapierre, S., Myrick, J., and Russell, G., 1999, The public health care planning problem: A case study using geographic information systems, *Journal of Medical Systems*, 23, 5, 401–417.

Lasker, R., 1997, *Medicine and Public Health: The Power of Collaboration*, Committee on Medicine and Public Health, Interinstitutional Relations, New York: The Academy, New York Academy of Medicine.

LaVenture, M., 2002, Integration of NEDSS and AI projects at the state level, *Proceedings from Data Management, Integration, and Dissemination for Public Health Action Conference,* Minneapolis, MN, January 2002.

Lawson, A.B., 2001, *Statistical Methods in Spatial Epidemiology,* New York: John Wiley & Sons.

Lawson, A.B. et al., 2000, Disease mapping models: An empirical evaluation, *Statistics in Medicine*, 19, 17–18, 2217–2241.

Lee, C.V. and Irving, J., 1999, Sources of spatial Data For Community Health Planning, *Journal of Public Health Management and Practice*, 5, 4, 7–22.

Logan, S.L. and Freeman, E.M., Eds., 2000, *Health Care in the Black Community: Empowerment, Knowledge, Skills, and Collectivism,* New York: Haworth Press.

Longley, P.A. et al., Eds., 1999, Introduction, *Geographical Information Systems, Principles and Technical Issues*, Vol. 1, 2nd ed., New York: John Wiley & Sons.

Lorence, D.P., Spink, A., and Richards, M.C., 2002, EPR adoption and dual record maintenance in the U.S.: Assessing variation in medical systems infrastructure, *Journal of Medical Systems*, 26, 5, 357–367.

Maantay, J., 2002, Mapping environmental injustices: Pitfalls and potential of geographic information systems in assessing environmental health and equity, *Environment Health Perspectives,* 110, Suppl. 2, 161–171.

Martinez, R., 2002, Exploring HIPAA, *Proceedings of the NACo Annual Conference,* July 2002, New Orleans, LA.

McDermott, T., 1998, A Change Detection Model for Evaluating Access to Public Health Services, *Proceedings Annual Conference, URISA '98.*

McFaul, E.J., 2002, LandView IV, A GIS application with the Missouri Information for the Community System, *Proceedings from Data Management, Integration, and Dissemination for Public Health Action Conference,* Minneapolis, MN, January 2002.

Melnick, A. and Fleming, D., 1999, Geographic information systems — Promise and pitfalls, Geographic information systems in public health, Part 1, *Journal of Public Health Management and Practice*, 5, 2, viii–x.

Melnick, A. et al., 1999, Clackamas County Department of Human Services community health mapping engine (CHiME) geographic information systems project, *Journal of Public Health Management Practice*, 5, 2, 64–69.

Meuser, M., 2001, MapCruzin™ map-tutorial and atlas, http://www.mapcruzin.com/learn_to_map/.

Miller, P., 1994, Medical center uses desktop mapping to cut costs and improve efficiency, *Geo Info Systems*, 6, 4, 40–41.

NACCHO, 1996, *GIS, pollution prevention, and public health guide*, pdf file available at http://www.naccho.org/downloadfile2.cfm?filenamex=General152.pdf.

NACCHO, 1999, *Geographic information systems, pollution prevention case studies,* pdf file available at http://www.naccho.org/downloadfile2.cfm?filenamex=General154.pdf.

NACCHO, 2000, *Assessment and planning excellence through community partners for health (APEXCPH),* http://www.naccho.org/project47.cfm.

National Strategy for Homeland Security, The White House, Office of Homeland Security, July 2002.

NEDSS, National Electronic Disease Surveillance System, 2001, A standards-based approach to connect public health and clinical medicine, *Journal of Public Health Management Practice,* 7, 6, 43–50.

NSGIC, 2002, Saving lives and saving money: An urgent call to build the national spatial data infrastructure in support of public safety, http:www.nsgic.org

Nyman, L.W., 1997, Federal agencies share public health data, *GIS World*, 10, 10, 78.

Oleske, D., Ed., 2001, *Epidemiology and the Delivery of Health Care Services: Methods and Applications*, 2nd ed, New York: Kluwer Academic and Plenum.

Perkins, B.B., 1999, Re-forming medical delivery systems: Economic organisation and dynamics of regional planning and managed competition, *Social Science & Medicine*, 48, 2, 241–251.

Pickle, L. et al., 1996, *Atlas of United States Mortality,* U.S. Department of Health and Human Services, Public Health Service, CDC, Hyattsville, MD: National Center for Health Statistics, http://www.cdc.gov/nchs/products/pubs/pubd/other/atlas/atlas.htm.

Poage, J.F., 2000, Market areas for primary care health services: How does one determine them? How does one publish the information? Why does one care? *Proceedings of the 20th Annual ESRI User Conference*, July 2000, San Diego, CA.

Pollard, B., 2002, New directions in assessment and planning: Integration of GIS with census, public health and syndicated market research data, *Proceedings from Data Management, Integration, and Dissemination for Public Health Action Conference,* Minneapolis, MN, January 2002.

Proceedings of the 1976 Workshop on Automated Cartography and Epidemiology (HEW Publication No. [PHS] 79–1254), Hyattsville, MD: U.S. Department of Health and Human Services.

Proceedings of the International Symposium on Computer Mapping in Epidemiology and Environmental Health, February 12–15, 1995.

Ralston, B.A. and Xin, X., 2000, GIS-based public health analysis with map objects and SAS, *Proceedings of the Twentieth Annual ESRI User Conference*, July 2000, San Diego, CA.

Reissman, D.B., Staley, F., and Curtis, G.B., 2001, Use of geographic information system technology to aid health department decision making about childhood lead poisoning prevention activities, *Environmental Health Perspectives*, 109, 1, 89–94.

Richards, T.B., Croner, C.M., and Novick, L.F., 1999a, Getting started with geographic information systems (GIS), Part 1, *Journal of Public Health Management Practice*, 5, 2, 73–76.

Richards, T.B., Croner, C.M., and Novick, L.F., 1999b, Geographic information systems (GIS) for state and local public health practitioners, Part 2, *Journal of Public Health Management Practice,* 5, 4, 1–6.

Richards, T.B., Croner, C.M., and Novick, L.F., 1999c, Atlas of state and local geographic information systems (GIS) maps to improve community health, *Journal of Public Health Management Practice*, 5, 2, 2–8.

Richards, T.B. et al., 1999d, Towards a GIS sampling frame for surveys of local health departments and local boards of health, *Journal of Public Health Management and Practice*, 5, 4, 65–75.

Richards, T.B. et al., 1999e, Geographic information systems and public health: mapping the future, *Public Health Reports,* 114, 359–373.

Rodwin, V.G., 2002, Comparative health systems, in Kovner, A.R. and Jonas, S., Eds., *Jonas and Kovner's Healthcare Delivery in the United States,* 7th ed., New York: Springer Publishing.

Rogers, M., 1999a, Using marketing information to focus smoking cessation programs in specific census block groups along the Buford Highway corridor, DeKalb County, Georgia, *Journal of Public Health Management Practice*, 5, 2, 55–57.

Rogers, M., 1999b, Getting started with geographic information systems (GIS): A local health department perspective, *Journal of Public Health Management Practice*, 5, 4, 22–23.

Roper, W. and Mays, G., 1999, GIS and public health policy: A new frontier for improving community health, *Journal of Public Health Management and Practice*, 5, 2, vi–vii.

Rushton, G., 1999, Methods to evaluate geographic access to health services, Geographic Information Systems in Public Health, Part 1 (special issue), *Journal of Public Health Management and Practice*, 5, 2, 93–100.

Rushton, G. and Armstrong, M., 1997, Improving public health through geographical information systems: An instructional guide to major concepts and their implementation [CD-ROM], version 2.0, Iowa City: University of Iowa, Department of Geography, http://www.uiowa.edu/~geog/.

Rushton, G., Elmes, G., and McMaster, R., 2000, Considerations for improving geographic information research in public health, *URISA Journal*, 12, 2, 31–49.

Shull, K., Hsiu-Hura, L., and Lamon, P., 1998, A process for developing vital health information at census tract level, *URISA 98 Annual Conference Proceedings*, Charlotte, NC.

Singer, B.H. and Ryff, C.D., Eds., 2001, New horizons in health: An integrative approach, National Research Council (US), Committee on Future Directions for Behavioral and Social Sciences Research at the National Institutes of Health, Washington, D.C.: National Academy Press.

Stockwell, J.J. et al., 1993, The U.S. EPA geographic information system for mapping environmental releases of toxic chemical release inventory (TRI) chemicals, *Risk Analysis,* 132, 155–164.

Stoe, D. and Oberle, S., 1999, Data-sharing: Legal, ethical and cultural issues associated with a multi-agency GIS, *URISA 99 Annual Conference Proceedings*, Chicago.

Sultz, H.A. and Young, K.M., 2001, *Health Care USA: Understanding Its Organization and Delivery,* 3rd ed., Gaithersburg, MD: Aspen Publishers.

Tatham, B., Fiedler, R., and Pruss, S.L., 2000, Public health care: Changing the model, *Proceedings of the 20th Annual ESRI User Conference,* July 2000, San Diego, CA.

Thorpe, K.E. and Knickman, J.R., 2002, Financing for health care, in Kovner A.R. and Jonas, S., Eds., *Jonas and Kovner's Healthcare Delivery in the United States,* 7th ed., New York: Springer.

Thrall, G.I., 1999, The future of GIS in public health management and practice, *Journal of Public Health Management Practice*, 5, 4, 75–82.

Tim, U., 1995, The application of GIS in environmental health sciences: Opportunities and limitations, *Environmental Research*, 71, 2, 75–88.

Turner, T.L. and Bowers, R.T. 2000, ArcIMS — The solution to streamlining data collection, modeling, planning, and design, *Proceedings of the 20th Annual ESRI User Conference*, San Diego, CA.

U.S. Federal Geographic Data Committee, 1997, Framework introduction and guide, Washington D.C.: GPO.

U.S. Health Care Financing Administration, 1999, Geomapping, outreach and health promotions support, *Commerce Business Daily,* April 28, Washington D.C.: HHS, PSA #2334.

U.S. National Cancer Institute, 1999, Cancer surveillance implementation plan, Division of Cancer Control and Population Sciences, Surveillance Implementation Group, March 1999, Rockville, MD: National Cancer Institute.

U.S. Public Health Service, 1999, Core public health functions, USPHS Steering Committee, Public health in America, Washington, D.C.: GPO, http://www.health.gov/phfunctions/public.htm.

Vinod, A., 2002, The Application of the Unified Modeling Language in object-oriented analysis of healthcare information systems, *Journal of Medical Systems,* 26, 5, 383–397.

Vlassoff, C. and Garcia-Moreno, C., 2002, Placing gender at the centre of health programming: Challenges and limitations, *Social Science & Medicine*, 54, 11, 1713–1723.

Warnecke, L. et al., 1998, *Geographic Information Technology in Cities and Counties: A Nationwide Assessment,* Washington, D.C.: American Forests.

Weinstein, A., 1994, *Market Segmentation: Using Demographics, Psychographics and Other Niche Marketing Techniques to Predict Consumer Behavior,* revised ed., Chicago: Probus.

Weiss, M. J., 1999, *The Clustered World: A Guide to Lifestyles in America and Beyond,* New York: Little Brown.

Wennberg, J. and Cooper, M., Eds., 1999, The quality of medical care in the United States: A report on the Medicare program, in *The Dartmouth Atlas of Medical Care in the United States 1999,* Chicago: American Hospital Association.

Wennberg, J.E., 2002, When too much care can be bad for your health, *The New Scientist,* August 17.

White, G.F. and Cerny, K.C., 1999, Client demographics (age and gender) at low-income clinics in Austin/Travis County, Texas, 1995–1996, *Journal of Public Health Management Practice,* 5, 2, 47–48.

Williams, Robert C. et al., Eds., 1998, *Proceedings of the Third National Conference on Geographic Information Systems in Public Health,* San Diego, CA.

Wittie, P., Drane, W., and Aldrich, T., 1996, Classification methods for denominators in small areas, *Statistics in Medicine*, 15, 17–18, 1921–1926.

Wood, M.S. and Coggan, J.M., 2000, *Women's Health on the Internet*, New York: Haworth Press.

World Health Organization, 2000, The World Health Report, 2000, Health Systems: Improving Performance, Geneva.

Yasnoff, W. and Sondik, E., 1999, Geographic information systems (GIS) in public health practice in the new millennium, *Journal of Public Health Management and Practice*, 5, 4, ix–xii.

Zenilman, J.M. et al., 2002, Geographic epidemiology of gonorrhoea and chlamydia on a large military installation: Application of a GIS system, *Sexually Transmitted Infections,* 78, 1, 40–44.

Section 4

Data Protection and E-Governance Issues in Public Health

14 GIS and Public Health in the Information Society

Massimo Craglia and Alessandro Annoni

CONTENTS

14.1 INTRODUCTION

Where do Europeans turn when they want reliable information on health? A Eurobarometer survey published today [16th April 2003] by the European Commission (EC) shows that, across the European Union (EU), nearly one in four Europeans (23 percent) use the Internet to get health information. The picture varies considerably, though, between countries: in Denmark and the Netherlands around 40 percent of people use the Internet for health information, while in Greece, Spain, Portugal, and France usage is at 15 percent or less. Health professionals, such as doctors and pharmacists, are still by far the most important source of health information for Europeans and the traditional media — television, newspapers, and magazines — still outperform the Internet. Other key findings of the survey are that medical and health organisations achieve the highest trust rating on health issues (84 percent), while businesses and political parties receive the lowest (16 and 11 percent, respectively).

"This survey shows that there is a clear demand for online health information among Europe's citizens, but it also highlights issues of trust," said Health and Consumer Protection Commissioner David Byrne. "A large number of Europeans are still unaware of the amount and reliability of health information that can be found on the Web. The EU, via the Public Health Action Programme and the E-health initiative, is working

0-415-30655-8/04/$0.00+$1.50

> to ensure that Europeans have access to high quality, useful and trustworthy online health information." Improving health information and knowledge is one of the priorities of the EU's €312 million Public Health Action Programme for 2003–2008 launched by Commissioner Byrne on 18 March.[1]

The extracts above from the Public Health Directorate General of the European Commission encapsulate the current situation in Europe in respect to the drive to include health applications as a key component of the European Information Society. They also reference the challenges that lay ahead including issues of lack of awareness, widespread physical and social access to public sector information, and trust in content providers. Trusting content providers includes having a clear regulatory framework in place to ensure that privacy and confidentiality are protected and information is not misused.

This fourth section of this book addresses these themes in four chapters, which focus on the legal framework in respect to the protection of personal and health-related information (Chapter 15), public attitudes toward confidentiality and the use of health information (Chapter 16), and the opportunities and challenges opened up by recent technological developments (Chapter 17). The purpose of this introductory chapter is to:

- Provide the broad policy context for the development of the Information Society in Europe (Section 14.2)
- Outline the specific measures supporting European E-health and public health programs (Section 14.3)
- Discuss the recent developments in relation to environmental information that are of great significance given the important relationships between public health and environmental factors (Section 14.4)
- Review the recent initiatives to build the geographic information infrastructure necessary to support the policies and programs discussed above (Section 14.5)

14.2 DEVELOPING THE INFORMATION SOCIETY

The policy debate on the development of the Information Society in Europe can be traced back to the 1993 Maastricht Treaty that gave the Union responsibility in matters of trans-European networks in the transport, energy, and telecommunications sectors, thus providing the legal basis for the development of the Information Society.[2] The EC white paper on Growth, Competitiveness, and Employment (Commission of the European Communities (CEC), 1993) stressed the urgent need for a pan-European infrastructure to help boost economic growth and competitiveness at a time when Europe was facing significant problems of industrial restructuring, and long-term unemployment. The development of an information-based society was seen as the key to the development of new job opportunities in the medium term.

---

[1] *Source:* http://europa.eu.int/comm/health/index_en.htm.

[2] *Source:* http://europa.eu.int/en/record/mt/top.html.

Acting on the proposals made in the white paper, the European Council of December 1993 asked a group of high-level experts and industrialists under the chair of Commissioner Martin Bangemann to draft a report on the Information Society, suggesting practical ways that its objectives could be achieved. The Bangemann Report (Bangemann, 1994) was published in June 1994, and identified the need to speed up the process of liberalization of the telecommunications sector in Europe, hitherto largely in the hands of state monopolies, and to reinforce universal service through deregulation that would enhance competition and thus (it was assumed) drive down prices. The Bangemann Report proposed a list of ten initiatives to demonstrate the utility of new telematics applications, including teleworking, distance learning, telematic services for health, trans-European public administrations networks, and city information highways. The report argued that financing the information infrastructure should come from the private sector, while the role of the EC would be to help target long-term investment in the exploitation of available technology. These proposals were incorporated into an action plan entitled "Europe's Way to the Information Society" (CEC, 1994), and has been supported by a number of funding streams in successive Research and Development Framework Programs since 1994.

The political support behind the development of an Information Society in Europe continued through the 1990s; it was reaffirmed at the highest level in 1999 by the adoption by the European Council of a new political initiative named E-Europe (CEC, 1999). The key objectives of E-Europe are to:

- Bring all citizens, businesses, and administrations online
- Promote education and the availability of venture capital
- Ensure that the whole process is socially inclusive and strengthening social cohesion

E-Europe has been followed by two action plans for 2002 (CEC, 2000) and 2005 (CEC, 2002a) focusing on cheaper Internet access, education, and skills and key application areas, including E-commerce, health, and the delivery of government services and information. Of particular relevance for this discussion is the increased emphasis on E-government with binding agreements among member states to reach set targets for the delivery of public services online by 2005 and, as a corollary, increased access to public sector information by all citizens. The action plans are largely funded by national governments, with some core EU funding.

The EC initiatives to liberalize physical access have had some notable successes. Most national telecommunications monopolies have been privatized, greater competition has increased consumer choice and level of service, and the common standard for mobile telephony (GSM) promoted by the EC in 1994 has created a multibillion euro market giving Europe a competitive edge in this sector (Liikanen, 2002; Standage, 2001). As a result, the high penetration of mobile phones across many segments of society outstrips ownership of personal computers (PC) in Europe and promises an alternative way to access Internet-based information and services from the PC paradigm prevailing in the United States and Canada (Standage, 2001).

Another notable success has been the establishment of a regulatory framework for electronic communications networks and services to ensure transparency and avoid market distortions by players exploiting their dominant position. This regulatory regime, agreed in April 2002, includes a Framework Directive (CEC, 2002b), and Directives on Authorization (CEC, 2002c), Access (CEC, 2002d), and Universal Service (CEC, 2002e), in addition to the one on Personal Data Processing and Privacy enacted in 1997 (CEC, 1997) and revised in 2002 (CEC, 2002f). Aside from the details of these directives, the recognition that this aspect of economic and social life cannot be left exclusively in the hand of the market and requires a set of agreed rules, checks, and balances is of extreme importance.

Against this set of initiatives, limited success has been achieved in increasing and regulating access to information or content. A set of guidelines put forward by the EC in 1989 (CEC, 1989) to promote access to information, transparency, and a level playing field were largely ignored, partly because of a lack of enforceable legal backing, and partly because of the immaturity of the market at that stage. It took another ten years before the debate was relaunched with the publication in early 1999 of the green paper on Public Sector Information: A Key Resource for Europe (CEC, 1998). This consultation paper played a major role in raising the debate across Europe on the opportunities created by the increased availability of public sector information (PSI) in digital format for its reuse beyond the purposes for which it was originally collected. The paper recognized existing barriers to accessing PSI, including different legal frameworks and pricing regimes, and posed pertinent questions on the extent to which such frameworks ought to be harmonized across Europe differentiating between administrative and non-administrative data and essential versus value-added data.

After extensive consultation, the green paper was followed-up by a communication (CEC, 2001a), and a draft directive (CEC, 2002g). The draft directive argues the case for action at the European level to remove the barriers identified and creates a minimum level of harmonization on the commercial and noncommercial reuse of PSI. Disappointingly, it does not address issues of access to data, arguing that these are best dealt with at national, regional, and local levels. Instead, it focuses on ensuring a level playing field, transparency, and nondiscriminatory practices in the conditions for the reuse and exploitation of data that are already accessible. The European Parliament scrutinized the draft in February 2003, with a robust debate between those members who wished to extend the provision of the directive to include a wider definition of PSI and require that it should be made available at no more than marginal cost and those who opposed such measures. In the event, a small majority lead by the United Kingdom and Germany rejected the amendments proposed by the rapporteur, Wim Van Velzen, who then commented:

> This small majority in the European Parliament would rather see that the private sector, and in particular SMEs, keep on paying the public sector (i.e., via the return on investment on the re-use of public sector information) and that there is no transparency on the re-use. Also, this small majority seems to think that more bureaucracy is favourable in this matter: the text as adopted today still leaves room for public sector bodies to approve (or not) the re-use of public sector information, while we are talking here about information that is already generally accessible! Having to ask for approval for re-use for generally accessible information in many cases even means a step backwards.[1]

[1] *Source:* http://www.wimvanvelzen.nl/e_statement.php3?statementid=46.

The revised draft directive obtained unanimous approval in the Telecommunications Council of Ministers on March 27, 2003. Europe is, of course, not alone in pushing forward Information Society initiatives. In the United States in 2002, for example, the federal government passed the E-Government Act to develop electronic government services, promote the use of Internet and access to information to citizens, and promote interagency collaboration. The act has an allocation of over $350 million for the period of 2003 to 2006 (U.S. Congress, 2002, Section 3604).

The extent of developments worldwide in promoting E-government can be seen from a recent survey (Accenture, 2003) of E-government initiatives across 22 countries. The findings indicate that Canada, Singapore, and the United States are at the forefront of such developments, closely followed by Australia, Hong Kong, and a group of leading European countries (see Figure 14.1).

From a more global perspective, the United Nations (UN) General Assembly Resolution 56/183 endorsed the framework for the first world summit on the Information Society, which was held in Geneva on December 10–12, 2003. The resolution described the purpose of the summit as being the development of a common vision and understanding of the Information Society and the adoption of a declaration and plan of action for implementation by governments, international institutions, and all sectors of civil society. The plan of action will address the following issues:[1]

- Information and communication infrastructure
  - Financing and investment
  - Affordability
  - Development
  - Sustainability
- Access to information and knowledge
- The role of governments, the business sector, and civil society in the promotion of information and communication technologies (ICT) for development
- Capacity building
  - Human resources development
  - Education
  - Training
- Security
- Enabling environment
- Promotion of development-oriented ICT applications for all
- Cultural identity and linguistic diversity, local content, and media development
- Identifying and overcoming barriers to the achievement of the Information Society with a human perspective

The second phase of the World Summit will be held in Tunis in 2005.

[1] *Source:* http://www.itu.int/wsis/.

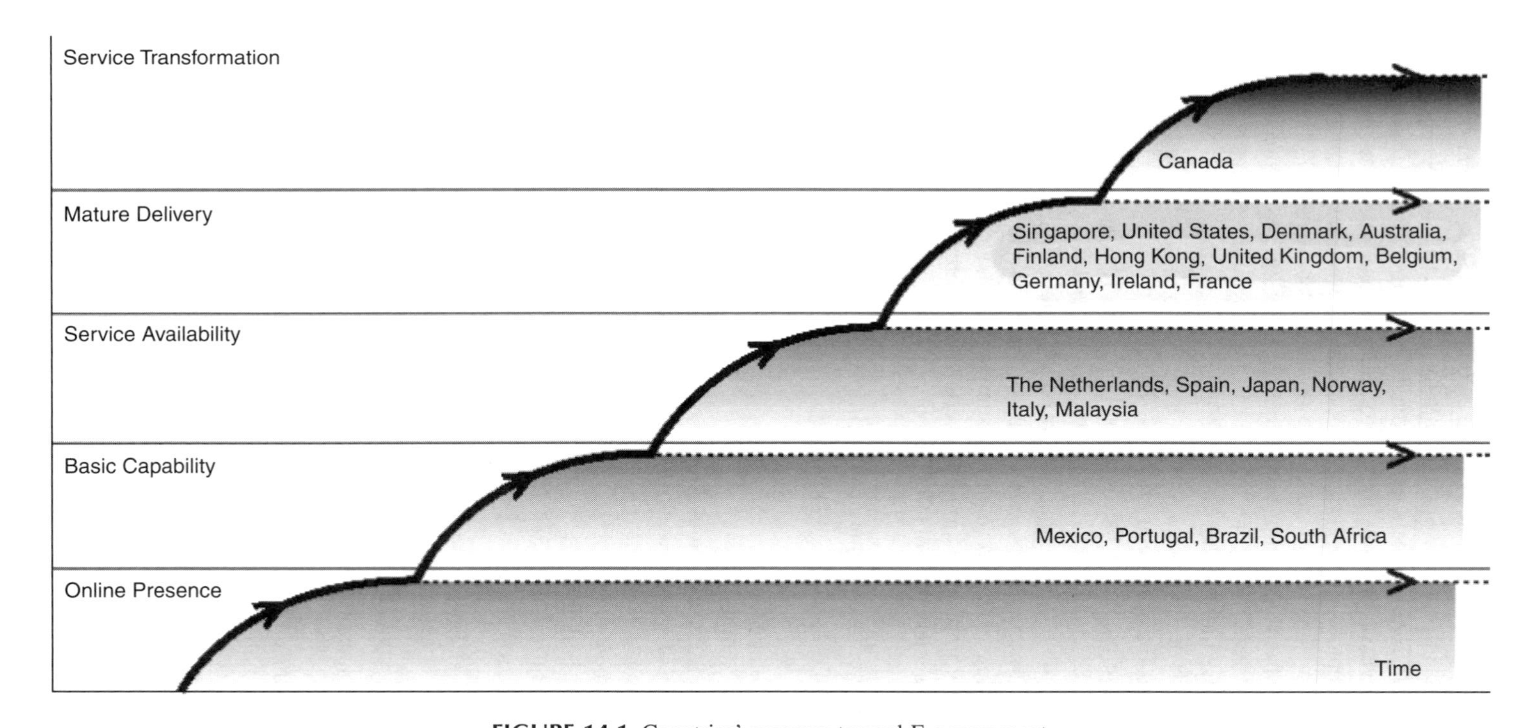

FIGURE 14.1 Countries' progress toward E-government.
Source: Accenture, 2003, *eGovernment Leadership: Engaging the Customer,* http://www/accenture.com/xdoc/en/industries/government/gove_capa_egov_leadership.pdf.

14.3 FOCUS ON HEALTH

14.3.1 E-HEALTH

As indicated in the previous section, there are a large number of initiatives worldwide to promote the use of ICT by citizens, governments, and businesses. As recognized by many commentators (Craglia and Masser, 2003; Niles and Hanson, 2003; Smith and Craglia, 2003) just promoting access to information electronically is not enough unless it is functional, responding to genuine needs, including the provision of more effective and efficient services to citizens. It is for this reason that even the earlier documents on the Information Society (Bangemann, 1994) placed great importance on citizen-centered applications such as E-government and E-health. In relation to the latter, the vision of ten years ago was for the following:

> Less costly and more effective healthcare systems for Europe's citizens: What should be done? Create a direct communication "network of networks" based on common standards linking general practitioners, hospitals, and social centres on a European scale. Who will do it? The private sector, insurance companies, medical associations, and Member State healthcare systems, with the European Union promoting standards and portable applications. Once telecom operators make available the required networks at reduced rates, the private sector will create competitively priced services at a European level, boosting the productivity and cost-effectiveness of the whole healthcare sector. Who gains? Citizens as patients will benefit from a substantial improvement in healthcare (improvement in diagnosis through online access to European specialists, online reservation of analysis and hospital services by practitioners extended on a European scale, transplant matching, etc.) (Bangemann, 1994).

That early vision has been slow to develop. However, health has remained one of the core streams of activity of the successive E-Europe action plans. For example, the 2002 Action Plan (CEC, 2000) focused on:

- Ensuring that primary and secondary healthcare providers have health telematics infrastructure in place including regional networks
- Identify and disseminate best practice in electronic health services in Europe
- Establish a set of quality criteria for health-related Web sites
- Establish health technology and data assessment networks
- Publish a communication on legal aspects of E-health

Similarly, the E-Europe 2005 Action Plan (CEC, 2002a) focused on electronic health cards, health information networks, and the further development of online health services.

In addition, the High-Level Committee on Health has established a Working Group on Health Telematics. This working group was asked to review the introduction of ICT in the health sector, the factors promoting or inhibiting its development, and areas where European Community legislation could be beneficial. The group considered particular applications of ICT in health, namely health cards, virtual hospitals, and provision of health-related information to health professionals and patients.

14.3.2 Promoting Public Health

The initiatives reviewed in the preceding section aim to develop the electronic delivery of health-related services. The EU, however, has also been pursuing a number of measures to promote public health across the Union and this section summarizes some of the main ones focusing in particular on those that either:

- Explicitly refer to the importance of geographic information to identify needs, target resources, and monitor outcomes
- Emphasize the role of better and more timely information flows to support health policy

The community action programs on health promotion and health monitoring aim to improve awareness of the benefits of healthy lifestyles and behavior. The health-monitoring program has led to the development of harmonized environmental health indicators. In particular, the European Community Health Indicators (ECHI) Project[1] has provided a framework for the development of these European Community public health indicators. It covers outdoor air quality, housing, drinking water supply, sewage systems, ionizing radiation, noise, physical and mental workplace exposures, accidents related to work, and occupational diseases. The ECHI project also includes indicators for the social and cultural environment, such as social support, social isolation, life events, and violence.

In the white paper on food safety (European Commission, 1999), the EC identified environmental sources as the origin of the presence of contaminants in the food chain. The paper called for mechanisms to control and enforce limits of contaminants and residues in foodstuffs. It also identifies surveillance, information gathering, and analysis as essential elements of food safety policy.

The new program of European Community action in the field of public health[2] (2003 to 2008) adopted by the European Parliament and the European Council on September 23, 2002, was launched in March 2003 with a budget of €312 million. The program puts into practice the integrated approach to public health advocated in the EC's May 2000 "Communication on Health Strategy" (European Commission, 2000). It replaces a series of eight EU programs that each focused on individual health issues:

1. Cancer
2. AIDS and other communicable diseases
3. Rare diseases
4. Pollution-related diseases
5. Injury prevention

[1] *Source:* http://europa.eu.int/comm/health/ph_projects/1998/monitoring/fp_monitoring_1998_frep_08_en.pdf.

[2] *Source:* http://europa.eu.int/comm/health/ph_programme/programme_en.htm.

6. Health monitoring
7. Health promotion
8. Drug abuse

The 2003 Work Plan contains a number of key "cross-cutting themes" that span the whole program:

- Developing work on health impact assessment
- Health in the applicant countries
- Inequalities in health
- Aging and health

These are issues of strategic and political importance and link the three strands of the program described below. In addition to work on these themes, there will be specific actions on the cooperation between health systems and on promoting best practice and effectiveness in the health sector. Projects launched under these actions will provide input for healthcare policy debates both at EU level and within member states. In particular, they will be relevant to discussions on intersectoral policymaking, patient mobility, and the future of care for the elderly. The three main strands of the program are:

1. *Improving health information and knowledge.* In this strand the program seeks to build on and develop the health data already gathered at European level, agreeing to list key health indicators on which to base the monitoring of health status, and creating the network of public health institutes around the EU that will operate an integrated EU health information system.
2. *Responding to health threats.* This part of the program builds on the "rapid alert" systems already in place at EU level: notably, the European Network on Communicable Diseases and the EU's rapid alert system for possible bioterrorist incidents. The program expands the geographical and disease coverage of the rapid response system and reinforces the member states's capability to respond to possible bioterrorism incidents. These include actions on the networking of laboratories and on building expertise in the field of chemical and biological pathogens.
3. *Addressing health determinants.* Health determinants are factors such as personal behavior, lifestyles, social conditions, environment, and working conditions that influence people's health. This part of the program allows health policy makers and nongovernmental organizations around the EU to pool their knowledge on various determinants by supporting EU-level networks, promoting exchange of experience, and financing innovative projects.[1]

The launch of this new public health program at the European level is clearly an important new development that will support the activities of researchers and

[1] *Source:* http://europa.eu.int/comm/health/index_en.htm.

practitioners across Europe and links in with other information pooling and integrating initiatives. Among them, the Community Action Program on pollution-related diseases identified two main objectives:

1. To improve information on pollution-related diseases
2. To enhance knowledge and understanding of the assessment and management of pollution-related diseases

The program launched interesting initiatives such as the development of GIS, allowing for a better health impact assessment of environmental living conditions such as the proximity to radioactive landfill sites or a better prevention of asthma and respiratory allergies depending on regional climatic and housing conditions. Moreover, in January 2003 the EC launched an Integrated Impact Assessment Tool (CEC, 2002h), which will identify health impacts of projects, policy proposals, and strategies not primarily meant to affect health and how these can be assessed. This will aid policy makers to assess trade-offs and compare different scenarios when deciding on a specific course of action. Impact assessment will be applied to the major initiatives presented by the EC in its annual policy strategy or its work program. There is considerable international experience in integrating health aspects into environmental impact assessments. This experience as well as the experience of health impact assessments should be drawn from when looking at potential health impacts of policy proposals in other areas than health, particularly when conducting extended impact assessments in the fields of health and the environment. The new procedure (i.e., implementing the new Integrated Impact Assessment Tool), provides an excellent opportunity for reviewing policy proposals in other areas and their potential impacts on health.

14.4 FOCUS ON THE ENVIRONMENT

Health has always been a major driver for environmental policy development. The European Community's environment legislation is based on safety standards, monitoring systems, and controls covering the vast majority of known health hazardous agents. The main areas are chemicals, including dioxins, endocrine disrupters, pesticides, air pollution, water protection and management, noise, waste, major industrial accidents, and ionizing radiation

As the EU has responsibilities in both the fields of environment and health as recognized by the Union Treaties Articles 152 and 174 (CEC, 2002i), there are numerous legal instruments adopted by the EU that address key issues in respect to environment and health.

In 2001, the EC adopted a white paper on the Strategy for a New Chemicals Policy (COM2001/88final). The need for a new strategy arose from wide acceptance that the existing legislation was not capable of responding adequately to public and political concern in Europe about the potential impact of chemicals on health and the environment. The proposed REACH system (registration, evaluation, and authorization of chemicals) provides for the stepwise collection of information on the estimated 30,000 chemical substances in the EU, including their toxicological properties and their uses, to provide for appropriate risk management measures. Registration will place the information submitted by industry in a central database. The information in the database will also be useful and validated for the establishment of a causal link between environmental factors and adverse health effects resulting from chemical production and use. To ensure a sound technical-scientific implementation across the EU, a chemicals agency may also be proposed.

One of the main thrusts of policy on air pollution is to reduce the amount of material deleterious to health that reaches the human body, whether directly or indirectly. EU air quality standards have been set since 1996, requiring member states to set up and maintain a system for assessing air quality, identifying areas where limit values are likely to be exceeded, and drawing up action plans to reduce the risk of exceedance as well as meeting the objectives of the EC directives. Limit values have been adopted for air concentrations of sulfur dioxide, nitrogen dioxide, particulate matter, lead, carbon monoxide, and benzene. In 2001, the EC launched the air quality program — Clean Air for Europe — that will lead to a long-term, integrated thematic strategy on air pollution.

The aim of EU water policy is to guarantee high safety standards for drinking water and to reduce adverse environmental effects of certain agricultural and industrial practices. The new Water Framework Directive 2000/60/EC highlights the need for protective measures for all water uses and aquatic ecosystems at the point where pollution occurs. It introduces a priority list of substances that are dangerous to the environment, to be phased out in the future. It also has provisions for monitoring and assessment measures to be applied in case of accidental water pollution.

Public concern about exposure to noise pollution remains high in spite of EU policies at EU and member state level. The EU Directive 2002/49/EC sets noise emission limits for products (e.g., cars, trucks, aircraft, and industrial equipment) and harmonizes the assessment and management of environmental noise. Both the Water Framework Directive and the Directive on Noise make explicit or implicit requirements for GIS data and analysis. Therefore, both directives are significantly relevant to the uptake of GIS in the organizations tasked with their implementation. Other examples of environmental legislation with a strong spatial component are the Seveso Directives (CEC, 2003), which were adopted following major industrial accidents with serious consequences for both man and the environment. Their aim is to reduce the risks arising from the production, transportation, and storage of dangerous chemicals and require location-specific plans and measures.

An important body of European Community legislation set up under Chapter III of the EURATOM Treaty (1957) ensures the protection of the health of workers and members of the public against ionizing radiation. The EU radiation protection Basic Safety Standards Council Directive 96/29 EURATOM includes specific provisions for the protection of the public from enhanced levels of radioactivity in the environment. Other important complementary European Community radiation protection legislation includes provisions on natural radiation sources (including radon gas), radioactive substances in the environment as a result of discharges of nuclear installations in normal operation and as a result of accidents. In addition, Article 35 to Article 38 of the EURATOM Treaty confer direct responsibilities to the EC with regard to environmental radioactivity.

Most of the initiatives reported above foresee the development of GIS applications. Here we can distinguish two main areas:

1. Issues to do with the provision of health-related services in natural or man-made disaster situations (floods, earthquakes, and major disaster such as Chernobyl, Toulouse, and Seveso)
2. The public health impacts related to the day-to-day exposure to inadequate environmental conditions such as:
   - Outdoor and indoor air pollution
   - Noise
   - Indoor environment and housing conditions
   - Water contamination
   - Electromagnetic fields and radiation
   - Chemical exposures

The importance of the relationship between environment and health and the need for good quality information to support European Community action is fully recognized by the Sixth Environmental Action Programme for 2002 through 2012 (CEC, 2001b). It includes environment and health as one of its four priorities. Specifically, it sets the following objectives:[1]

- Achieving better understanding of the threats to environment and human health and to take action to prevent and reduce these threats.
- Contributing to a better quality of life through an integrated approach concentrating on urban areas.
- Aiming to achieve within one generation (2020) that chemicals are only produced and used in ways that do not lead to a significant negative impact on health and the environment, recognizing that the present gaps of knowledge on the properties, use, disposal, and exposure of chemicals need to be overcome.
- Substituting chemicals that are dangerous with safer chemicals or safer alternative technologies not entailing the use of chemicals, with the aim of reducing risks to man and the environment.
- Reducing the impacts of pesticides on human health and the environment and more generally to achieve a more sustainable use of pesticides as well as a significant overall reduction in risks of the use of pesticides consistent with the necessary crop protection; pesticides in use that are persistent, bio-accumulative, or toxic or have other properties of concern should be substituted by less dangerous ones where possible.
- Achieving quality levels of ground and surface water that do not significantly impact and cause risk to human health and the environment, and to ensure that the rates of extraction from water resources are sustainable over the long term.

---

[1] *Source:* CEC (Commission of the European Communities), 2001b, *Communication on the 6th Environment Action Programme of the European Community: "Environment 2010: Our Future, Our Choice,"* COM (2001) 31 final, Article 7, Brussels: EC.

- Achieving levels of air quality that do not give rise to significant negative impacts on and risks to human health and the environment.
- Substantially reducing the number of people regularly affected by long-term average levels of noise, in particular from traffic which, according to scientific studies, causes detrimental effects on human health.

Of particular relevance to this book on GIS and public health is the increasing recognition that meeting these objectives, and more generally aiming at sustainable development, requires a much increased availability of good quality geographic information to assess the multiple impacts (i.e., environmental, social, and economic) of policies in different sectors, target resources, and monitor effects. An evidence-based and integrated approach to policy is emerging across EU (and national) polices (Craglia and Annoni, 2001), but particularly in the environmental field. As an example, the Sixth Environmental Action Programme discussed above requires in Article 10 that environmental objectives be pursued through:[1]

- Greater consultation with all stakeholders
- Greater public participation and access to information
- Extensive use of ex-ante and ex-post evaluation
- Reviewing and regularly monitoring information and reporting systems with a view to a more coherent and effective system to ensure streamlined reporting of high quality, comparable, and relevant environmental data and information
- Reinforcing the development and the use of earth monitoring (e.g., satellite technology) applications and tools in support of policy making and implementation

The political importance of the environment and health is captured by this quotation from the DG Environment Web site:

> It is estimated that around 20 percent of the burden of disease in industrialised countries can be attributed to environmental factors, with the bulk of this affecting children and vulnerable groups. The magnitude of the problem is also perceived by the majority of Europeans: in a recent survey,[2] some 89 percent are worried about the potential impact of the environment on their health. Furthermore, new technologies, changing lifestyles, work and life patterns, present new and sometimes unexpected impacts on the environment and its influence on health.[3]

The size and complexity of environment and health issues have reached calls for new ways to approach the sustainable development dimension of EU policies. These approaches need to match the scale of the problems in all their dimensions.

---

[1] *Source:* CEC (Commission of the European Communities), 2001b, *Communication on the 6th Environment Action Programme of the European Community: "Environment 2010: Our Future, Our Choice,"* COM (2001) 31 final, Article 10, Brussels: EC.

[2] *Source*: Eurobarometer 58: http://europa.eu.int/comm/environment/barometer/barometer_2003_en.pdf.

[3] *Source:* http://europa.eu.int/comm/environment/health/index_en.htm.

With this in mind, the EC recently adopted a new Communication on the Environment and Health Strategy (European Commission, 2003), thereby setting the scene for the EU contribution to this challenge. The benefit of this proposal is the development of a community system integrating all the information on the state of the environment, the ecosystem, and human health. This intends to make the assessment of the overall environmental impact on human health more efficient by taking into account the full complexity of the effects (e.g., cocktail effects, combined exposure, accumulative effects, etc.) and interrelations between environment and health. The goal of the proposed strategy is therefore to develop an environment and health "cause-effect framework" that will provide the necessary information for the development of European Community policy.

The integrated approach advocated by the Environment and Health Strategy makes explicit reference to the need to integrate information (i.e., to pool and to link available knowledge and experience across the European Community, providing a strategic overview of environmental threats to health), irrespective of the type of burden involved or the environmental compartment through which that burden is transmitted. To achieve the long-term objectives of this strategy, the strategy proposes to set up an integrated environment and health monitoring system for the systematic and comprehensive collection of data over time. Because of existing European legislation, member states are already involved in data collection on a national basis. The value added at the European level is to generate synergies and facilitate the sharing of data and methodologies with a view to increasing understanding of the relationship between environment and health. As a result, health data is to be linked to the full range of environmental data, including all the different environmental compartments and the whole ecosystem, to obtain a picture of the exposure of populations to environmental contaminants and their adverse health effects. The strategy in particular links the forthcoming Health Monitoring and Information System, with two other major initiatives discussed later: INSPIRE and GMES. What is important for both researchers and practitioners is that the strategy recognizes that the impediments are not only technological or data-related in nature, but also policy-related in the extent to which many of the barriers to increased information sharing have to do with variable government policies on access, lack of standards and comparability.

14.5 EUROPEAN INFRASTRUCTURE INITIATIVES

14.5.1 Infrastructure for Spatial Information in Europe

The Infrastructure for Spatial Information in Europe (INSPIRE) initiative (www.ec-gis.org/inspire) was launched at the end of 2001 with the aim of making available relevant, harmonized, and quality geographic information for the purpose of formulation, implementation, monitoring, and evaluation of European Community policy making. To achieve its aim, INSPIRE has been addressing a broad set of issues including common reference data and metadata, architecture and standards, legal aspects and data policy, funding and implementation structures, and impact analysis. The objective is to arrive at an agreed-upon European legal framework that focuses on the needs of environmental policy and subsequently extends to other areas of European Community concern, such as agriculture, regional policy, and transport. INSPIRE is governed by the following principles:

- Data should be collected once and maintained at the level where this can be done most effectively.
- It must be possible to combine seamlessly spatial data from different sources across the EU and share it between many users and applications.
- It must be possible for spatial data collected at one level of government to be shared between all levels of government.
- Spatial data needed for good governance should be available on conditions that are not restricting its extensive use.
- It should be easy to discover which spatial data is available, to evaluate its fitness for purpose, and to know which conditions apply for its use.

INSPIRE will be built on top of existing and future national and regional spatial data infrastructures (SDIs). For this reason, the implementation of these principles is not a trivial task and requires further investigation and research on how to harmonize access to scattered and heterogeneous spatial data; for a review of SDIs, see, e.g., Craglia et al. (2000–2002), Masser (1998, 1999, 2002), and Wiliamson et al. (2003).

The importance of INSPIRE rests on a series of considerations. First, it marks the recognition that policy formulation, implementation, and evaluation require good information, which is up-to-date and at a territorial scale congruent with the focus of the policy being considered. As argued earlier, there is an increasing recognition that subnational and regional levels are the most appropriate levels to assess policy requirements and impacts. Hence, it is information that is referenced to these geographical scales that is becoming increasingly important for European policy. Second, it also recognizes that to maintain up-to-date local or regional information, it is important to involve providers at these levels and leave it to them to manage their information resources rather than attempt to centralize information at the European level. Consequently, this decentralized model of information management requires agreed rules to harmonize data collection and management methods and to access the information so that it can be shared and integrated. Third, although the first focus of INSPIRE is on environmental information, much of this information and the core geographic themes that underpin it are extremely relevant for research on public health and on the spatial relationship between health and the physical and social environment.

14.5.2 Global Monitoring for Environment and Security

The Global Monitoring for Environment and Security (GMES) initiative aims to implement an integrated European approach for the collection, dissemination, and analysis of space information and to coordinate the structures of the systems that produce space information (CEC, 2001c). As such, GMES is a framework, federating a number of national and European systems, projects, and services that have to be broadly organized and interrelated in line with users' needs. The key tasks of the GMES initiative are to:

- Contribute to the understanding and command of global change using models fed by satellite data.
- Enhance the study of various processes that put pressure on the environment, in particular due to the growth of urban or industrial areas.
- Support the work of civil protection and town planning agencies in respect to the prevention and evaluation of catastrophes or disasters of human or natural origin, from forest fires and floods to pollution by hydrocarbons.
- Make a contribution to the common foreign and security policy (CFSP) to which the EU is now clearly committed.

The list of themes that could find a place under the GMES umbrella is long and constantly growing. Initial actions are concentrated on the delivery of services for a range of environment-related topics, including:

Environmental stress
Urban and regional development
Soil erosion
Nature and landscape
Coastal areas
Ozone and UV radiation
River basin management
Agro-environment
Global change and environmental conventions
Terrestrial and marine carbon
Marine organic pollution
Desertification
Sustainable forest management
Atmospheric chemistry
Climate change
Natural hazards and crises
Fires, floods, earthquakes, and landslides
Crisis management
Humanitarian aid

The contribution that GMES will be able to make to the analysis of health outcomes and the relationships between the physical and human environment and health is potentially significant. Being strongly linked to the use of satellites, GMES will benefit from the development of the EU's Galileo program (Council Regulation (EC) No 876/2002). GMES will also benefit from the development of INSPIRE, which will provide the platform on which EU spatial data requirements resulting from the implementation of existing and new thematic strategies will be coordinated and structured. These infrastructure developments coupled with the efforts toward integrated health-related information systems reviewed in

Section 14.3 give an indication of the concerted action in Europe toward addressing health and environment issues.

14.6 CONCLUSIONS

This chapter has provided a broad view of the policy framework within which we are likely to see an increased role of GIS in public health research and practice. In particular, it has highlighted the following:

- The continued development of the Information Society in Europe provides new opportunities for the delivery of health-related information and services through ICTs.
- The increasing recognition that the complexity of urban society requires more-integrated approaches to policy analysis and policy making is supporting more and more local and regional spatial perspectives to assess impacts, target intervention, and evaluate outcomes. This in turns supports wider use of spatial analytical perspectives and methods and increased access to geographically referenced data.
- Public health is increasing its importance on the European political agenda with targeted programs addressing social, environmental, and economic impacts.
- An infrastructure for spatial information in Europe is coming into being to support the policy needs identified above. This includes technologies, data, policies, people and skills, and coordinated approaches.
- International and European legislation is putting increased emphasis on wider access to information for justice and public participation, as well as better-informed policy and wider business opportunities.

With these considerations in mind, it could be argued that the future for GIS and public health in Europe is better than ever. There are, however, a number of important challenges to be addressed:

- Although increased access to environmental and geographic information is likely to become available, there is still a debate raging on the terms and conditions for access, including pricing models and copyright, whether differential conditions will apply for public sector organizations, research and education, the private sector, and citizens. The continuing instability of business models for electronic content, and the natural tendency of organizations to eschew change suggest that there is little hope for this debate to be settled soon to the satisfaction of all concerned.
- Access to health-related information then raises another set of issues. First, there are issues about privacy and confidentiality that are crucial to building and maintaining trust between information providers, researchers, and users. Some of these are discussed in the following chapters of this section, but clearly much research and public debate continues to be necessary. Second, an important issue is that with rights come obligations

on all the stakeholders. If citizens have the right to confidentiality and privacy, what obligation do they have to ensure that the wider "public good" is achieved? What are the obligations on health professionals, public servants, and researchers on the sharing of personal information that may save lives? What are the obligations on the private sector in the handling and reuse of personal data? It could be argued that existing legislation such as the Data Protection Act addresses all that, but in reality the paucity of cases taken up for investigation by Information Commissioners across Europe suggest that much unreported activity goes on in the shadow of legislation.

- There is an underlying assumption that more information is better for all concerned, including citizens, government, and business, but is that really the case? Particularly in the context of health services online, what is the evidence for this? What are the costs of maintaining such services in relation to the benefits they provide?
- Education and skills are the other major issue, not only with respect to the increased use of GIS and spatial analysis in public health research and practice, but to support the cross-departmental and interagency integrated approach to policy and research as well. This approach is advocated by many, but is very difficult to achieve in practice (see, e.g., Signoretta and Craglia, 2002). Education and skills are required not just at the technical level, but also at the organizational and institutional levels.

These major issues will continue to require the attention of all involved. Noticeably they are not technical, but ethical, organizational, and economic as these are the real areas where more discussion and research is needed.

References

Accenture, 2003, *eGovernment Leadership: Engaging the Customer,* http://www.accenture.com/xdoc/en/industries/government/gove_capa_egov_leadership.pdf.

Bangemann, M., 1994, *Europe and the Global Information Society: Recommendations to the European Council (26 May 1994),* High-Level Group on the Information Society, European Commission [cited October 19, 2000], http://europa.eu.int/ISPO/docs/basics/docs/bangemann.html.

CEC (Commission of the European Communities), 1989, *Guidelines for Improving the Synergy between the Public and Private Sectors in the Information Market,* Brussels: European Commission, ftp://ftp.cordis.lu/pub/econtent/docs/1989_public_sector_guidelines_en.pdf.

CEC (Commission of the European Communities), 1990, *Council Directive 90/313/EC of 7 June 1990 on the Freedom of Access to Information on the Environment,* June 7, European Commission, [cited November 6 2002], http://europa.eu.int/scadplus/leg/en/lvb/l28091.htm.

CEC (Commission of the European Communities), 1993, *Growth, Competitiveness and Employment: The Challenges and Ways Forward into the 21st Century,* Brussels: European Commission, http://europa.eu.int/en/record/white/c93700/contents.html.

CEC (Commission of the European Communities), 1994, *Europe's Way to the Information Society: An Action Plan,* Brussels: European Commission, http://europa.eu.int/ISPO/infosoc/backg/action.html.

CEC (Commission of the European Communities), 1997, *Directive 97/66/EC of the European Parliament and of the Council of 15 December 1997 Concerning the Processing of Personal Data and the Protection of Privacy in the Telecommunications Sector* (December 15), European Commission, [cited November 6 2002], http://europa.eu.int/smartapi/cgi/sga_doc?smartapi!celexapi!prod!CELEXnumdoc&lg=EN&numdoc=31997L0066&model=guichett.

CEC (Commission of the European Communities), 1998, *Public Sector Information: A Key Resource for Europe*, Brussels: European Commission, http://europa.eu.int/ISPO/docs/policy/docs/COM(98)585/.

CEC (Commission of the European Communities), 1999, *An Information Society for All. Communication on a Commission Initiative for the Special European Council of Lisbon, 23 and 24 March 2000.* Luxembourg: European Commission, http://europa.eu.int/ information_society/index.en.

CEC (Commission of the European Communities), 2000, *eEurope 2002 Action Plan,* http://europa.eu.int/ information_society/index.en.

CEC (Commission of the European Communities), 2001a, *eEurope 2002: Creating an EU Framework for the Exploitation of Public Sector Information*, Brussels: European Commission, ftp://ftp.cordis.lu/pub/econent/docs/2001_607_en.pdf.

CEC (Commission of the European Communities), 2001b, *Communication on the 6th Environment Action Programme of the European Community: "Environment 2010: Our Future, Our Choice,"* COM (2001) 31 final, Brussels: EC.

CEC (Commission of the European Communities), 2001c, *Global Monitoring for Environment and Security,* COM(2001)609, http://europa.eu.int/comm/space/prog/gmes/gmes_en.html.

CEC (Commission of the European Communities), 2002a, *eEurope 2005: An Information Society for All: An Action Plan to Be Presented in View of the Sevilla European Council, 21/22 June 2002,* Brussels: European Commission, http://europa.eu.int/ information_society/index.en.

CEC (Commission of the European Communities), 2002b, *Directive 2002/21/EC of the European Parliament and of the Council of 7 March 2002 on a Common Regulatory Framework for Electronic Communications Networks and Services (Framework Directive),* Brussels: European Commission, p. 18.

CEC (Commission of the European Communities), 2002c, *Directive 2002/20/EC of the European Parliament and of the Council of 7 March 2002 on the Authorisation of Electronic Communications Networks and Services (Authorisation Directive),* Brussels: European Commission, p. 12, http://www.etsi.org/public-interest/Documents/Directives/Standardization/Authorisation_Directive.pdf.

CEC (Commission of the European Communities), 2002d, Directive 2002/19/EC of the European Parliament and of the Council of 7 March 2002 on Access to, and Interconnection of, Electronic Communications Networks and Associated Facilities (Access Directive), Brussels: European Commission, p. 14.

CEC (Commission of the European Communities), 2002e, Directive 2002/22/EC of the European Parliament and of the Council of 7 March 2002 on Universal Service and Users' Rights Relating to Electronic Communications Networks and Services (Universal Service Directive), Brussels: European Commission, p. 27.

CEC (Commission of the European Communities), 2002f, Directive 2002/58/EC of the European Parliament and of the Council Of 12 July 2002 Concerning the Processing of Personal Data and the Protection of Privacy in the Electronic Communications Sector (Directive on Privacy and Electronic Communications), Brussels: European Commission, p. 11.

CEC (Commission of the European Communities), 2002g, Proposal for a European Parliament and Council Directive on the Re-Use and Commercial Exploitation of Public Sector Documents, Brussels: European Commission, p. 20.

CEC (Commission of the European Communities), 2002h, Communication from the Commission on Impact Assessment, COM (2002) 276 final of 5.06.2002, Brussels: European Commission.

CEC (Commission of the European Communities), 2002i, European Union: Consolidated Versions of the Treaty on European Union and of the Treaty Establishing the European Community (2002). Official Journal C 235/1 24–12–2002.

CEC (Commission of the European Communities), 2003, Common Position (EC) No 15/2003 Adopted by the Council on 20 February 2003 with a View to the Adoption of a Directive of the European Parliament and of the Council Amending Council Directive 96/82/EC on the Control of Major-Accident Hazards Involving Dangerous Substances. Official Journal (2003/C 102 E/01).

Craglia, M. and Annoni, A., 2001, *The Spatial Impact of European Union Policies*, Ispra: Joint Research Centre, EUR 20212lEN.

Craglia, M., Annoni, A., and Masser, I., 2000, *Geographic Information Policies in Europe: National and Regional Perspectives*, Ispra: European Commission, EUR19552EN.

Craglia, M., Annoni, A., Smits, P., and Smith, R., 2002, *Spatial Data Infrastructures: Country Reports,* Ispra: Joint Research Centre, EUR 20428EN.

Craglia, M. and Masser, I., 2003, *Access to Geographic Information: A European Perspective,* URISA Vol. 15 APA-1, http://www.urisa.org.

Craglia, M., Masser, I., and Dallemand, J-F., 2001, *Geographic Information and the Enlargement of the European Union,* Ispra: European Commission, EUR19824EN.

EC (European Commission), 1999, White Paper on Food Safety, COM (1999) 719, final, Brussels: European Commission.

EC (European Commission), 2000, Communication on the Health Strategy of the European Community, COM (2000) 285, Brussels: European Commission.

EC (European Commission), 2003, Communication on Environment and Health Strategy, COM (2003) 338, Brussels: European Commission.

Liikanen, E., 2002, *The Vision of a Mobile Europe,* March 18, European Commission, [cited March 18 2002], http://europa.eu.int/rapid/start/cgi/guesten.ksh?p_action.gettxt=gt&doc=SPEECH/02/111|0|RAPID&lg=EN.

Masser, I., 1998, *Governments and Geographic Information*, London: Taylor and Francis.

Masser, I., 1999, All shapes and sizes: The first generation of national spatial data infrastructures, *International Journal of Geographical Information Science,* 13, 67–84.

Masser, I., 2002, A Comparative Evaluation of NSDIs in Australia, Canada, and the United States, GINIE Report D 5.4, http://www.ec-gis.org/ginie/documents/.

Niles, S. and Hanson S., 2003, *A New Era of Accessibility?* URISA Vol. 15 APA-1, http://www.urisa.org.

Signoretta, P. and Craglia, M., 2002, Joined-up government in practice: A case study of children's needs in Sheffield, *Local Government Studies*, 28, 1, 59–76.

Smith, R.S., and Craglia, M., 2003, *Digital Participation and Access to Geographic Information: A Case Study of U.K. Local Government*, URISA Vol. 15, APA-1, http://www.urisa.org.

Standage, T., 2001, The Internet, untethered, *The Economist*, October 11 [cited October 13 2001], http://www.economist.com/surveys/displaystory.cfm?story_id=811934.
United States Congress, 2002, E-Government Act 2002, H.R. 2458, Washington, D.C.
Williamson, I., Rajabifard, A., and Feeney, M.E., 2003. *Geospatial Data Infrastructures: From Concepts to Reality*, London: Taylor and Francis.

15 Data Protection and Medical Research

Deryck Beyleveld and David Townend

CONTENTS

15.1 INTRODUCTION

There are many misconceptions about data protection and research, including research in the GIS field. The most common is that processing data for research purposes is exempt from data protection law. The second is that anonymized data is equally exempt from the requirements of data protection legislation. As in most cases, these misconceptions are grounded in confusion. It is true that there is a limited provision for a research exemption from certain of the requirements of the legislation and it is equally true that anonymous data or data once anonymized are outside the provisions of the law. However, it is equally clear that data protection law imposes considerable regulation upon the processing of personal data in research contexts. This chapter explores the extent of data protection under European law in relation to medical research, focusing in particular on issues of consent, the research exemption, and anonymization. These aspects are particularly relevant to geocoded data on individuals. While the chapter is primarily concerned with European law, contentious issues in the U.K. implementation of Directive 95/46/EC will be considered. The purpose of this chapter is to show that while those who conduct medical research may see data protection requirements as damaging to their ability to ensure

0-415-30655-8/04/$0.00+$1.50

comprehensive samples and highest-quality research, the contrary is true. Such regulation ensures trust between the patient, clinician, and research. The failure of trust threatens medical research.

Data protection law is harmonized across the European Union (EU) and the European Economic Area (EEA) through the requirements of Directive 95/46/EC on the protection of individuals with regard to the processing of personal data and on the free movement of such data (Official Journal L281, 23/11/1995, P. 0031–0050 — hereafter, "the Directive"). Implementation of the Directive will be required in each of the newly associated states (or accession states) on their entry into the EU. Further, the transfer of data from the EU and EEA is regulated, such that data (without the specific consent of the data subject to the transfer) may only be transferred to states with equivalent data protection in place (Articles 25 and 26, and Recital 56 to Recital 60). (Articles and recitals are sections within, or associated with, laws and legal directives). The Directive, therefore, has considerable influence and authority in data processing in international as well as national or European contexts. The United Kingdom has implemented the Directive in the Data Protection Act 1998 (1998 Act), and in relation to data protection in medical research, the Health and Social Care Act 2001 is important. Neither the Directive nor the 1998 Act specifically include provisions for data protection in medical research. However, it is clearly covered in the general operation of the Directive and 1998 Act in the operation of their provisions concerning "sensitive personal data."

15.2 THE PURPOSE OF THE DIRECTIVE

The Directive is addressed to member states, requiring implementation of certain provisions of the Directive while giving some limited discretion in the implementation of other provisions. The processing of personal data (including "sensitive personal data") must not violate "the fundamental rights and freedoms of natural persons, and in particular their right to privacy" (Article 1.1; see also Recital 10 and Recital 11). Two things must be noted immediately. First, the Directive is not simply a privacy directive; rather it is concerned with the protection of all fundamental rights and freedoms "and in particular privacy." Thus, it concerns the rights found in the laws of the member states, the European Convention for the Protection of Fundamental Rights and Freedoms, and other internationally recognized rights and freedoms. Second, the Directive is not concerned with balancing economic rights and the development of the European free market with fundamental rights and freedoms; it is in place to protect the latter. The initial recitals of the Directive indicate the context that the European Parliament and Council had to address, namely that personal data concerning the individual has considerable economic value and information technology allows for greater transfer and processing of such data and requires greater data flow between states. However, the purpose of the EU is to facilitate these developments within a context of human rights and fundamental freedoms (Recital 1 to Recital 23). Indeed, the protection of such rights in part facilitates the ends of the EU, as, having safeguarded the rights and freedoms across the EU, member states "shall neither restrict nor prohibit the free flow of personal data between member states for reasons" of protection of the fundamental rights (Article 1.2).

These purposes are fundamental to medical ethics and high-quality medical research. Medical research has a high priority in the EU and requires free information flows; the purposes of the Directive assist to ensure the continued development of medical research. Patients must have confidence in their clinicians and that they are treated with dignity and respect. Recent high-profile events have shaken that trust and it must be restored as without confidence in clinicians and researchers, patients will withhold information or not seek medical assistance. This would clearly be catastrophic for patients' well being and for research. Strong data protection can go some way to strengthening confidence and ensuring full disclosure of information from patients.

15.3 GENERAL REQUIREMENTS OF THE DIRECTIVE

The Directive requires member states to safeguard the fundamental rights and freedoms of individual data subjects through two mechanisms. The first places duties on the conduct of those who process such personal data — "data controllers" and any "data processors" working on their behalf — (Article 2(d) and Article 2(e)). The second mechanism for the protection of data subjects is by giving them direct rights to access their personal data (Article 12) and to object to the processing of their personal data (Article 14 and Article 15).

Under the 1995 Directive and current law, data processing is "any operation or set of operations which is performed upon personal data, whether or not by automatic means, such as collection, recording, organization, storage, adaptation or alteration, retrieval, consultation, use, disclosure by transmission, dissemination or otherwise making available, alignment or combination, blocking, erasure or destruction" (Article 2(b)). The concept of processing must cover anything done to personal data, so the list of processes given is not exhaustive. Further, processing can be automatic or manual, applying to personal data that forms part of a structured "filing system," (Article 2(c) and Article 3, and Recital 15 and Recital 27). "Personal data" under the Directive is "any information relating to an identified or identifiable natural person" (Article 2(a)). "Sensitive personal data" is "data which are capable by their nature of infringing fundamental freedoms or privacy" (Recital 33). This special category includes "racial or ethnic origin, political opinions, religious or philosophical beliefs, trade-union membership," and "data concerning health or sex life" (Article 8(1)). Thus, medical research will undoubtedly concern the processing of sensitive personal data.

The fundamental rights and freedoms of the data subject are safeguarded in the Directive (with a requirement that the principles are implemented in member states' legislation) by three central elements imposing duties upon data controllers:

1. The data protection principles (which relate to data quality)
2. The general and the special data processing provisions (making processing of data legitimate and defining fair and lawful processing of data)
3. The information provisions

15.3.1 The Data Protection Principles

The data controller must ensure that personal data must be (Article 6(1)):

- Processed fairly and lawfully
- Collected for specified, explicit, and legitimate purposes and not further processed in a way incompatible with those purposes [further processing for historical, statistical, or scientific purposes not being considered incompatible provided that the member state provides proper safeguards to ensure this]
- Adequate, relevant, and not excessive in relation to the purposes for which they are collected or further processed
- Accurate and, where necessary, kept up to date [with a requirement of reasonable effort, considering the purpose of the processing, to rectify inaccuracy]
- Kept in a form that permits identification of data subjects for no longer than is necessary for the purposes for which data were collected or for which they are further processed

Further, data must be processed with "appropriate technical and organizational measures" given the nature of the processing and the nature of the data to protect the data from "accidental or unlawful destruction or accidental loss, alteration, unauthorized disclosure or access, and against all other unlawful forms of processing" (Article 17).

The data protection principles, with these important additional safeguards, are enforced through a duty owed by the controller to notify the supervisory authority (the information commissioner in the United Kingdom) of processing of personal data (Article 18). The notification includes the controller's details, the purpose of the processing, a description of the type of data subjects whose details are to be processed, the recipients or type of recipient to receive the data, any third country transfers of the data, and an indication of the measures taken to ensure the security of the data (Article 19). The Directive provides that failure to register must give rise to a judicial remedy (Article 22 to Article 24). Further, the Directive attaches to the notification process a requirement that supervisory authorities should assess if the proposed processing poses a particular threat to data subjects' rights and freedoms, and, where it poses such a threat, to examine the processing operations prior to their start (Article 20, the prior checking provisions). The Directive also requires that processing should be publicized and a register of processing be kept by the authority (Article 21).

15.3.2 When Is it Lawful to Process Personal Data or Special Personal Data?

The first of the data protection principles in the Directive is amplified in part by Article 7 and Article 8. Processing of any personal data can only be legitimate if (Article 7):

- The data subject has unambiguously given his consent
- Processing is necessary for the performance of a contract to which the data subject is party
- Processing is necessary for compliance with a legal obligation to which the controller is subject
- Processing is necessary to protect the vital interests of the data subject
- Processing is necessary for the performance of a task carried out in the public interest or in the exercise of official authority vested in the controller or in a third party to whom the data are disclosed
- Processing is necessary for the purposes of the legitimate interests pursued by the controller or by the third party or parties to whom the data are disclosed, except where such interests are overridden by the interests for fundamental rights and freedoms of the data subject

The processing of the special categories of personal data (Article 8(1) outlined above) can only be processed legitimately where (Article 8(2)):

- The data subject has given explicit consent to the processing of those data [unless this is not allowed in a member state's law]
- Processing is necessary [for the controller's employment law obligations in, and adequately safeguarded by, national law]
- Processing is necessary to protect the vital interests of the data subject or of another person where the data subject is physically or legally incapable of giving his consent
- Processing is carried out [with appropriate guarantees] by a nonprofit-seeking body of which the data subject is a member and for the purposes of that membership and without disclosure to a third party
- Processing relates to data manifestly made public by the data subject or is necessary for the establishment, exercise, or defence of legal claims

Or, "where processing of the data is required for the purposes of preventive medicine, medical diagnosis, the provision of care or treatment or the management of health-care services, and where those data are processed by a health professional subject [to professional regulation at national law]" (Article 8(3)). Member states may make further provisions for "reasons of substantial public interest," and processing of these data for the process of criminal law may be undertaken only under the control of an official authority or under suitable safeguards in national law, notifying the European Commission (EC) of such provisions (Article 8(4) to Article 8(6)). Member states must also determine the conditions for the processing of data identifiable from national identification numbers or other general identifiers (Article 8(7)).

15.3.2.1 The Problem of Consent

This produces a most interesting set of questions around the importance of "consent" in both Article 7 and Article 8. The first question is the relationship of the first condition, the data subject's consent to processing, to the others in each list. There is no indication in the Directive as to whether the conditions in Article 7 and Article 8 lists are all equal in standing. However, when one considers the requirements of the European Convention on Human Rights (ECHR), one sees that the Directive's Article 7 and Article 8 cannot be read as an equal list. Article 8(1) of the ECHR establishes a right to privacy. Article 8(2) ECHR gives the conditions when that right can be qualified:

> There shall be no interference by a public authority with the exercise of this right except such as is in accordance with the law and is necessary in a democratic society in the interests of national security, public safety or the economic well being of the country, for the prevention of disorder or crime, for the protection of health or morals, or for the protection of the rights and freedoms of others.

These could legitimately be described as emergency supervening situations.

This must establish that the basic assumption is that consent of the data subject is required, as that indicates the individual's permission for the interference with his or her right to privacy, except in circumstances where the violation of that privacy right would be justified by Article 8(2) ECHR. Here we can see that the remainder of the list can, and should, be read in that basic human rights way. Therefore, we submit that it is not lawful under ECHR (and now the Human Rights Act 1998 in the United Kingdom) to avoid getting consent in medical research and relying upon one of the other grounds for mere convenience or to ensure a 100 percent sample. Rather, the starting position must be one of obtaining consent unless there are Article 8(2) ECHR compelling reasons for violating the data subject's rights to control their data.

There is a further difficulty in consent as it appears in both Article 7 and Article 8: its definition. By Article 2(h), consent must be "any freely given specific and informed indication of his wishes by which a data subject signifies his agreement to personal data relating to him being processed." Article 7(a) strengthens this by requiring that the data subject "unambiguously" gives consent. It is then a matter of evidence to find an indication of agreement from the data subject to the proposed processing. Article 8 (and Recital 33) of the Directive requires a further level of consent when seeking to process special personal data lawfully and fairly: "explicit consent." This is not defined, but is clearly seen as a higher standard for dealing with sensitive data. Indeed, member states in implementing Article 8, may elect not to allow consent for use by the data subject, providing for use only in the emergency supervening situations discussed above (Article 8(2)(a)).

In the absence of a positive definition of explicit consent, certain things are clear. Explicit consent will not be sufficient to permit processing of the data for illegitimate purposes, nor when the data includes personal data on third parties. Nonobjection does not constitute any form of consent. Where the requirements of consent are active, unambiguous, explicit indications of agreement, a claim inferring consent from the inaction of the data subject is insufficient. Arguably, where it can be shown that the subject knows about the processing and of his or her right to object to the processing and yet makes no objection, this could constitute consent. However, this line of argument is difficult in the face of the Directive's definitions of consent.

Taking this line, one must be confident that there is no other reasonable interpretation of the facts. Thus, where the data subject presents for a blood test, is informed of the purpose of the test and the uses for the personal data in the collected sample and he or she presents his or her arm for the test without coercion, this will be sufficient indication of consent (if properly supported in evidence). Likewise, if the data subject having presented his or her arm does not remove it from the table having heard the details, this could be sufficient.

In medical research then, consent to the processing of personal data must be the basic procedural standard. However, there are a number of possible exceptions to the requirement to obtain explicit consent under Article 8(2). Where the vital interests of any person are threatened, if the data subject cannot give consent personal data can be processed. Further, by Article 8(4) if the processing of such data is in the substantial public interest the member state, either by law or by a supervisory authority's decision and subject to suitable safeguards, may introduce further exemptions to Article 8(2). The EC must be notified of such an exercise of power (Article 8(6)). The United Kingdom has exercised this power in Statutory Instrument 417 of 2000.

By Article 8(3) and Recital 33, special data may be processed for medical purposes without explicit consent. However, it is arguable that these purposes do not include medical research purposes, because the key element in the drafting of Article 8(3) is the requirement of a treatment need in the data subject that cannot be delayed to gain the explicit consent of the data subject (or for the management of healthcare services). If, however, medical research is accepted as a medical purpose under Article 8(3) (as the U.K. act does), then the processing of the personal data is acceptable if undertaken by health professionals subject to national regulatory authorities' rules on secrecy or others subject to a similar duty of secrecy. As special data remains personal data for the purposes of Article 7, one of its conditions must be satisfied, namely consent, or that the processing is in the vital interests of the data subject or in the public interest.

15.3.3 Fair and Lawful Processing and the Provision of Information

In many respects, the most important protection afforded to the data subject is through the requirement to provide the data subject with information about the processing and this again defines fairness towards the data subject. This could be said to be a right of the data subject to information, however, it is treated by the Directive as an obligation on the data controller to provide the information to the data subject regardless of whether or not it is requested. Without the information, data subjects are most unlikely to know of the proposed processing of their data. It, therefore, allows the data subject to give informed consent, to seek access to the data, and to exercise a right to the correction or removal of data from the record (the right to object). The provisions can be separated into three scenarios:

1. Where the controller obtains the information directly from the data subject
2. When the information is not obtained from the data subject

3. Where the data was obtained from the data subject, but disclosures to third parties or other new processes were not anticipated at the point of data collection

Where the data controller collects data from the data subject directly and at the outset, then the requirements are clear. Article 10 of the Directive requires that data controllers are compelled to ensure that data subjects are given certain fundamental information about the proposed processing of their data. This information includes the identity of the data controller (and his representatives if applicable), the purposes of the proposed processing, and anything else that is required for the processing to be fair to the data subject (Article 10 and Recital 38). Where the information is not obtained directly from the data subject, but is provided by a third party, then Article 11(1) of the Directive requires that new data controllers be compelled to provide the same information. However, Article 11(2) (and Recital 40) provides that Article 11(1) does not apply "where, in particular for statistical purposes or for the purposes of historical or scientific research, the provision of such information proves impossible or would involve a disproportionate effort, or if recording or disclosing is laid down by law." Disproportionate effort must mean disproportionate to the risks to the data subject's fundamental rights and freedoms. Where the purposes have changed from those envisaged at the time of collection of the data by the data controller, including the disclosure of the data to a third party, then Article 11(2) applies (Recital 39 and Recital 40).

These provisions apply regardless of whether or not consent was the provision used under Article 7 or Article 8 to establish when processing could occur. Clearly, the information contained in Article 10 and Article 11 is fundamental to informed consent, but the information must also be provided to an individual whose data is processed in his or her vital interests or in a medical emergency. The most interesting element to observe is that in the Directive, the Article 10 situation envisages no Article 11(2) type provision. It is not possible for data controllers at the point of collecting the data from a data subject to evade the requirement to give full information to the best of their knowledge at that time. Further, Article 11(2) provides an exclusion only where it is impossible to provide the information, for example where the data has been received in an anonymized form, or where the risks to the fundamental freedoms and rights of the data subject do not outweigh the effort required to provide the information.

The implementation of these provisions in U.K. law does not reflect the Directive. First, the interpretation of Article 11(2) in the U.K. statute is "so far as practicable" rather than "impossible" or with some element of balance relating to the fundamental rights and freedoms (DPA 1998, Schedule 1, Part II, Paragraph 2 (1)(a) and Paragraph 2(1)(b)). Second, the Article 11(2) exemption is applied not only to Article 11(1) but also to Article 10 situations (DPA 1998, Schedule 1, Part II, Paragraph 2(1)(a)).

If a data controller is exempt from providing information under the Directive, because of impossibility or other, then there is still a need for adequate safeguards for the data subject's rights. This could be provided through the supervisory authority and the prior checking provisions (Article 20). Further, Article 6(1)(b) requires that further processing should not be incompatible with the initially specified, explicit, and legitimate purposes stated under the Article 10 scenario. Where further processing occurs for historical, statistical, or scientific purposes, although it is not to be considered as incompatible with the original purposes, it must be in a context of safeguards provided by the member states and these must ensure that further processing is not used for decision-making about the particular data subject (Article 6(1)(b) and Recital 29).

15.4 THE RESEARCH EXEMPTION

At a number of points, the Directive makes limited exemptions in relation to historical, statistical, and scientific purposes, but in all cases, the exemption is based on a requirement that member states provide adequate safeguards to protect the fundamental rights and freedoms of the data subject. The final point in Section 15.3 clearly shows the balance held concerning research in the Directive. There must be safeguards, especially preventing the use of processing undertaken for historical, statistical, and scientific purposes to make decisions about the data subject. However, processing for historical, statistical, and scientific purposes is not to be considered incompatible with further processing. This simply indicates a presumption in favor of the purpose.

Personal data further processed solely for historical, statistical, and scientific purposes may be kept for longer than is necessary and allowed for any other purposes for which the data might have been collected (Article 6(1)(e)). When processing is "solely for scientific research" or data are kept in a personal form for such time as is necessary for "the sole purpose of creating statistics," then the data subject's right of access to the data may be removed. Under Article 13(2), that right can only be removed if:

- The derogation from the right is by legislative measure of the member state
- There is "clearly no risk of breaching the privacy of the data subject"
- Other adequate legal safeguards of the data subject's fundamental rights and freedoms are in place, particularly guarding against the use of that data for decision-making about the data subject

In the United Kingdom, the "clearly no risk" element is interpreted as "unlikely to cause substantial damage or distress" (DPA 1998, s.33(1)(b)).

The prohibition on the processing of sensitive personal data may be lifted, as discussed earlier, if that purpose is seen as a subcategory of the broader treatment categories that are expressed in Article 8(3). Article 8(4) allows for the processing of sensitive personal data for reasons of the substantial public interest. Recital 34 includes scientific research within this if an "important" public interest is a "substantial" one. The data subject's rights are safeguarded under Article 8(3) by the regulation of the medical professional or other researcher within a professional obligation of secrecy; under Article 8(4), the processing must be sanctioned by national law or the supervisory authority and notification to EC.

Whereas the safeguards for the individual data subject are to protect that person's individual rights and freedoms, Article 13(1)(g) provides for a situation where the provisions of Article 6(1) (that processing should be fair and lawful), Article 10 and Article 11 (the information provisions), Article 12 (the data subject's right of access), and Article 21 (concerning the publication and maintenance of the register of processing) may be modified. Generally, this is where the processing is necessary to safeguard the data subject or the rights and freedoms of others. By implication, medical research could be such a process in some circumstances. However, these circumstances do not produce a blanket exemption for medical research from the requirements to process fairly and lawfully, including Article 7 and Article 8, and the requirements of the information provisions.

In the U.K. legislation, the research exemption is set up explicitly in Section 33 of the Data Protection Act 1998. In Section 33(1), two general "relevant conditions" must be met in all processing seeking the research exemptions:

1. That research processing does not affect measures or decision making about the individual data subject (s. 33(1)(a))
2. That the data is not processed in "such a way that substantial damage or substantial distress is, or is likely to be, caused to any data subject" (s. 33(1)(b))

The scope of the latter is very difficult to judge, but it must include a protection of the individual with reasonable and known sensibilities. Given that the opportunity for medical research on the data may arise after the data's initial collection and that it may be impossible to contact data subjects individually to notify them of the processing or to gain their consent, the prior checking duties of the supervisory authorities could, and arguably must, be used to ensure that reasonable and known sensibilities are not likely to be violated by the further research processing. Arguably, this is necessary to ensure continued confidence in medical treatment.

15.5 ANONYMIZATION

Holding data in an anonymous form and anonymizing data is clearly one of the strongest safeguards for the practical protection of the data subject's identity and certain aspects of their privacy. As a matter of good practice, research should be conducted with anonymized or anonymous data unless the rights of the data subject require that it is processed in a personal form. However, anonymization is not without its difficulties and it does not guarantee, in itself, the privacy of the subject. Rendering personal data anonymous may remove the immediate danger of identification and, therefore, the likelihood of causing substantial damage to the data subject (strengthening the use of other justifications for processing than consent under Article 7 and Article 8). However, in a situation where, for example, one's data is processed, albeit anonymously, for purposes opposed to one's moral or religious sensibilities, then one's fundamental rights and freedoms can still be violated and substantial distress may still be caused.

It is clear that personal data is information from which an individual natural person is "identified or identifiable." Recital 26 of the Directive is explicit in saying that the "principles of protection shall not apply to data rendered anonymous." Anonymous data are outside the scope of the Directive. However, personal data collected in an identifiable form that is subsequently anonymized will be within the protection of the Directive at least until it is completely unidentifiable, as removing identifiers must be a "process" operating on personal data under the Directive. The U.K. legislation and courts, however, have not taken this view.

The U.K. courts considered the status of anonymized data in the case of *R* v *Department of Health, ex parte Source Informatics Ltd.* ([2000] 1 All ER 786, CA; see Beyleveld and Histed (2000)). To establish marketing strategies for particular drugs, medical data about prescription habits of general practitioners (GPs) was purchased from GPs by Source Informatics in a form anonymized by the GPs. The GPs had not gained the consent of their patients to process their data for this purpose and one of the key questions before the court was whether the data came within the ambit of data protection legislation. Recital 26 of the Directive, however, states that data protection principles must apply to any information concerning personal data and Article 2(b) of the Directive defines processing as "any" operations performed on personal data. Further, the Article 13(2) exemption for the creation of anonymous statistics from personal data does not exempt the data controller from the requirements of Article 7, Article 8, Article 10, and Article 11. The Article 12 exemption provided is still conditional on adequate safeguards and there being no risk of breaching the privacy of the data subject. These three elements clearly indicate that the operation of rendering identifiable personal data anonymous (i.e. the process of anonymization) is itself a process under the Directive and subject to the regulations of processing.

When considering anonymous data and anonymization and anonymized data, it is only once the data is rendered fully anonymous that the processing of the data is outside the ambit of the Directive. When data is processed by those who receive the data in personal, identifiable form (either directly from the data or indirectly with a key (Article 2(d) and Recital 26) that processing is subject to the data protection principles, including Article 10 (unless that is subject to an exemption for other reasons).

This was not the position accepted in Source Informatics, where the Court of Appeal held that where personal data was collected with a view to anonymization then the data protection principles did not apply. This is where the United Kingdom is arguably in violation of EC law. The most legally satisfactory response to the decision from the government and the Department of Health would have been to appeal the decision to the House of Lords. However, the response employed tried to deal with the matter through the Health and Social Care Act 2001, Section 60, which was intended to grant the secretary of state powers to render, through regulations:

- Processing of anonymized data unlawful
- Processing of confidential patient identifiable data without consent lawful, where this would be in the public interest

Pressure of time in the House of Lords and opposition from the Conservative Party in the Lords led to the dropping of the provisions relating to anonymized information.

Section 60 of the Health and Social Care Act provides that the secretary of state has powers, in the public interests or for medical purposes, to render not unlawful processing that would otherwise be unlawful for breaching patient confidentiality, if consent was not practicable to obtain. This power has been exercised through the Health Services (Control of Patient Information) Regulations (SI 2002 No. 1438). By these regulations, confidential information of patients presenting for diagnosis or treatment may be processed for various specified medical purposes including medical research approved by research ethics committees (Regulation 2(1)(d)). Such data may be processed by persons approved by the secretary of state and authorized by the person who legally holds the data (Regulation 2(3)). The secretary of state may require by notice, in the public interest, any person so approved to process personal data within the timescale set out by the notice (Regulation 2(4)). The regulations also allow for the processing of confidential patient information in relation to communicable diseases and other risks to public health (Regulation 3). Regulation 6 allows for the transfer of any confidential patient data for the creation of a register, for example a cancer register.

The striking element in all these regulations is that the data can be processed for these purposes without the consent of the patient. In all of these cases, Regulation 4 states that the processing of data for the purposes outlined in the regulations will not breach any duties of confidentiality owed in respect of the information. However, the regulations cannot make legal acts that would violate the Data Protection Directive. The Directive requirements concerning information to be given to a data subject and the requirements of consent to the processing of data could be violated by the regulations. For example, the regulations allow data to be placed onto cancer registries without patient consent or disclosure of purpose to the patient even where the information is gathered directly from the data subject. Even under the 1998 Act, which allows for this where it is impracticable to meet the Article 10 requirements, it is difficult to see how it will be impracticable to inform the patient of the purpose and to gain consent in line with the Human Rights Act requirements. The regulations arguably stand at odds with the Directive.

15.6 CONCLUSIONS

As can be seen, the variations in the implementation of the Directive in U.K. law cause difficulties in the interpretation of duties. Undoubtedly, other member states will have interesting interpretations of the duties created by the Directive. These variations may be tested in legal action to clarify the extent of the duties under the law across Europe. Alongside these problems of implementing the Directive, there are many interest groups that see the Directive as too intrusive for the purposes of security, commerce, and research, especially medical research. The call is for a wide reform of the Directive to reduce the duties imposed upon data controllers. However, these voices must be set against the underpinning purpose of the Directive, which is to ensure an environment of trust within which personal data is protected, freely offered, and safely transferred to ensure the continued benefits of the EU to the commercial and research purposes. If the Directive is weakened, then the weakness will extend into the trust and confidence of data subjects, with potentially serious implications.

References

Beyleveld, D. and Histed, 2000, Betrayal of confidence in the Court of Appeal, *Medical Law International*, 4, 277–311.

16 Public and Patient Attitudes Toward the Use of Their Health Information: A Review of the Literature

Rupert Suckling, Darren Shickle, and Susan Wallace

CONTENTS

16.1 INTRODUCTION

Data protection legislation and professional guidelines in a number of countries have been criticized by researchers and epidemiologists who claim that there will be disastrous consequences for epidemiological activities such as cancer registration and communicable disease surveillance (see, e.g., Doll and Peto, 2001; Helliwell, 2001; U.K. Association of Cancer Registries, 2000). There is an expectation that if the public are asked to give consent, then they will either explicitly refuse or not

0-415-30655-8/04/$0.00+$1.50

respond to requests for consent. Consequently, this would introduce significant volunteer bias into databases and limit the utility for public health purposes. The Data Protection Act 1998 does limit the requirement to obtain consent or to inform data subjects according to what is practicable, reasonable, or requires disproportionate effort. Empirical evidence of adverse consequences and the difficulties involved in approaching patients would be required to justify use of personal data without seeking consent or giving data subjects an opportunity to object. This chapter is based on a review of the literature to assess public attitudes to privacy and use of personal health information. Although the attitudes examined in this chapter are generic in nature, they are equally applicable to the use of health information in the public health GIS field.

16.2 SEARCH STRATEGY

The following electronic databases were searched: Medline 1966 to 2002/02, CINAHL 1982–2002/02, and Embase 1980–2002/02. Searches were restricted to English language papers and the keywords used were "attitude," "health information" or "medical records," "public" or "patient," and "privacy" or "confidentiality."

Of the 110 references found, the titles and abstracts were reviewed to identify 26 suitable papers. Hand searching, searching of grey literature, and canvassing of expert opinion identified a further 18 papers, so in total 44 papers were reviewed. Papers were included only if they reported original research that explored public or patient attitudes to the use of, or limits to, the use of their own health information. Theoretical discussion papers were excluded. In view of the small number of original research papers found, all papers were reviewed irrespective of sample size or methodology. A qualitative analysis of the studies was undertaken.

16.3 RESULTS

Public attitudes to the use of their own health information are related to their attitudes to confidentiality and privacy, together with their attitudes toward and expectations of healthcare and other professionals who might access their information. These attitudes may vary depending on the sensitivity of the information, the mechanism of recording this information, the healthcare setting, and the potential uses to which their information may be put. There is no evidence from the published literature as to which of these factors the public perceive to be the most important.

16.3.1 Knowledge of Rights, Privacy, and Confidentiality

Constitutional rights, including rights to privacy are a key concern to 85 percent of Americans (Gostin et al., 1993) and much of the literature on public attitudes to data protection has been conducted in the United States. Thirty percent of Americans were termed "privacy fundamentalists," those people who place high value on privacy, and 55 percent "privacy pragmatists," who were able to trade off privacy for other goods (Detmer, 2000). The Internet has highlighted differences between individual attitudes to health information compared to other information. Fifty-four percent of Internet users have shared information and yet of those defined as health seekers only 21 percent have provided an e-mail address, 17 percent a name or other identifying information, because 80 percent want to obtain health information anonymously (Pew Internet and Life Project, 2000). Individuals were particularly concerned that their health insurers might find out about their online health activities (California Health Care Foundation, 2000).

Although 89 percent of American high school pupils could correctly identify the principle of confidentiality, this was simply identifying the correct definition of the word confidential from four alternative definitions without any assessment of ability to use the principle correctly (Cheng et al., 1993). A third of the pupils were aware of a right to confidentiality for specific health issues, but at least half of the pupils admitted they did not know their rights. In the United Kingdom, 92 percent of teenagers agreed with the definition of confidentiality as "what you tell your doctor should not be discussed with other people without you knowing" (Churchill et al., 2000). Although only two thirds believed this is what their GP did, this had no effect on their consultation behavior.

Among American physicians, 53 percent reported discussing confidentiality with their adolescent patients, 21 percent discussed confidentiality with all their young patients and 11 percent did not discuss it at all (Ford and Millstein, 1997). Female doctors were more likely to discuss confidentiality than their male counterparts were.

Not only adolescents struggle with confidentiality. Psychiatric patients in Oregon valued medical confidentiality highly, but lacked adequate information as to their rights (Kinzie et al., 1985). They were much more likely to approve release of information for medical purposes than for other purposes. Only a third of patients had an accurate knowledge of who had access to their records, many thought erroneously that only doctors and nurses had access, and fewer still knew of any legal protections of confidentiality. Many felt that the release of health information was mandatory prior to receiving healthcare and almost all patients felt the release of health information was mandatory for other purposes and only a third signed for the release of information without any sense of coercion. Parents also struggle, with only 22 percent of Minnesota parents knowing their parental rights and responsibilities when it came to access to information and medical records of their children (Cutler et al., 1999).

16.3.2 Health Professional Groups and Need to Know

Public attitudes toward who should have access to health information is closely linked with the "need to know" of the individual and the perceived extent to which that individual is bound by confidentiality (Carmen and Britten, 1995). In one U.K. general practice, all the 39 patients interviewed agreed that all the doctors in the practice should have some degree of access to their medical records, but only their usual general practitioner (GP) should have unlimited access. A minority felt that other primary care staff (e.g., nurses and midwives) should have no access whatsoever, because they were not perceived to be bound by confidentiality to the same extent as doctors. In some cases, it was felt that the doctor should decide whether the nurse was responsible enough to have access to the records.

A larger U.K. study involving 1000 patients replicated these findings (Wardman et al., 2000). Over 94 percent of respondents thought their usual doctor had access and 98 percent felt they should have access to all their medical records. These figures were lower (76 and 84 percent) for other doctors in the practice. However, when it came to other staff, less than half (43 percent) thought the practice nurse had access to their records and even fewer (34 percent) believed that they should have access to all their notes, with 40 percent feeling that access to part of the record would be acceptable. Again, patients were less enthusiastic at other professional members of the primary healthcare team (e.g., district nurse, health visitor, midwife, physiotherapist, and occupational therapist) having access to their records. Twelve to fourteen percent of individuals thought other professional members currently had access to their notes, with 11 to 20 percent agreeing that other professional members should have access to all their records, and 22 to 37 percent agreeing with access to part of their record. Seventy-five percent of men believed that the midwife does not and should not have access to their medical records. Receptionists were felt to have more access than they should, but medical secretaries were perceived to have had special training and therefore were bound by the same professional rules of conduct as medical staff (Carmen and Britten, 1995).

Australian chemists were perceived by adolescents to raise particular concerns over their ability to maintain confidentiality where sexual health information and condoms are involved (Warr and Hillier, 1997). These concerns may arise from the small communities that the chemists in this study were working in, where chemist staff may be family friends or relatives, rather than anything intrinsic to chemists. In Belgium, worries about confidentiality breaches to parents were also cited as a reason for teenagers delaying attending a doctor for contraceptive advice (Peremans, 2000). For this reason, 25 percent of American high school pupils would forgo healthcare (Cheng et al., 1993).

16.3.3 Doctors and Nonclinicians

This compares with experience in South Australia where 85 percent of 3000 people asked reported that they were confident or very confident that doctors and hospitals were responsible data custodians, but almost 10 percent were not very or not at all confident in their ability (Mulligan, 2001). South Australian patients were less likely to share their patient-held record information with nonclinicians (Liaw, 1993). Doctors are thought to protect personal information (and therefore confidentiality) better than other nonclinical professional groups (i.e., the insurance industry, banks, the government, the news media or any other institution) (News and Notes, 1979). However, of the 2131 Americans surveyed, 17 percent thought that doctors and 23 percent thought that hospitals should be doing more to protect the confidentiality of their information.

16.3.4 Expectations of Patients

From eight countries (Denmark, Germany, Israel, Norway, Portugal, Sweden, The Netherlands, and United Kingdom), 3540 patients were asked about their priorities with regard to general practice. Of the patients in the countries surveyed, 77 to 91 percent felt that a GP should be able to guarantee confidentiality of information of all his patients (Grol et al., 1999). The doctor-patient relationship may also be threatened by questioning the doctor, which may arise from issues of privacy or confidentiality (Carmen and Britten, 1995; Ornstein and Bearden, 1994).

The perceived level of anonymity is important for patients (e.g., sperm donors) (Robinson et al., 1991), but also for the perceived content of the health record (Carmen and Britten, 1995). In many cases, confidentiality is maintained by "indifference to anonymous patients." This may account for the public being less worried about information in hospitals than in general practice, because general practice records tend to carry much more personal and social information (Carmen and Britten, 1995). Many of those concerned about the content of the information were not concerned by who has access to it, providing factual rather than subjective information was recorded (Carmen and Britten, 1995). However, Siegler demonstrated in a university-affiliated teaching hospital in the United States that at least 25 and up to 100 healthcare professionals and administrative staff had access to a patient's medical record (Siegler, 1982). If the public were aware of the large number of people who have access to their information, they might be more concerned about both access and content.

Patients have different expectations of confidentiality than "house staff" and medical students. Either patients have a stricter definition of confidentiality than medical staff or they expect a tighter adherence to the principle (Weiss, 1982). When 108 patient-reported confidentiality breaches were investigated, 48 were legally defensible breaches (i.e., information passed from one treating practitioner to another without patient authorization), 32 were legally indefensible disclosures and 28 disclosures could not be analyzed (Mulligan, 2001). Of those who had suffered a breach, legitimate or not, 58 believed that direct harm to them had resulted from the breach including embarrassment, arguments, and loss of trust in medical services.

16.3.5 Content of Records and Sensitivity of Information

Most patients think that the decision as to what health information was recorded rested with the doctor (Carmen and Britten, 1995). There is a perceived need for negotiated entries over sensitive issues, as 11 percent of respondents in a (U.S.) Louis and Harris Associates survey thought that doctors' questions were too personal (News and Notes, 1979). This perception may arise because doctors are asking personal questions (e.g., about relationships), which are not perceived as necessary for clinical care or because patients do not appreciate how personal information may be used in their care or the care of other people. Sensitive information is more likely to be disclosed if confidentiality is assured (Ford et al., 1997).

Sexual health issues seem to be a particular concern. Of 102 self-identified gay, lesbian, and bisexual individuals aged between 18 and 23, two thirds never discussed sexual orientation with healthcare providers, less than half remembered being informed about confidentiality, but those who did remember being informed were three times as likely to have discussed issues of sexual orientation (Allen et al., 1998). Of those not informed, over 70 percent said they would discuss issues to do with sexuality if informed.

The information may be so sensitive that patients feel unable to give information to their usual healthcare provider and may seek healthcare from other providers or give false information. Whereas 86 percent of high school pupils in the United States would seek healthcare from their family physicians for physical illnesses, this fell to 57 percent for care related to pregnancy, HIV, or substance misuse, because they felt their doctors were unable to maintain confidentiality (Cheng et al., 1993). Of men at high risk from HIV, 63 percent would not test if name-based reporting were required (Woods et al., 1999). If the benefits of name-based testing were explained, this was reduced to 50 percent. However, even of those who were tested, 42 percent would give a false name. In Germany, Kochen found in his sample of over 400 individuals diagnosed with HIV that although for the majority (91 percent) of individuals the GP was aware of their HIV status, over a third of patients did not routinely inform other doctors or medical staff about their status (Kochen et al., 1991). Individuals had more confidence in specialist centers than general practices to maintain confidentiality and this was related to the level of anonymity and confidence in the medical practitioner. In Uganda, confidentiality breaches are a major concern for women considering voluntary counseling and testing for HIV (Pool et al., 2001). In Maryland, 50 percent of blood donors indicated they would provide less accurate medical and personal information if the blood-donating agency were required to divulge previously confidential information (Banks et al., 1993).

There has only been limited research on the acceptability of communicable disease contact tracing for the index patient, the contact, and the staff involved. Cowan et al. (1996) summarized the research by suggesting that acceptability seemed determined by two factors: maintenance of confidentiality and availability of treatment. For example, Cowan et al. quoted a U.S. study (Chervenak and Weiss, 1989) of 25 women with HIV infection, which found that 68 percent were willing to disclose the names of their sexual partners to the health department if confidentiality was ensured. In practice, however, only 24 percent of the women in the study had informed partners that they had had prior to their HIV diagnosis and 52 percent had told partners subsequent to diagnosis. Another U.S. study with 132 partners of HIV-infected patients used an anonymous, self-completion questionnaire to assess their attitudes to being told by the public health department that they were at risk. Most (87 percent) thought that the public health department was correct in disclosing their exposure risk and 97 percent thought that notification should continue. Pavia et al. (1993) noted that partner notification was less successful in white men who have sex with men, compared with other groups. They concluded that this may be due to distrust of public health authorities and that homosexual and bisexual men preferred to notify partners without the involvement of public health workers. Fenton et al. (1997) surveyed senior consultants in 59 genitourinary medicine clinics in England. There was concern that partner notification, if handled inappropriately, could lead to identification and ostracization of individuals from their communities. Although 77 percent of consultants stated that HIV partner notification had become an accepted part of their clinic's practice, all respondents thought that there were factors that hindered this process. The most common limiting factor (mentioned by 73 percent) was healthcare workers' concerns about the unacceptability of HIV partner notification to patients.

16.3.6 Use of Health Information

The public may be happy about their information being used for research in general terms, with 77 percent of a health maintenance organization (HMO) membership agreeing to the use of their information in this way (Purdy et al., 2000). Most of those who agreed were highly educated and predominantly white and felt that participation in research had a positive effect on their healthcare. However, the subject area for research is crucial. When study-specific consent was required for an epilepsy study using medical records, the rates of consent fell to 19 percent (McCarthy et al., 1999), as opposed to in excess of 90 percent where study-specific consent was not required (Yawn et al., 1998). Refusal rates were highest in patients with mental health concerns, trauma or eye care, and among women aged 39 or older.

Health information is used as part of physician peer-review. Of 648 patients surveyed, 64 percent disapproved of their records being read by outside physicians without their permission, as there was no attempt to seek individual patient consent or to anonymize the records prior to the review (Dodek and Dodek, 1997). Yet when asked about an audit of their medical records the same percentage (64 percent) agreed (Neuhaus et al., 1976). Agreement to be audited varied markedly and depended on the physician involved and individuals with intimate diagnoses (e.g., gynecological diagnoses and examinations) were more likely to consent to a review of their records than those with less intimate diagnoses (e.g., tonsillitis and hypertension).

Over 20 percent of Swedish patients found it difficult to decline being involved in medical student teaching (Westbeg et al., 2001). Yet in New Zealand, 73 to 96 percent of members of the public were strongly in favor of taking part in medical student teaching depending on the medical setting (Grant, 1994). The percentage who would agree fell if the setting were a sexually transmitted disease clinic. Almost all the women and a third of the men would expect to be told about teaching involvement at booking if they were receiving care from the private sector. In the United Kingdom, consent to have a medical student at the consultation was more likely to be granted for less sensitive consultations, but also when there was only to be limited discussion between the doctor and the student once the patient had left the room (O'Flynn et al., 1997).

Cancer registries use information for public health monitoring. A natural experiment of white middle-aged women in the United States found that enrollment rates for a clinical trial were no different if information from a cancer registry was used to identify women compared with an indirect approach via a physician (Sugarman et al., 1999). Only 2 of 351 women approached directly complained about the approach, although 2 potential subjects of the 65 women approached indirectly felt pressured to participate because the approach came through their physician.

16.3.7 Electronic Records

Computerized methods of recording information are felt to present a much greater threat to privacy and confidentiality than written records (Carmen and Britten, 1995). Although many of the issues are the same for paper and electronic records, the public appears to be more engaged with the electronic debate.

16.3.8 Areas where Confidentiality May Be Unwittingly Breached

Although patients value confidentiality highly, Luke suggested that it may be overlooked for the sake of improved quality of care. The majority of parents of children on a pediatric ward were happy for their children's notes to be kept at the end of their beds, despite the fact that the issue of confidentiality was not specifically raised (Luke et al., 1999). There are potential breaches of confidentiality that patients might not realize, such as overhearing patient-specific information on ward rounds or in elevators (Rylance, 1999; Ubel et al., 1995). A minority of parents (10 out of 24) had concerns over confidentiality within a pediatric grand round (Birtwistle et al., 2000). Publication of identifiable information in medical journals has in the past caused distress to individuals (Smith, 1996).

16.4 DISCUSSION AND CONCLUSIONS

The search strategy employed found relatively few original research papers. Moreover, the majority of the research is from America and applying these findings to other countries is difficult and exacerbated by the fact that American HMOs rely on health information for billing information. Other drawbacks of the research are that many of the studies are small and nonresponse rates are high and nonresponders may have markedly different attitudes toward health information than responders. The majority of excluded literature focused on the doctor's role in disclosing confidential information to third parties, together with hypothetical attitudes taken by the public to their health information. There has been an increase in published literature on public attitudes toward health information in recent years through issues surrounding HIV and, in part, the emergence of electronic methods of information recording, which has brought this issue to greater prominence (Whetten-Goldstein et al., 2001). Obvious gaps in the research remain, particularly concerning the effects of age, gender, and social group on public attitudes. The debate has been restricted to attitudes toward those with more-traditional roles in healthcare — doctors and nurses — as opposed to the role of public health practitioners, managers, and those with close partnerships with health services.

Public attitudes to the use of their own health information are related to attitudes toward confidentiality and privacy, together with their attitudes toward and expectations of healthcare and other professionals who might access their information. Attitudes vary depending on the sensitivity of the information, the mechanism of recording the information, the healthcare setting, and the potential uses to which the information may be put. However, there is no evidence from the published literature as to which of these factors the public perceives to be the most important. Public attitudes to their health information may be different to professional attitudes to patient information, which may be a cause for conflict. In many cases, the public may not even have considered the issues surrounding their health information.

References

Allen, L. et al., 1998, Adolescent health care experience of gay, lesbian, and bisexual young adults, *Journal of Adolescent Health*, 23, 212–220.

Banks, H. et al., 1993, Changes in intention to donate blood under hypothetical condition of reduced confidentiality, *Transfusion*, 33, 671–674.

Birtwistle, L., Houghton, J., and Rostil, H., 2000, A review of a surgical ward round in a large teaching hospital: Does it achieve its aims? *Medical Education*, 34, 398–403.

California Health Care Foundation, 2000, Ethics survey of consumer attitudes about health Web sites, *California Health Care Foundation 2000,* 2nd ed., http://www.chcf.org/topics/view.cfm?itemID=12493.

Carmen, D. and Britten, N., 1995, Confidentiality of medical records: The patient's perspective, *British Journal of General Practice*, 45, 485–488.

Cheng, T. et al., 1993, Confidentiality in health care: A survey of knowledge, perceptions and attitudes among high school pupils, *Journal of the American Medical Association,* 269, 11, 1404–1407.

Chervenak, J.L. and Weiss, S.H., 1989, Sexual partner notification: Attitude and actions of HIV-infected women, presented at the 5th International Conference on AIDS, Montreal, June 8, 1989, Abstract Th.D.P.4, p. 759.

Churchill, R. et al., 2000, Do the attitudes and beliefs of young teenagers towards general practice influence actual consulting behaviour? *British Journal of General Practice*, 50, 953–957.

Cowan, F.M., French, R., and Johnson, A.M., 1996, The role and effectiveness of partner notification in STD control: A review, *Genitourinary Medicine*, 72, 4, 247–252.

Cutler, E. et al., 1999 Parental knowledge and attitudes of minnesota laws concerning adolescent medical care, *Pediatrics*, 103, 3, 582–587.

Detmer, D.E., 2000, Your privacy or your health: Will medical privacy legislation stop quality healthcare? *International Journal for Quality in Health Care*, 12(1), 1–3.

Dodek, D. and Dodek, A., 1997, From Hippocrates to facsimile: Protecting patient confidentiality is more difficult and more important than ever before, *Canadian Medical Association Journal*, 156, 6, 847–852.

Doll, R. and Peto, R., 2001, Rights involve responsibility for patients, *British Medical Journal*, 322, 730.

Fenton, K.A. et al., 1997, HIV partner notification policy and practice within GUM clinics in England: Where are we now? *Genitourinary Medicine*, 73, 1, 49–53.

Ford, C. and Millstein, S., 1997, Delivery of confidentiality assurances to adolescents by primary care physicians, *Archives of Pediatric Adolescent Medicine*, 151, 505–509.

Ford, C. et al., 1997, Influence of physician confidentiality assurances on adolescent's willingness to disclose information and seek future health care: A randomised controlled trial, *Journal of the American Medical Association,* 278, 12, 1029–1034.

Gostin, L. et al., 1993, Privacy and security of health care information in a new health care system, *Journal of the American Medical Association*, 270, 20, 2787–2493.

Grant, V., 1994, Patient involvement in clinical teaching, *Journal of Medical Ethics*, 20, 244–250.

Grol, R. et al., 1999, Patients' priorities with respect to general practice care: An international comparison, *Family Practice*, 16, 4–11.

Helliwell, T., 2001, Need for patient consent for cancer registration creates logistical nightmare, *British Medical Journal*, 322, 730.

Kinzie, J., Holmes, J., and Arent, J., 1985, Patients' release of medical records: Involuntary, uninformed consent, *Hospital and Community Psychiatry*, 36, 843–847.

Kochen, M. et al., 1991, How do patients with HIV perceive their general practitioners? *British Medical Journal*, 303, 1365–1368.

Liaw, S.T., 1993, Patient and general practitioner perceptions of patient-held health records, *Family Practice*, 10, 4, 406–415.

Luke, S., Gallagher, A., and Lloyd, B., 1999, Staff and family attitudes to keeping joint medical and nursing notes at the foot of the bed: Questionnaire survey, *British Medical Journal*, 319, 735.

McCarthy, D. et al., 1999, Medical records and privacy: Empirical effects of legislation, *Health Services Research*, 34, 1, 417–425.

Mulligan, E., 2001, Confidentiality in health records: Evidence of current performance from a population survey in South Australia, *Medical Journal of Australia*, 174, 637–640.

Neuhaus, E., Lyons, T., and Payne, B., 1976, Patient responses to request for written permission to review medical records, *American Journal of Public Health*, 66, 11, 1090–1092.

News and Notes, 1979, Most people think doctors do a good job of protecting the privacy of their records, *Hospital and Community Psychiatry*, 30, 12, 860–861.

O'Flynn, N., Spencer, J., and Jones, R., 1997, Consent and confidentiality in teaching in general practice: Survey of patient's views on the presence of students, *British Medical Journal*, 315, 1142.

Ornstein, S. and Bearden, A., 1994, Patient perspectives on computer-based medical records, *Journal of Family Practice*, 38, 6, 606–610.

Pavia, A.T. et al., 1993, Partner notification for control of HIV: Results after two years of a statewide program in Utah, *American Journal of Public Health*, 83, 1418–1424.

Peremans, L. et al., 2000, Contraceptive knowledge and expectations by adolescents: An explanation by focus groups, *Patient Education and Counseling*, 40, 133–140.

Pew Internet and Life Project, 2000, The online health care revolution: How the Web helps Americans take better care of themselves, *Pew Internet and Life Project*, http://www.pewinternet.org/reports/toc.asp?Report=26.

Pool, R., Nyanzi, S., and Whitworth, J., 2001, Attitudes to voluntary counselling and testing for HIV among pregnant women in rural southwest Uganda, *AIDS Care*, 13, 5, 605–615.

Purdy, S. et al., 2000, Patient participation in research in the managed care environment: Key perceptions of members in an HMO, *Journal of General Internal Medicine*, 15, 492–495.

Robinson, J. et al., 1991, Attitudes of donors and recipients to gamete donation, *Human Reproduction*, 6, 2, 307–309.

Rylance, G., 1999, Privacy, dignity and confidentiality: Interview study with structured questionnaire, *British Medical Journal*, 318, 301.

Siegler, M., 1982, Confidentiality in medicine: A decrepit concept, *New England Journal of Medicine*, 307, 1518–1521.

Smith, R., 1996, The importance of patient's consent of publication, *British Medical Journal*, 313, 16.

Sugarman, J. et al., 1999, Ethical ramifications of alternative means of recruiting research participant from cancer registries, *Cancer*, 86, 4, 647–651.

Ubel, P. et al., 1995, Elevator talk: Observational Study of inappropriate comments in a public space, *American Journal of Medicine*, 99, 2, 190–194.

U.K. Association of Cancer Registries, 2000, Statement by the UKACR on the General Medical Council (GMC) Guidance on Confidentiality, 2000, *British Medical Journal*, 321, 854.

Wardman, L. et al., 2000, Patient's knowledge and expectations of confidentiality in primary health care: A quantitative study, *British Journal of General Practice*, 50, 901–902.

Warr, D., and Hillier, L., 1997, "That's the problem with living in a small town": Privacy and sexual health issues for young rural people, *Australian Journal of Rural Health*, 5, 132–139.

Weiss, B.D., 1982, Confidentiality expectations of patients, physicians, and medical students, *Journal of the American Medical Association*, 247, 2695–2697.

Westbeg, K. et al., 2001, Getting informed consent from patients to take part in the clinical training of students: Randomised trial of two strategies, *British Medical Journal*, 323, 488.

Whetten-Goldstein, K., Nguyen, T., and Sugarman, J., 2001, So much for keeping secrets: The importance of considering patients' perspectives on maintaining confidentiality, *AIDS Care*, 12, 4, 457–466.

Woods, W. et al., 1999, Name-based reporting of HIV-positive test results as a deterrent to testing, *American Journal of Public Health*, 89, 1097–1100.

Yawn, B. et al., 1998, The impact of requiring patient authorization for use of data in medical records research, *Family Practice*, 47, 5, 361–365.

17 Mobile Phone Positioning Systems and the Accessibility of Health Services

Markku Löytönen and Clive E. Sabel

CONTENTS

17.1 INTRODUCTION

In this chapter, we outline our vision of how new emerging technologies in both mobile communications and GIS research areas will combine in the near future to provide a multitude of opportunities within the healthcare field. We start by discussing some relevant aspects of the new technologies, then review current remote health service provision, before combining the discussion to give examples of how new mobile geographically aware technologies could aid better healthcare provision in the future.

17.2 GEOGRAPHY AND GEOGRAPHIC INFORMATION SYSTEMS

One of the most rapidly developing branches of geography is that concerned with GIS and its applications. Although the subdiscipline extends back almost 40 years,

0-415-30655-8/04/$0.00+$1.50

the range of applications has expanded rapidly since the first commercial GIS software became available at the workstation level in the early 1980s. Nowadays, GIS applications are in use in almost all walks of life, e.g., in the planning of retail areas, transportation, national defense, environmental protection, and healthcare.

The key idea behind GIS is in principle a simple one. Two kinds of data, positional data and attribute data, are integrated. The positional data can be any form of data identifying points (e.g., map coordinates) or defining larger areas (or polygons), such as municipalities or hospital districts. The attribute data can consist of statistics on almost anything that happens to be of interest to the user, such as smoking habits, taxable incomes, or the prevalence of a given disease within the population. When these attribute data (variables) are linked to the positional data, the result is a powerful means of analyzing the geographical distribution of the phenomenon in question. Although the idea in itself is a simple one, individual GIS applications can be of considerable complexity, especially when provisions are made for functions such as spatial calculations, route optimization, the analysis of satellite images, or the statistical testing of spatial clusters.

17.3 GIS AND MOBILE COMMUNICATIONS

The last decade of the previous millennium will be remembered as the age of mobile communications. Small, highly versatile mobile phones achieved enormous popularity and revolutionized the telecommunications market. The next breakthrough is about to begin, based on the notion of locating the position of the receiver. New generation mobile (or cellular) phones or perhaps personal digital assistants (PDAs) will be capable of identifying their own position with a high degree of accuracy, by reference to a satellite (the American global positioning system [GPS] or the European equivalent [Galileo]), a relay mast (perhaps using the global system for mobile communication, GSM), or some other system. When other new technical innovations, such as Bluetooth® wireless technology, WLAN (wireless local area network) applications, real-time speech recognition (Kumagai, 2002), proactive data processing, and learning computer environments and smart materials are added to this, a whole new range of spatial analytical opportunities is likely to emerge in the immediate future. Bluetooth is a new wireless personal area networking (PAN) technology that allows diverse information technology (IT) devices (such as mobile communicators, PDAs, laptops, MP3 players, and digital cameras) to connect together within a range of approximately ten meters using radio waves (Erasala and Yen, 2002). It includes built-in security such as authentication and encryption to prevent eavesdropping.

GIS and its associated technologies form one of the main building blocks in the new positioning and navigating concept for mobile communications. GPS and CD-ROM-based in-car navigation has been around for some years. However, the relatively recent development of handheld PDA devices can incorporate mobile communications, computing power, memory cards, and, importantly, access to the Internet to accurately locate the handset within a geographical context on maps downloaded on demand. In Finland, the Personal Navigation Spearhead

Programme[1] was established precisely to encourage the integration of GPS, electronic maps and mobile communications on a handheld microprocessor. Anticipated services included traffic jam notification and traveling services, such as locations of hotels, automatic teller machines (ATMs), or perhaps a local weather forecast for the vicinity of the handset. The Benefon GPS-GSM mobile phone already enables precise personal navigation by means of a map that appears on its screen. We believe that in the future the system will be based on the combination of a GPS and a mobile phone with maps no longer needing to be locally stored either in memory or on storage devices. The maps will be downloaded when necessary through the operator along with other navigation tools such as route optimization. Another application area is that of indoor pedestrian navigation based on Bluetooth technology or WLAN, such as the implemented prototype IRREAL system (Baus et al., 2002). Although Bluetooth is becoming more common in mobile phones, the best option for precise positioning and navigations systems may require a combination of GPS, Bluetooth, and WLAN technology. Accurate base maps with geocoded street addresses are needed for a successful navigation system. The 3D City Info project (Rakkolainen and Vainio, 2001) is one example of an operating prototype system using accurate digital maps. The Virtual Reality Modeling Language (VRML)-based prototype application, based in the Finnish city of Tampere, incorporates a GPS receiver, built-in compass, and either a laptop or handheld mobile device to enable pedestrian navigation with accurate 3D rendering of the surrounding buildings, albeit for limited geographical coverage in Tampere city center. Once such a system is available worldwide, it will be possible in the future for tourists, for instance, to navigate their way through the art collections of the Palazzo Pitti in Florence and receive commentary in their own language direct to their mobile phones that focuses on the particular work that they are standing nearest to at the time.

17.4 NETWORK SERVICES EXTENDED TO MOBILE COMMUNICATION DEVICES

Currently the situation is changing yet again in response to technological advances. Although many IT companies are finding themselves in serious financial difficulties, astronomical sums of money have been paid in advance for third-generation UMTS (universal mobile telecommunications system) mobile operator licenses. Although much uncertainty prevails on the high-tech investment market, we are convinced that the new technologies now envisaged will become a part of our lives and sooner than we could ever imagine. The situation resembles in many ways the advent of personal computers 20 years ago. We understand the possibilities ahead and are able to construct scenarios, but the innovations themselves are shrouded in uncertainty. The following is one possible scenario.

It is already the case that the majority of processors manufactured are installed in devices other than computers. With the spread of Bluetooth technology, WLAN

[1] Personal Navigation Spearhead Programme in Finland, http://www.vtt.fi/tte/samba/projects/navigointi/navigation_en.html, accessed .30 January 2004.

technology, and proactive and self-teaching computer environments, processors are now communicating with each other, analyzing their users' behavior and functioning on the strength of what they have learned. Thus, it will not be long before going to work might involve a scenario where our mobile phones will communicate with the building's computer systems to let us in the main door, eliminating the need for security swipe cards and simultaneously turning on the main lighting system for our personal safety. As we approach our own offices, the mobile phones will also communicate with our desktop or laptop computers in our offices, boot them up, and start the applications that we most commonly use. With the use of intelligent room processors that learn the habits and patterns of users, we might also envisage an office that adjusts the heating system as we approach and perhaps switch on table lamps automatically.

The next generation of mobile communicators will be combinations of computer, positioning system, and telephone; in effect, "universal machines" of an open architecture that we will learn to use just as effortlessly as we do a computer nowadays, possibly even more so. These devices will be of a far greater capacity than the present ones and will have for all practical purposes real-time network interfaces, regardless of the technology by which they are implemented. People will expect positioning services from their mobile phones on an everyday basis and it will come as naturally to them as electric current or running water.

In other words, the Web and its services will be a part of our everyday lives to the extent that we will not need to do anything in particular to switch it on. We will be online all the time and use the services as needs arise. Nor will our mobile phones necessarily need to be separate instruments that we carry around with us, for looking further into the future. They could just as well be integrated into our overcoats or belts. We may well start seeing clothing advertisements for "a sale of last spring's 2000-GHz jogging suits with the new soft solar panels."

17.5 REMOTE PROVISION OF HEALTH SERVICES

Although the concept of telemedicine is already a few decades old, the field has developed slowly. Telemedicine might be considered as the use of communication technologies to provide healthcare when distance separates the caregiver and receiver (Cutchin, 2002). The most common form traditionally has been a satellite-linked video-consultation between a distant specialist, perhaps in the United States, and a local doctor and patient, perhaps located in one of the remote Antarctic bases. Numerous telemedicine services now exist worldwide, such those based in Alaska, Queensland, Australia, and India. The various traditional services that have been developed are based on closed systems: single-purpose closed networks and specifically designed hardware for a small group of users. This has made them expensive both to construct and to use. The lack of established standards has also hampered the progress of this development work, so that the resulting systems have never achieved any great popularity. Admittedly, the major actors in the field of healthcare, both private and public, were cautious and wary about committing themselves to projects that would have involved considerable investment. According to Cutchin (2002), remotely accessed healthcare can offer many advantages to traditionally neglected populations, such as poor people, older people, and those based in rural areas. By establishing virtual medical care regions, quality improvements and cost savings can be achieved, but there will always be some communities and sectors of society excluded from virtual supply regions just as there are today with the more traditional healthcare services. A recent United Kingdom-based study supports these potential quality and cost improvements (Wallace et al., 2002). The study utilized virtual outreach facilities to include video consultations between general practitioners (GPs) or family doctors, hospital-based specialists, and patients, with reported higher levels of satisfaction among patients together with cost efficiencies with significantly fewer tests and investigations being carried out, when compared to traditional GP consultations and separate specialist referrals.

In the early 1990s, the slow development of telemedicine changed, largely because of a spread in one of the services offered by the Internet, the Web. The Internet itself was created in the 1960s and rapidly gained popularity within scientific circles, but it was some time before it was appreciated by the public. Once the public accepted the Internet and the Web, the range of services offered by these channels, the numbers of servers linked to the network, and the numbers of users began to increase exponentially. Now, at the dawn of the new millennium, the Web is a part of everyday life in industrialized countries.

As no doubt the majority of readers will know, the Web can provide virtually anything imaginable. It is an excellent tool for many people, as it can give access to a vast quantity of high-quality services everywhere and for everyone, once the user has a network interface available. However, it can also be a bottomless barrel containing a mass of confused, undifferentiated, and uncontrollable information and services. It is somewhat a matter of luck whether one finds the information that one is looking for. Conversely, it is possible to claim that the absence of control enables the free dissemination of information, which is the greatest strength of the Web.

In spite of all its problems, the Web contains vast amounts of useful, relevant information and services of proven quality and one of the best of these has already been appreciated extensively in the healthcare sector. Web services have become an irreplaceable aid for healthcare professionals. Among the many applications available, the Web can enable a researcher to check and update the bibliography to a paper in minutes, obtain an electronic copy of a published paper, consult a reference database for the interpretation of x-rays or practice various professional skills through Internet courses. The net services provided by the Finnish medical association Duodecim,[1] for example, with their journal reviews, reference databases, and treatment recommendations are of the highest quality. It is now also possible to carry out online surgery with a surgeon thousands of kilometers from a remote patient and local performing doctor who carries out the operation with the aid of a live camera feed and real-time patient monitoring data relayed over the Internet back to the surgeon.

[1] Duodecim, http://www.duodecim.fi, accessed 30 January 2004.

17.6 WHAT ABOUT FUTURE HEALTH SERVICES?

An enormous selection of health services is already available on the Web and these will be transferred to the screens of mobile communicators or PDAs in the course of time. It will also be easy to invent new applications. A future Bluetooth PDA device could possibly monitor the bodily functions of a user who has a heart complaint, warn him to take his medicine at the right times, relay his heart monitor information to his local hospital's monitoring system, and automatically phone the rescue services for help if something goes wrong (Erasala and Yen, 2002). The request will be accompanied by a precise indication of the device's position, which can be read in the control room and transferred automatically to the ambulance's computerized navigation system. The system could then assess the traffic situation in terms of the various potential routes and their current traffic flows and supply the driver with a proposal for the optimal route.

Many of these individual components are operational. For example, a prototype ambulance-management system has been built based in Attica, Greece, which incorporates GIS, GPS, and GSM technologies to route ambulances to emergency calls using shortest-path algorithms and taking account of traffic conditions (Derekenaris et al., 2002). Some ambulance services in the United Kingdom are already moving a step further, by anticipating potential demand — an emergency call — by using historical call patterns through varying times of the day or days of the week to move their empty ambulances to positions (or way-points) where they can best respond to anticipated demand. Then they constantly reevaluate these positions in relation to real-time traffic congestion and the relative coverage of other ambulances to provide as optimal a service as possible. These ambulance dispatch applications require accurate mobile positioning systems to determine where ambulances are, digital maps to provide routing information, and mobile communications to link to their dispatch computers and operators.

The Web is currently able to provide information on self-care possibilities, regional differences in health behavior, and locations of health services of various kinds. This same information could be relayed in the near future to handheld devices. There is a growing plethora of online doctor services, such as the United Kingdom-based Netdoctor,[1] which provides ask-the-doctor services both electronically and by phone, together with resources such as online disease, ailments, and medicine encyclopedias. Also in the United Kingdom, the online and telephone service NHS Direct[2] has been introduced, provided by the U.K. government in an effort to make medical advice both more accessible and cheaper to supply and to relieve pressure on doctors' surgeries and hospitals. Such services have the advantage of convenience for those with Internet access, at the same time containing a degree of anonymity, enabling perhaps wider access to medical information without the need to be physically present, which might be attractive to certain (perhaps younger or disillusioned) sectors of society. Counts of visits made to Web pages indicate that the public makes avid use of these services.

[1] Netdoctor, http://www.netdoctor.co.uk, accessed 30 January 2004.

[2] NHS Direct, http://www.nhsdirect.nhs.uk, accessed 30 January 2004.

Technology can be directly applied to reduce exposure to known or suspected sources. One of the specific health concerns regarding the ever-increasing use of mobile phones over the past decade has been the supposedly high level of radiation exposure near to the user's brain caused by the mobile phone's transmitter. With Bluetooth devices, the public perception of the health risk (and indeed any real health risk) can be reduced by using a low radiation emitting Bluetooth headset, linked to the mobile communicator stored elsewhere on the body, in a car, or in a room (Erasala and Yen, 2002).

It will also be possible to use a mobile communicator for data acquisition purposes. Accurately estimating an individual's exposure to an environmental exposure that might be implicated in the etiology of a disease has been an inexact science up to now. Often the place of residence or work is used as a surrogate location. However, individuals have complex daily activity spaces where they are constantly exposed to a variety of pathogens that cannot be accurately represented by just one location. In our future scenario, users would carry the mobile device with them and it could be fitted with a sensor, e.g., for measuring levels of noise, air pollution, or some other exposure of interest in their surroundings and the data collected could be transmitted along with precise geographical coordinates. It could also, if required, record at the same time features of his or her bodily functions that might be expected to react to these external conditions. It might make sense technically to not provide sensors to each mobile device, but to make use of regularly placed, but fixed environmental sensors. Rebolj and Sturm (1999) have implemented such a prototype system, based in Austria, to integrate road traffic pollution monitoring with GIS modeling of exposure patterns in the immediate vicinity. If this air pollution and GIS modeled data were joined together with accurate pedestrian locations (obtained via their handheld devices) this would provide invaluable information to epidemiologists attempting to identify the causes of diseases in addition to the obvious personal benefits to the individual concerned.

It is also easy to envisage many situations in which a mobile communicator could be used proactively. People with asthma living or working in San Francisco might be willing to pay for a service that informs their PDAs of advance warnings of temperature inversion situations and the associated increases in air pollution by connecting to Californian meteorological Web sites. Perhaps the service will suggest that they wait a couple of hours longer before going home from work so that an anticipated coming low-pressure system would have dispersed the inversion and hence cleared the pollution.

17.7 IS BIG BROTHER WATCHING YOU?

The things we have been talking about above may seem as if they are taken out of a science fiction book and it is easy to imagine that the new technology could be used to subject individuals to round-the-clock surveillance. In fact, every one of the examples mentioned represents a service that is already available, a system that is at the testing stage, or a project for which the basic ideas are maturing fast. In any case, the fear of universal surveillance is already a reality, as it is possible with present-day technology to monitor accurately where a mobile phone is at a particular point in time, although few users have probably realized this yet.

Many valid ethical and data confidentiality issues remain that should not be overlooked and need to be addressed. We write from an affluent, developed world perspective, but we should also consider how accessible these services would be in the developing world. There are also many sectors of the community that lie in information deserts within the developed world, both metaphorically among the less well educated, socioeconomically disadvantaged, or elderly population, as well as physically, perhaps in rural or remote areas. Ethically we must address who owns, controls, and accesses individuals' locational health information to protect individual privacy where appropriate. We should not overlook potential medical licensing and associated legal issues. Doctors are currently licensed and able to practice in certain geographical regions and have legal protection within these areas. The Internet by its nature, removes these artificial boundaries and consequently, there is a fuzzy or grey area, where doctors based, say, in the United States might give advice through the Internet to someone in China. Which national laws apply or are new international protocols or licensing agreements needed?

17.8 BASIC RESEARCH IS NEEDED

Although we chiefly entertain favorable expectations of future developments in mobile communications, we also think that we still need a lot of research-backed information on the building of such systems starting out from people's real needs. We also need results to show how these systems can be made to serve their users in the best ways possible and in accordance with jointly agreed rules. This is a task that can be expected to be devolved most of all to the scientific community, for it is difficult to conceive who else would carry out this form of basic research. In this respect, our gaze turns upon the representatives of geography and other social sciences, as well as disciplines such as the medical sciences, the humanities, and, naturally, the computer sciences. There is plenty of work to be done and we can be sure that it will be interesting and challenging.

ACKNOWLEDGMENTS

We wish to thank Åke Sivertun for his most valuable comments and suggestions.

References

Baus, J., Krüger, A., and Wahlster, W., 2002, A resource-adaptive mobile navigation system, *Proceedings of IUI2002: International Conference on Intelligent User Interfaces 2002*, San Francisco, CA: ACM Press.

Cutchin, M.P., 2002, Virtual medical geographies: Conceptualizing telemedicine and regionalization, *Progress in Human Geography,* 26, 1, 19–39.

Derekenaris, G. et al., 2002, Integrating GIS, GPS, and GSM technologies for the effective management of ambulances, *Computers, Environment and Urban Systems*, 25, 267–278.

Erasala, N. and Yen, D.C., 2002, Bluetooth technology: A strategic analysis of its role in the global 3G wireless communication era, *Computer Standards & Interfaces,* 24, 193–206.

Kumagai, J., 2002, Talk to the machine, *IEEE Spectrum*, 60–64.

Rakkolainen, I. and Vainio, T., 2001, A 3D city info for mobile users, *Computer & Graphics,* 25, 619–625.

Rebolj, D. and Sturm, P.J., 1999, A GIS-based component-oriented integrated system for estimation, visualization, and analysis of road traffic air pollution, *Environmental Modelling & Software*, 14, 531–539.

Wallace, P. et al., Virtual Outreach Project Group, 2002, Joint teleconsultations (Virtual Outreach) versus standard outpatient appointments for patients referred by their general practitioner for a specialist opinion: A randomised trial, *The Lancet*, 359, 1961–1968.

18 Conclusions and Future Prospects

Massimo Craglia and Ravi Maheswaran

CONTENTS

0-415-30655-8/04/$0.00+$1.50

18.1 CONCLUSIONS

Public health by its nature covers a wide field ranging from scientific and technical issues to sociological aspects, accountability of government agencies, and empowerment of populations. This book has focused on aspects of public health in which the spatial dimension is a particularly important element, hence the sections on communicable disease control and environmental health and healthcare planning and policy. Section 1 described some of the methodological aspects of GIS underpinning applications in these areas of work, highlighting progress and new developments. Section 4 on data protection and E-governance issues has addressed broader policy-related, societal, and developmental issues that have a direct impact on the spatial aspects of public health work. These issues also impact on the scope for, and desirability of, further integration of GIS within the public health field.

To draw together the many threads and issues arising from the preceding chapters, we found it useful to undertake an analysis of the strengths, weaknesses, opportunities, and threats (SWOT analysis) of the current state of GIS and public health.

18.2 STRENGTHS

18.2.1 Technology

A major strength is the increased availability, affordability, and performance of GIS software and supporting hardware. This has greatly facilitated the diffusion of GIS in a wide range of fields, including public health, to an extent that was previously not possible. In addition, developments in relation to the Internet and Web mapping are increasingly facilitating the access to and sharing of information to the benefit of researchers, practitioners, and the public. Although not yet the main form of access to health-related information, the increased usage of the Internet in this field reported by the Eurobarometer survey is worthy of note (see Chapter 14).

18.2.2 Visualization

The ability to show on a map the distribution of needs and services, disease rates, and composite factors such as those related to the underlying population at risk or environmental conditions has many advantages over a nonspatial, tabular format. These advantages relate to not only the representation and communication of information to different audiences, but also to the ability to use visualization as a first step in the analytical process of enquiry, described in Chapter 2 in relation to exploratory spatial data analysis and illustrated in Chapter 6 in relation to the analysis of the *Salmonella* Brandenburg infection. Furthermore, the combination of visualization techniques with the Internet and Web mapping technologies is increasing the importance of this aspect by a considerable degree.

18.2.3 Data Availability

Although far from being entirely satisfactory (see Section 18.3) there is little doubt that the much increased availability of spatially referenced data pertaining to population and socioeconomic factors, health, and the environment has substantially enhanced the application of GIS to public health research and practice. Environmental information in particular is becoming much more widely available and enshrined in international agreements such as the Aarhus Convention and European legislation. Similarly, socioeconomic data such as that provided by population censuses or public registers, now easily accessible through the Internet, supports a wide range of applications of relevance to needs assessment and service provision, or the estimation of underlying populations at risk. Health-related information is also becoming increasingly available via national statistics offices and international organizations, such as the World Health Organization, although the sensitive nature of this information requires additional safeguards before public release. In more general terms, the trend toward the development of spatial data infrastructures at regional, national, and international levels noted in Chapter 14 is important for a number of reasons. These infrastructures enable access to many data resources of direct relevance to public health. They enable the development of broad frameworks of practice to identify existing data resources and data custodians for these resources, avoiding duplication of data collection. The frameworks of practice include shared policies for accessing and sharing information and the development of technologies and standards. Such developments should ensure that any investment made by organizations with respect to data management has long-term benefits.

18.2.4 Integration

One of the main benefits of exploiting the geographic dimension of spatial data relates to the ability to integrate data from different sources and systems that often have little in common in the way they are collected and structured, except for their common location. Although location may be expressed in many different ways, implicitly via an address, postcode, or area, or explicitly via coordinates, the strength of a GIS is its ability to handle any of these identifiers and link the data attributes. This integrative function is critical not only for linking composite factors, such as air pollution, the population at risk, and health outcomes as described in Chapter 8, but also for facilitating the joint analysis of problems and the formulation of solutions among different agencies with responsibilities for a defined territory. Data integration is thus as critical to joined-up government as it is to multidisciplinary or multilevel analysis. This important organizational support function is highlighted in Chapter 10 and Chapter 11, both of which report on the strengths of GIS in regional and district operational settings.

18.2.5 Analytical Functions

GIS has specific areas of strength compared with traditional databases. One in particular is that it enables a set of operations (e.g., querying and buffering) to be used on attributes of data that are often implicit (i.e., locations) and not explicit (i.e., fields in the databases). The chapters in Section 2 and Section 3 provide many examples of such operations and the benefits derived by users. These analytical functions may be applied to vector or raster data for communicable disease control (Chapter 5), infection surveillance (Chapter 6), and exposure assessment (Chapter 7), as well as to network data as in the case of the accessibility analysis (Chapter 12). The analytical strengths of GIS for supporting public health research and practice are succinctly summarized in Table 5.2, which gives examples of specific applications for each key analytical function. Although most applications in public health practice only make use of the operations available in most commercial GIS products, we have started to see the emergence of dedicated software to support more-advanced spatial and temporal analyses, as described in the chapters in Section 2. These dedicated software and methods require a high level of knowledge for appropriate use. Their increasing availability and scope for integration with the main commercial GIS products are indications of the potential for reaching maturity in this field.

18.2.6 Body of Knowledge

Public health GIS is the convergence of a well-established body of sciences underpinning public health with the emerging body of knowledge and theory now recognized as geographic information science. The latter brings together and reinterprets in a contemporary context many of the scientific endeavors of the past centuries, together with the new challenges posed by technological advances. The community of researchers with an interest in geographic information as a science is steadily growing and refocusing from a purely application-orientated effort to one that recognizes the interplay between systems, science, and society (see Longley et al., 2001). As such, questions posed by public health researchers and practitioners should receive more careful and considered attention from counterparts in the GIS community leading to new insights into research and practice, rather than only a set of applications for a technology.

18.3 WEAKNESSES

18.3.1 Data Quality

Although the availability of spatial data has increased substantially, there are several weaknesses in relation to data quality. The first weakness is the lack of documentation about data quality itself, which then makes it difficult to understand the propagation of errors when integrating different data sets and using analytical operations. Second, much of the data is aggregated for confidentiality or administrative reasons, which leads to the familiar problems of matching data at different scales and area boundaries (the modifiable areal units problem) and inferring the characteristics of individuals from those of the area they live in (ecological fallacy). These problems in GIS are exacerbated in the context of public health applications by the need to link individual-level outcomes with area-level data. Additional problems in the field of GIS and public health have been highlighted in several chapters. They include the extent to which data refer to the place of residence rather than place of potential exposure, such as the workplace or school and the static nature of much of the data, which limits temporal and spatiotemporal analysis. Ideally, individual-level data over time is required so that the effects of short distance (e.g., travel to work) and long distance (e.g., migration) movements of the population at risk can be properly considered. Such data are only available in few countries (e.g., Finland) and Chapter 4 demonstrates some of the benefits that this level of detail can offer. On the other hand, detailed information raises other issues such as inadequate methods of analysis and societal concerns over confidentiality.

18.3.2 Analytical Functions

Although current GIS probably addresses most of the operational requirements most of the time, the chapters in Section 2 and Section 3, in particular, have indicated the limitations of current software with respect to more advanced spatial and temporal analysis. Dedicated software has been developed but its integration into mainstream GIS packages is limited, largely because vendors do not see enough of a market to do so.

18.3.3 Methodology

A number of limitations exist with respect to the methods that have been developed over the last few years. They include the lack of satisfactory integration of time and space variables into models and inadequate methods for linking physical models (e.g., for air and water) to models of social behavior and characteristics and individual level health outcomes. In a broader context, the full understanding of the complex relationship between the physical and social environments and health is still poorly developed as recognized in individual chapters in this book and in the recent European Communication on the environment and health (Commission of the European Communities, 2003).

18.3.4 Organizational Issues

The weaknesses here are still numerous and include the poor integration of GIS and spatial perspectives into the information technology (IT) systems of organizations and into the routine analysis of problems, strategies, and resources. In Figure 13.1, Gregory Elmes indicates the type of strategic planning cycle that one would expect organizations to adopt as a generic mechanism for resource allocation. GIS would have a major role to play if such a framework were to be deployed but the evidence to date is that most countries have yet to adopt similar approaches. In more-general terms, most public sector organizations, including those in the health sector, still have some way to go in developing and implementing organizational strategies that view information as a strategic asset. By this, we mean developing information strategies that are about the value of information and its place in the organization and beyond, including access and dissemination, rather than IT strategies that are about hardware and software procurement. In the absence of such strategies, we will continue to see haphazard deployment of GIS-informed methods and technologies and poor integration within the mainstream activities of the organization. As a corollary of this lack of information strategies, we will also continue to witness barriers to accessing and sharing information among organizations, which are more often than not based on lack of awareness, fear of loss of control, or misunderstanding of the legal framework.

18.3.5 Education and Training

This is a major barrier across the public sector at central and local levels and internally among managerial and technical staff. Public health organizations also suffer from similar weaknesses and in the context of the deployment of GIS in practice, the lack of education and skills is particularly restrictive. The needs are for not only the development of IT skills, but also more crucially for education about the limitations of data sources and the appropriateness of different analytical and visualization methods depending on the problems at hand. Equally crucial is the lack of education and awareness of senior managers regarding the added value that a spatial perspective brings to public health problems. As a result, they cannot ask the right questions nor mobilize staff and resources to fill the gaps in skills.

18.4 OPPORTUNITIES

18.4.1 Data and Technology

The strengths and weaknesses of these aspects have been highlighted above, but in the future, we are likely to see a much greater development of spatial data infrastructures at all levels and increased interoperability and harmonization of data based on agreed standards and Web-enabled services. This will present enormous opportunities for greater access to data and services and the integration of spatial perspectives into public health work. Therefore, for example, it will no longer be necessary to have GIS software on users' machines, but it will be possible to access spatial data on the Web, overlay it with other data, and invoke Web-based services to undertake specific analytical functions. This is already becoming possible but the full uptake across public sector organizations will take time. In addition, new data sources and technologies are likely to support a much greater use of GIS in public health. For example, the use of remotely sensed data including high-resolution aerial photography and satellite data, GPS signals, and mobile technologies will open up vast new data resources, as indicated in Chapter 17. In Europe alone, the Galileo Project (European Commission, 2002) and the Global Monitoring and Environment System (European Commission, 2001) will be of great significance to public health in relation to the environment.

18.4.2 Political Agenda

A number of strands come together under this heading. They include the high political priority given to health as one of the largest areas of government expenditure, which is increasing due to demographic change. Public health has raised its profile in the collective consciousness due to recent scares, such as variant Creutzfeldt-Jakob disease (the human form of mad cow disease) and severe acute respiratory syndrome (SARS) and potential scares related to genetically modified organisms. Because of these factors, there has been increased pressure to adopt a more evidence-based approach to resource allocation and public information. These provide opportunities for technologies and methods that facilitate the integration and sharing of data and the analysis of inequalities in the distribution of services and clusters of events. Moreover, the increasing drive in Europe for more integrated policy at all levels and the pursuit of environmental objectives, including the better understanding of the relationship between the environment and health, lend further support to the uptake of GIS as a routine method of analysis.

18.4.3 Organizational Awareness

Despite the weaknesses in the current uptake of GIS in public health, there is little doubt that significant progress has been made over the last few years. The current situation can be turned into an opportunity for further expanding and embedding GIS into routine organizational practice. Further support for change is going to come from other areas of policy, such as the push toward E-government and E-health. Combined with new opportunities from technology and engineering methods, these are likely to move organizations to recast their models of information handling from a stand-alone, desk-centered paradigm to a more Web-centered and distributed one. Web-enabled service delivery and analysis will require more-accurate geographic information to work effectively and organizations will pay a lot more attention as a result to the quality of their geographic identifiers and to the formulation and implementation of their information strategies.

18.4.4 Public Health GIS Community

This community is growing rapidly from a pure research-led group of medical geographers to a wider multidisciplinary community of researchers and practitioners meeting regularly at local, national, and international levels. The First European Conference on GIS and Public Health held in Sheffield in 2001 drew over 250 people;[1] in the United States, such events are now regularly held. As the exchange between researchers and practitioners increases, so will examples of good practice in methods and applications that will come about as a result of cross-fertilization of ideas particularly among spatial statisticians, public health practitioners, and GIS researchers. The importance of building a critical mass for this community is also underlined by the growth in special interest groups on GIS and health among professional GIS associations and the development of dedicated centers of excellence such as the Informatics Collaboratory for the Social Sciences in the United Kingdom.

18.5 THREATS

18.5.1 Confidentiality

As more and more detailed, personal-level information is collected through an array of administrative systems and technologies, there is growing public anxiety regarding the erosion of the individual's right to privacy. Spatial privacy is becoming an area of concern in its own right, for example, through the use or publication of detailed aerial photographs of individual properties (see for example Letham, 2003) or through the collection of spatial information via mobile phones and closed circuit

[1] http://gis.sheffield.ac.uk.

television. When combined with sensitive personal information, such as that relating to health, this raises serious societal issues that need to be carefully addressed through the consistent enforcement of legal protection. Confidentiality protection, however, also raises concerns among researchers and practitioners who are either unclear about what can or cannot be done in data analysis or that major sources of data valuable for research may be eroded by confidentiality restrictions.

18.5.2 Erosion of Trust

Breaches of confidentiality or perceptions of intrusion will potentially have major implications for the relationship of trust that underpins most data collection through administrative processes. If that trust is broken, then collecting reliable and consistent data becomes virtually impossible with major consequences for public policy. A taste of such events occurred in the United Kingdom with the poll tax and in Germany in relation to the 1981 census. The relationship between doctor and patient is a particularly sensitive one and must be protected for the benefit of all. Thus, the development of fully integrated spatially enabled public health systems must be careful to balance what is technologically possible with what is socially desirable at any given period.

18.5.3 Loss of Credibility

Public health may raise emotional issues, such as concern surrounding suspected clusters of disease. GIS can be of significant help as identified throughout the book. However, the limitations in data and methodology that still characterize this field mean that there is always the possibility of making mistakes, particularly when the analysis is undertaken under pressure or uncritically. If the expectations raised by the use of GIS in public health are not carefully managed, the loss in credibility of the results may cast a wider shadow on the methods deployed. Some echoes of such loss in credibility as reported in Chapter 13 may pose a threat to further development of the public health GIS field.

18.5.4 Political Environment

Although high political visibility may be seen as providing opportunities for public health GIS, it may also be a significant threat. Political pressures put demands that may be unrealistic or not achievable within the time and resources available. Endless reorganizations of units of service and administration may disrupt the activities of teams that have taken time to develop expertise. The sheer size of health organizations makes any change in organizational practice and culture difficult to achieve. All these factors need to be realistically taken into account when considering the future development of public health GIS.

18.6 FUTURE PROSPECTS

Table 18.1 summarizes the key aspects identified. As the analysis indicates, there are multiple factors in each of the four areas that may influence the future

TABLE 18.1
Strengths, Weaknesses, Opportunities, and Threats in the Public Health GIS Field

Strengths	Weaknesses	Opportunities	Threats
Technology	Data quality	Data and technology	Confidentiality
Visualization	Analytical functions	Political agenda	Erosion of trust
Data availability	Methodology	Organizational awareness	Loss of credibility
Integration	Organizational issues	Public health GIS community	Political environment
Analytical functions	Education and training		
Body of knowledge			

development of the public health GIS field. There are many weaknesses and threats, but also major opportunities to build on current strengths. Some elements appear in more than one box, as there is more than one facet to them. This is to be expected in a developing field where the issues are interconnected in multiple ways. The community of interest in this field must learn to work together in addressing all the facets of this complex web of related issues.

The purpose of this book was to highlight major areas of intersection between the GIS and public health fields. We hope that by drawing attention to these key areas, public health researchers and practitioners will become more aware of the potential for GIS. It can then be applied to other aspects of public health in which the spatial dimension, although not a key aspect,will nevertheless bring added value. Examples of such areas include communication of health information to the wider public and the promotion of public participation in health policy and planning. A reasonably robust set of GIS-based methodologies already exists, as illustrated in this book, for addressing at least the basic spatial aspects of public health. These methods can be applied to a wide range of practical applications, building capacity, and raising awareness.

There is much to be gained from the widespread use of GIS within the public health field. Sustained effort is required to achieve this goal from all parties concerned, but especially from public health organizations, researchers, and practitioners. In this respect, we hope that this book will make a positive contribution, facilitating the efforts of individuals and organizations.

References

Commission of the European Communities, 2003, A European environment and health strategy, Brussels: European Commission, COM (2003) 338.

European Commission, 2001, Global monitoring for environment and security (GMES): Outline GMES EC Action Plan, Brussels: European Commission, COM (2001) 609.

European Commission, 2002, Council Regulation (EC) No 876/2002 of 21 May 2002, Setting up the Galileo Joint Undertaking, Brussels: Official Journal L 138/1 28 May 2002.

Letham, G., 2003, Streisand seeks court help to remove aerial photographs, *SpatialNews*, http://spatialnews.geocomm.com/features/bsphotos.

Longley, P. et al., 2001, *Geographic Information Systems and Science,* Chichester, U.K.: Wiley and Sons.

Index

C

D

E

F

G

H

I

K

L

M

N

O

P

Z

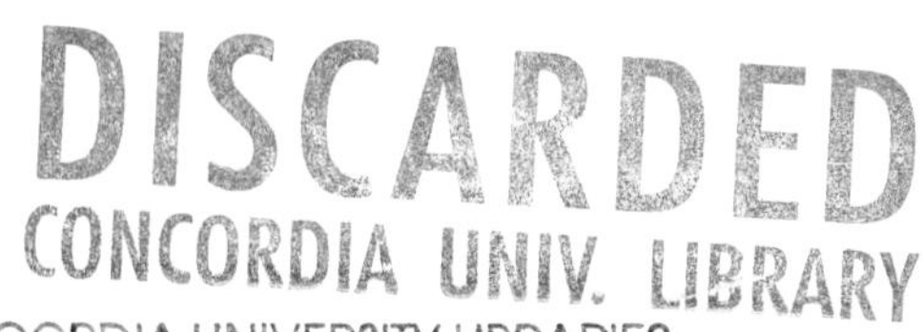